The Practice of Sleep Medicine Around The World: Challenges, Knowledge Gaps and Unique Needs

Edited By

Hrayr P. Attarian
Northwestern University Feinberg School of Medicine, Chicago, IL, USA

Marie-Louise M. Coussa-Koniski
Division of Pulmonary Diseases, Lebanese American University, Beirut, Lebanon

&

Alain Michel Sabri
Department of Otolaryngology-Head & Neck Surgery, SSMC-Mayo Clinic, Abu Dhabi, UAE

The Practice of Sleep Medicine around the World: Challenges, Knowledge Gaps and Unique Needs

Editors: Hrayr Attarian, Marie-Louise M. Coussa-Koniski and Alain Michel Sabri

ISBN (Online): 978-981-5049-36-7

ISBN (Print): 978-981-5049-37-4

ISBN (Paperback): 978-981-5049-38-1

need for a court order if at any point you breach any terms of this License Agreement. In no event will any delay or failure by Bentham Science Publishers in enforcing your compliance with this License Agreement constitute a waiver of any of its rights.

3. You acknowledge that you have read this License Agreement, and agree to be bound by its terms and conditions. To the extent that any other terms and conditions presented on any website of Bentham Science Publishers conflict with, or are inconsistent with, the terms and conditions set out in this License Agreement, you acknowledge that the terms and conditions set out in this License Agreement shall prevail.

Bentham Science Publishers Pte. Ltd.
80 Robinson Road #02-00
Singapore 068898
Singapore
Email: subscriptions@benthamscience.net

BENTHAM SCIENCE

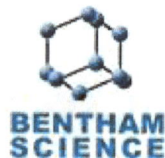

CONTENTS

PREFACE

The art and science of sleep medicine have evolved significantly over the past several decades. Both diagnostic and therapeutic advancements have led to a multidisciplinary approach to the field. Impactful research as well as technological innovations have been major catalysts in the rapid development of this important specialty.

Despite the above, those advancements have predominantly manifested in high and some middle-income countries. Meanwhile, there have been wide disparities in the delivery of care in economically disadvantaged parts of the world. When considering the entirety of sleep health and the wide range of sleep disorders, even within the same geopolitical areas, city, country, or continent, the ability to properly diagnose and, more importantly, manage sleep disorders by medical professionals and healthcare systems varies greatly.

Because of the multidisciplinary nature of the field, each editor of this publication comes from a different primary specialty. Dr. Marie-Louise M. Coussa-Koniski is a pulmonologist, Dr. Alain Michel Sabri is an otolaryngologist-head and neck surgeon and Dr. Hrayr P. Attarian is a neurologist. Similarly, the authors of the individual chapters cover a wide range of specialties, including the aforementioned ones as well as paediatrics, psychiatry, occupational medicine, internal medicine and others.

This textbook seeks to highlight the above by elucidating the particularities within each country, as well as the challenges encountered and the potential for improvement in the management of sleep disorders. The latter has a high impact on the healthcare of the individual, the healthcare system and various notions in terms of morbidity, mortality and overall well-being and quality of life. The impact of sleep disorders carries important economic implications. Leading healthcare experts describe the differences in the healthcare systems, available resources, patient population, accessibility as well as teaching and research in the field. Future directions and suggestions for improvement are also discussed.

We hope that you will find this textbook informative and that it will stimulate ideas for growth and development in the field of sleep disorders around the world.

Alain Michel Sabri, MD, MPH, FACS
Department of Otolaryngology-Head & Neck Surgery,
SSMC-Mayo Clinic,
Abu Dhabi, UAE

INTRODUCTION

Sleep is a biological imperative and one of the four pillars of health along with nutrition, physical activity and relaxation. Yet, sleep medicine has only recently become an individual discipline. Even then it is more developed in high-income countries than in middle or low-income ones. Although a large proportion of the world's population suffers chronically from poor sleep, addressing it is not a major priority. This is also true for economically disadvantaged populations even in the wealthiest of nations. The limitations to this are greatly due to a lack of resources for both screening for poor sleep health as well as for appropriate interventions. There is, however, a lack of knowledge about the impact of poor sleep on overall health. A fair proportion of healthcare workers both here and in other countries I have visited as part of my global health education work think of sleep medicine as only treating sleep apnea or a rare disease such as narcolepsy. Both are viewed as not essential for populations who have difficulty obtaining basic healthcare. Sleep medicine, however, could be much more than this. As different chapters in this book will show, sleep is one of the first bodily functions to be affected when people are displaced, or live in crowded tenements, or when they become homeless. Not getting sufficient and quality sleep can lead to both poorer cardiovascular health, increased risk of accidents and lower cognitive functioning. It can help prevent any type of upward mobility for the working poor in the developed world.

In mid October 2019 while in Lebanon, I ran the idea of this book by two colleagues, the pulmonologist Dr. Marie-Louise Coussa and the otolaryngologist Dr. Alain Michel Sabri. We all decided on the need for such a publication and decided to collaborate on it. Given my own background in neurology, we hoped our approach would be multidisciplinary. Political turmoil in Lebanon delayed the start of the project by a few months. At the beginning of 2020, we had already queried PubMed, Medline and Google Scholar for publications in English on sleep medicine, sleep health and overall sleep science. We identified 51 representative countries that had produced peer-reviewed papers on these topics. We spent the first 2 months of the, now infamous, year confirming authors. Thirty-five authors agreed. However, with the advent of the COVID-19 pandemic, the medical communities' priorities changed around the globe. This resulted not only in a delay in compiling this volume but also in the further withdrawal of seven of the original authors.

The final tally of 28 chapters covers most if not all the regions of the world, perhaps a bit heavy on North America and the Middle East, given our own origins. Figure **1** shows in green the countries of the world that we cover in the book. The big five, the most populous nations, are there. These are China, India, Russia, USA and Brazil. We also have examples from southern, western, eastern and northern Europe as well as North and Sub-Saharan Africa. In addition, we have chapters from Australia, Hong Kong, Thailand and Nepal.

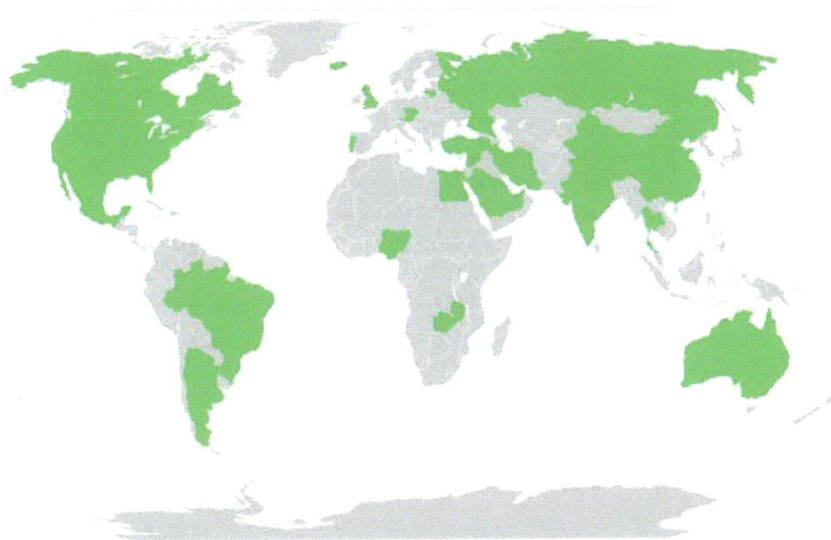

Fig. (1). In green are highlighted the areas of the world discussed in this book.

Each chapter addresses the following questions

1) The current practice of sleep medicine: This includes answers as to what type of facilities provide care, the type of practitioners involved in sleep medicine, any practice guidelines, professional societies or regulatory bodies, etc. In this subsection, there is a description of the kind of clinics and specialists who are primarily tasked with the care of patients with sleep complaints. A description of their educational backgrounds and any regulatory bodies that assure their continued competency in the area is given. Practice guidelines and who puts them in place are also mentioned with the availability of diagnostic tools and medications to treat common sleep disorders. We would also explore cultural nuances affecting sleep disorder care. Lastly, a description of payment systems for sleep diagnostic services and treatments is given.

2) Challenges to the practice of sleep medicine: This includes information about patient access to care, and barriers to appropriate care. In this subsection, the respective authors discuss what challenges they and their patients deal with in obtaining and delivering appropriate care. These include educational barriers, resource limitations and financial hardships. For instance, do primary care doctors and patients know much about sleep disorders? And what to do about sleep complaints? Are there clinics that can deal with the situation or are they overwhelmed with scant resources and have barely time to deal with more common medical problems?. Can patients even afford testing and treatment if these are even available? Are there regional differences in accessing care? For instance, a lot of developing nations may have excellent services in the cities but not in rural areas. Lastly, we would discuss cultural barriers to receiving appropriate sleep care.

3) Clinical and research knowledge gap: Unique needs of the field in that particular country and what can make the situation better and close these gaps and overcome barriers. In this

subsection, the respective authors address the presence or absence of country-specific epidemiological data on various sleep disorders and how it affects the clinical and educational efforts. They also discuss any limitations of the existing research as it applies to their unique regions. Lastly, they mention what educational opportunities are lacking among healthcare providers and what can be done to improve those.

We hope that this book will increase collaboration between countries of different economic quartiles and increase awareness of needs in lower-income regions and open up avenues by which these needs can be met. Especially with the acceleration of telecommunication in the age of COVID-19, these cooperative efforts are both more urgent and easier to accomplish. Lastly, we hope to raise awareness of the importance of sleep and facilitate ways to address its deficits for overall better health for all people of the world.

Hrayr P. Attarian
Northwestern University Feinberg School of Medicine,
Chicago,
USA

DEDICATION

To my students who taught me the value of academic medicine and, as always, to my wife and soulmate Diana Monaghan

Hrayr P. Attarian

To my country Lebanon, may the hard times end soon and may it return to its past glory

Marie-Louise M. Coussa-Kosinski

To my late parents, Michel and Berthe Sabri
To my wife and daughter, Pascale and Raphaelle Sabri
To my brothers Dr. Roy and Rony Sabri
To my uncle Dr. Joseph Sabri
To my patients and my mentors

Alain Michel Sabri

List of Contributors

Abdul Ghani Sankari   Professor at Wayne State, University in Michigan, USA

Ahmad Abefe SANUSI   Department of Medicine, Obafemi Awolowo University Teaching Hospitals Complex, Ile-Ife, Osun State, Nigeria

Ahmed Omokayode IDOWU   Department of Medicine, Obafemi Awolowo University Teaching Hospitals Complex, Ile-Ife, Osun State, Nigeria

Ahmed S. BaHammam   Department of Medicine, Riyadh, Saudi Arabia, University Sleep Disorders Center and Pulmonary Service, King Saud University, Riyadh, Saudi Arabia
The Strategic Technologies Program of the National Plan for Sciences and Technology, Innovation in the Kingdom of Saudi Arabia (08 MED511 02), Riyadh, Saudi Arabia

Akintunde Adeolu ADEBOWALE   Department of Medicine, Obafemi Awolowo University, Ile-Ife, Osun State, Nigeria

Alain Michel Sabri   Department of Otolaryngology-Head & Neck Surgery, SSMC-Mayo Clinic, Abu Dhab, UAE

Alexander Sweetman   National Centre for Sleep Health Services Research, Bedford Park, South Australia, Australia
Adelaide Institute for Sleep Health/FHMRI Sleep, College of Medicine and Public Health, Flinders University, Bedford Park, South Australia, Australia

A.M. Li   Department of Pediatrics, Prince of Wales Hospital, The Chinese University of Hong Kong, Hong Kong SAR, China

Amélia Feliciano   Portuguese Association of Chronobiology and Sleep Medicine, Portugal

Anatoly Alekhin   Herzen State Pedagogical University of Russia, St Petersburg, Russia

Andrew Vakulin   National Centre for Sleep Health Services Research, Bedford Park, South Australia, Australia
Adelaide Institute for Sleep Health/FHMRI Sleep, College of Medicine and Public Health, Flinders University, Bedford Park, South Australia, Australia

Arezu Najafi   Occupational Sleep Research Center, Baharloo Hospital, Tehran University of Medical Sciences, Tehran, Iran

Aroonwan Preutthipan   Sleep Society of Thailand, Bangkok, Thailand
Ramathibodi Hospital Sleep Disorder Center, Ramathibodi, Ramathibodi, Bangkok, Thailand
Division of Pediatric Pulmonology, Department of Pediatrics, Ramathibodi Hospital, Mahidol University, Bangkok, Thailand

Avatar Verma   Department of Pulmonary, Critical Care & Sleep Medicine B.P., Koirala Institute of Health Sciences (BPKIHS), Dharan, Nepal

Ayesha Ahmed   Neurological Institute, Cleveland Clinic Abu Dhabi, Abu Dhabi, United Arab Emirates

Brian J. Murray	Division of Neurology, Department of Medicine, Sunnybrook Health Sciences Centre, University of Toronto, Toronto, Ontario, Canada
Caner Sahin	Department of ENT, School of Medicine, Alanya Aladdin Keykubat University, Alanya/Antalya, Turkey
Carmen Type-Roberts	Northwestern Feinberg School of Medicine, Chicago, IL, USA
Chairat Neruntarat	Department of Otolaryngology, Faculty of Medicine, Srinakharinwirot University, Bangkok, Thailand Sleep Apnea Association, Bangkok, Thailand
Chenyang Li	Division of Sleep Medicine, Peking University People's Hospital, Beijing, China
Ching Li Chai-Coetzer	National Centre for Sleep Health Services Research, Bedford Park, South Australia, Australia Adelaide Institute for Sleep Health/FHMRI Sleep, College of Medicine and Public Health, Flinders University, Bedford Park, South Australia, Australia Southern Adelaide Local Health Network, SA Health, Bedford Park, South Australia, Australia
Christy Costanian	School of Medicine, Lebanese American University, Beirut, Lebanon
Cláudio D' Elia	Portuguese Association of Chronobiology and Sleep Medicine, Portugal
Dalia Matačiūnienė	Kardiolita Hospital, Vilnius, Lithuania
Dalva Poyares	Department of Psychobiology, Universidade Federal de Sao Paulo, Sao Paulo, SP, Brazil
Daniel Ninello Polesel	Department of Psychobiology, Universidade Federal de Sao Paulo, Sao Paulo, SP, Brazil
Deebya Raj Mishra	Department of Pulmonary, Critical Care & Sleep Medicine B.P., Koirala Institute of Health Sciences (BPKIHS), Dharan, Nepal
Eglė Sakalauskaitė-Juodeikienė	Department of Neurology and Neurosurgery, Institute of Clinical Medicine, Faculty of Medicine, Vilnius University, Vilnius, Lithuania
Erna Sif Arnardottir	Reykjavik University Sleep Institute, School of Technology, Reykjavik University, Reykjavik, Iceland Landspitali University Hospital, Reykjavik, Iceland
Evelina Pajėdienė	Department of Neurology, Academy of Medicine, Lithuanian University of Health Sciences, Kaunas, Lithuania
Fang Han	Division of Sleep Medicine, Peking University People's Hospital, Beijing, China
Franceschini Carlos	Sleep Medicine-Mechanical Ventilation, Hospital Cosme Argerich, Ciudad de Buenos Aires (CABA), Argentina

Garay Arturo Sleep Medicine-Neurology, Centro de Estudios Médicos e Investigaciones Clínicas "Norberto Quirno" (CEMIC), Ciudad de Buenos Aires (CABA), Argentina

Gozde Orhan Kubat Department of ENT, School of Medicine, Alanya Aladdin Keykubat University, Alanya/Antalya, Turkey

Hadie Rifai Surgical Subspecialities Institute, Cleveland Clinic Abu Dhabi, Abu Dhabi, United Arab Emirates

Haykuhi Hovakimyan Department of Neurology and Neurosurgery, National Institute of Health, Yerevan, Armenia
Sleep Disorders Center, Somnus Neurology Clinic, Yerevan, Armenia

Helena Hachul Department of Psychobiology, Universidade Federal de Sao Paulo, Sao Paulo, SP, Brazil

Horacio Balám Álvarez García Sleep Disorder Clinic, Faculty of Medicine, Research Division, National Autonomous University of Mexico, 04510 Ciudad de México, CDMX, Mexico

Jana Vyskocilova EUC Clinic, Pilsen, Czech Republic

Jordan Cunningham Landspitali University Hospital, Reykjavik, Iceland

Josephine Eniola A. EZIYI Department of Otorhinolaryngology, Obafemi Awolowo University, Ile-Ife, Osun State, Nigeria

J.W. Chan Department of Psychiatry, Faculty of Medicine, The Chinese University of Hong Kong, Shatin, N.T., Hong Kong SAR, China
Department of Psychiatry, Faculty of Medicine, The Chinese University of Hong Kong, Hong Kong SAR, China

Karen Tieme Nozoe Department of Psychobiology, Universidade Federal de Sao Paulo, Sao Paulo, SP, Brazil

Kelly L Huffman Neurological Institute, Cleveland Clinic Abu Dhabi, Abu Dhabi, United Arab Emirates

Khosro Sadeghniiat-Haghighi Occupational Sleep Research Center, Baharloo Hospital, Tehran University of Medical Sciences, Tehran, Iran

Khunying Nanta Maranetra Sleep Society of Thailand, Bangkok, Thailand

Kikelomo Adebanke KOLAWOLE Department of Child Dental Health, Faculty of Dentistry, Obafemi Awolowo University, Ile-Ife, Osun State, Nigeria

K.L. Choo Department of Medicine, North District Hospital, Hong Kong SAR, China; Past President, Hong Kong Society of Sleep Medicine, Hong Kong SAR, China

Kondwelani John Mateyo Department of Internal Medicine, University Teaching Hospita Nationalist Road, Lusaka, Zambia

Kolawole S. MOSAKU Department of Mental Health, Obafemi Awolowo University, Ile-Ife, Osun state, Nigeria

Liyue Xu Division of Sleep Medicine, Peking University People's Hospital, Beijing, China

Lyudmila Korostovtseva	Almazov National Medical Research Centre, St Petersburg, Russia
Marie-Louise M. Coussa-Koniski	School of Medicine, Lebanese American University, Beirut, Lebanon
Michael Bimbola FAWALE	Department of Medicine, Obafemi Awolowo University, Ile-Ife, Osun State, Nigeria
Mikhail Bochkarev	Almazov National Medical Research Centre, St Petersburg, Russia
Michael T. Saletu	Department of Sleep Medicine, State Hospital Graz II, Location South, 8036 Graz, Austria
Miguel Meira e Cruz	Portuguese Association of Chronobiology and Sleep Medicine, Portugal
Mikhail Agaltsov	National Medicine Therapy and Preventive Centre, Moscow, Russia
Mohammed Zaher Sahloul	Clinical Associate Professo, the University of Illinois, Chicago, USA
Monica Levy Andersen	Department of Psychobiology, Universidade Federal de Sao Paulo, Sao Paulo, SP, Brazil
Morenikeji Adeyoyin KOMOLAFE	Department of Medicine, Obafemi Awolowo University, Ile-Ife, Osun State, Nigeria
Naiphinich Kotchabhakdi	Sleep Society of Thailand, Bangkok, Thailand Research Center for Neuroscience and Salaya Sleep Research Laboratory, Institute of Molecular Biosciences, Mahidol University Salaya, Nakornpathom, Thailand
Narendra Bhatta	Department of Pulmonary, Critical Care & Sleep Medicine B.P., Koirala Institute of Health Sciences (BPKIHS), Dharan, Nepal
Naricha Chirakalwasan	Division of Pulmonary and Critical Care Medicine, Department of Medicine, Faculty of Medicine, Chulalongkorn University, Bangkok, Thailand Excellence Center for Sleep Disorders, King Chulalongkorn Memorial Hospital, Thai Red Cross Society, Bangkok, Thailand Sleep Society of Thailand, Bangkok, Thailand
Natalya Leonenko	Herzen State Pedagogical University of Russia, St Petersburg, Russia
Nitika Dang	Consultant Sleep Medicine, Naõ Health (Fellow, World Sleep Federation - Indian Society of Sleep Research; American Academy of Sleep Medicine), New Delhi, India
Nicole Lovato	National Centre for Sleep Health Services Research, Bedford Park, South Australia, Australia Adelaide Institute for Sleep Health/FHMRI Sleep, College of Medicine and Public Health, Flinders University, Bedford Park, South Australia, Australia
Nishad Bhatta	Department of Pulmonary, Critical Care & Sleep Medicine B.P., Koirala Institute of Health Sciences (BPKIHS), Dharan, Nepal

Nevin Fayez Zaki — Sleep Research Unit, Department of Psychiatry, Faculty of Medicine, Mansoura University, Mansoura, Egypt

Nicole Grivell — National Centre for Sleep Health Services Research, Bedford Park, South Australia, Australia
Adelaide Institute for Sleep Health/FHMRI Sleep, College of Medicine and Public Health, Flinders University, Bedford Park, South Australia, Australia

Nesreen Elsayed Morsy — Pulmonary Medicine, Sleep Disordered Breathing Unit (SDB), Mansoura University Sleep Center (MUSC), Mansoura, Egypt

Olufemi K. OGUNDIPE — Department of Oral Maxillofacial Surgery, Obafemi Awolowo University Ile-Ife, Osun State, Nigeria

Ondrej Ludka — Department of Internal Medicine – Cardioangiology, Faculty of Medicine, Masaryk University and Teaching Hospital St. Anna, Brno, Czech Republic

Oluwatosin E. OLORUNMOTENI — Department of Paediatrics and Child Health, Obafemi Awolowo University, Ile-Ife, Osun State, Nigeria

Prapan Yongchaiyudh — Sleep Society of Thailand, Bangkok, Thailand

Preeti Devnani — Neurological Institute, Cleveland Clinic Abu Dhabi, Abu Dhabi, United Arab Emirates

Rainer Popovic — Department of Internal Medicine, Franziskusspital, 1050 Wien, Austria

Reinhold Kerbl — Department of Pediatrics and Adolescent Medicine, LKH Hochsteiermark, 8900 Leoben, Austria

Rejina Shahi — Department of Pulmonary, Critical Care & Sleep Medicine B.P., Koirala Institute of Health Sciences (BPKIHS), Dharan, Nepal

Samson Khachatryan — Department of Neurology and Neurosurgery, National Institute of Health, Yerevan, Armenia
Sleep Disorders Center, Somnus Neurology Clinic, Yerevan, Armenia

Sergio Tufik — Department of Psychobiology, Universidade Federal de Sao Paulo, Sao Paulo, SP, Brazil

Shaden O. Qasrawi — Sleep Disorders Service, Kingdom Hospital, Riyadh, Saudi Arabia

Sion Hangma Limbu — Department of Pulmonary, Critical Care & Sleep Medicine B.P., Koirala Institute of Health Sciences (BPKIHS), Dharan, Nepal

Sobia Farooq — Respiratory Institute, Cleveland Clinic Abu Dhabi, Abu Dhabi, United Arab Emirates

Sona Nevsimalova — Department of Neurology and Clinical Sciences, 1st Faculty of Medicine, Charles University and General Teaching Hospital, Prague, Czech Republic

Srijan Katwal — Department of Pulmonary, Critical Care & Sleep Medicine B.P., Koirala Institute of Health Sciences (BPKIHS), Dharan, Nepal

Tayard Desudchit Excellence Center for Sleep Disorders, King Chulalongkorn Memorial Hospital, Thai Red Cross Society, Bangkok, Thailand
Sleep Society of Thailand, Bangkok, Thailand
Division of Pediatric Neurology, Department of Pediatrics, Chulalongkorn University, Bangkok, Thailand

Thuan Dang Northwestern Feinberg School of Medicine, Chicago, IL, USA

Timothy G. Quinnell Royal Papworth Hospital Foundation NHS Trust, Cambridge, UK

Ulises Jiménez Correa Sleep Disorder Clinic, Faculty of Medicine, Research Division, National Autonomous University of Mexico, 04510 Ciudad de México, CDMX, Mexico

Valeria Amelina Herzen State Pedagogical University of Russia, St Petersburg, Russia
Almazov National Medical Research Centre, St Petersburg, Russia

Valiensi Stella Sleep Medicine-Neurology, Hospital Italiano, Ciudad de Buenos Aires (CABA), Argentina

Vivian Leske Sleep Unit-Pediatric Pulmonology, Hospital de Pediatría S.A.M.I.C. "Prof. Dr. J.P. Garrahan", Ciudad de Buenos Aires (CABA), Argentina

V.K.H. Lam Department of Psychiatry, Faculty of Medicine, The Chinese University of Hong Kong, Hong Kong SAR, China

Y.K. Wing Department of Psychiatry, Faculty of Medicine, The Chinese University of Hong Kong, Shatin, N.T., Hong Kong SAR, China
Department of Psychiatry, Faculty of Medicine, The Chinese University of Hong Kong, Hong Kong SAR, China

Yotin Chinvarun Sleep Society of Thailand, Bangkok, Thailand
Neurology division, Department of Medicine, Phramongkutklao Royal Army Hospital and Medical College, Bangkok, Thailand

Yurii Sviryaev Almazov National Medical Research Centre, St Petersburg, Russia

Zachary L. Adirim Division of Neurology, Department of Medicine, unnybrook Health Sciences Centre, University of Toronto, Toronto, Ontario, Canada

Current Practice of Sleep Medicine in the USA

Thuan Dang[1,*] and **Carmen Taype-Roberts**[1]

[1] *Northwestern Feinberg School of Medicine, Chicago, IL, USA*

Abstract: Sleep medicine and its practice in the United States of America (USA) has grown from the first center focusing on sleep disorders established at Stanford University in 1964 to more than 2,500 American Academy of Sleep Medicine (AASM) accredited sleep centers and numerous professional organizations supporting sleep health professionals including board-certified sleep medicine physicians, behavioral sleep specialists, advance practice registered nurses and/or physician assistants and sleep technologists. As sleep medicine continues to grow in the USA, multiple challenges including widening economic inequality, racial/ethnic inequities, and limited healthcare access directly affects the patient setting. Limited sleep medicine education in medical school restricts the ability to educate patients as well as primary care providers on the importance of identifying sleep disorders early on to improve access. The financial burdens of diagnosing and treating sleep disorders, particularly obstructive sleep apnea is seen in an estimated cost of $16 billion annually. Research and data collection includes surveillance surveys conducted by the Sleep and Sleep Disorders Team from the Centers for Disease Control and Prevention (CDC) as well as continuing research in the diagnosis and treatment of obstructive sleep apnea. Additional studies addressing sleep issues and racial disparities in the US are prudent in highlighting this crucial area. Continued efforts in clinical and research knowledge gaps are necessary to support the growing need for sleep medicine providers and services in the USA.

Keywords: Academy of Dental Sleep Medicine, American Academy of Sleep Medicine, Board-certified sleep physicians, Centers for Disease Control and Prevention, Durable Medical Equipment, Medicare, Positive airway pressure, Sleep disparities, Training programs.

BACKGROUND

The first electrocephalogram (EEG) patterns were documented by Loomis in the US describing NREM sleep [1], which paved the way for sleep medicine to grow as a profession. This led to the development of various professional societies to serve the requirements of individual sleep medicine practitioners and sleep disor-

* **Corresponding author Thuan Dang:** Northwestern Feinberg School of Medicine, Chicago, IL, USA; Tel: +1 312-227-5595; Fax +1 312.227.9419; E-mail: tdang@luriechildrens.org

Hrayr P. Attarian, Marie-Louise M. Coussa-Koniski & Alain Michel Sabri (Eds.)

der centers. In 1964, Stanford University introduced a narcolepsy clinic, which was the first sleep disorders center established. There are currently more than 2,500 American Academy of Sleep Medicine (AASM) accredited sleep centers in the U.S. These centers are directed by a board-certified sleep medicine physician who coordinates care with a group of providers which may include otolaryngologists, behavioral sleep medicine specialists often with training in psychology, qualified dentists with sleep training, advanced practice registered nurses and/or physician assistants and sleep technologists.

Board-certified sleep medicine physicians are required to complete medical school and residency training in one of the seven approved programs including anesthesiology, family medicine, internal medicine, neurology, otolaryngology, pediatrics, or psychiatry programs before matching into and completing an ACGME 12-month sleep medicine fellowship program to become board eligible. There are currently 95 sleep medicine fellowship training programs in the US. In addition to ACGME-accredited sleep medicine fellowship programs, there are two pilot programs in the Advancing Innovation in Residency Education (AIRE) initiative. A part-time model allows a trainee to continue additional employment during training. A combined model incorporates sleep training into an established specialty training program which allows graduates to become board eligible in both specialties upon completion. Previously board certification was administered by the American Board of Sleep Medicine which is now currently offered through the Sleep Medicine Certification Program developed by the American Board of Internal Medicine (ABIM), American Board of Family Medicine (ABFM), the American Board of Pediatrics (ABP), the American Board of Psychiatry and Neurology (ABPN), and the American Board of Otolaryngology (ABOto).

The AASM endorses three different types of accreditations. The first accreditation is for sleep facilities that manage patients, perform home sleep apnea testing, and provide a laboratory for in-center sleep studies. A second accreditation is for independent sleep practices to manage patients and conduct home sleep apnea testing. The last accreditation is for Durable Medical Equipment (DME) organizations to provide sleep-related DME to patients. Accreditation is not mandatory, however, many insurers require accreditation for sleep-related services reimbursement [2].

Professional organizations that support the practice and accreditation of sleep medicine in the US include the American Academy of Sleep Medicine (AASM), the Sleep Research Society, the American Board of Sleep Medicine, the Associated Professional Sleep Societies, and the Academy of Dental Sleep Medicine (ADSM). The historical development of these organizations is beyond the scope of this chapter but the growth of each organization contributes directly to the current practice of sleep medicine in the US as we know it.

CHALLENGES TO THE PRACTICE OF SLEEP MEDICINE IN THE USA

The challenges to accessing and delivering optimal management for sleep medical conditions in the USA can be divided into 3 major areas: patients, healthcare systems, and healthcare providers. In the patient setting, the main barriers include affordability, racial and ethnic inequities, lower socioeconomic status, decreased health literacy, and limited healthcare access during the COVID-19 pandemic due to clinical operation restrictions.

Economic inequality in the USA has been associated with inequality in health. Americans with lower incomes have deficits in healthcare than wealthy Americans, in part, due to limited access to health insurance [3]. The implementation of healthcare reform through the Affordable Care Act or Obamacare, has increased healthcare access to more Americans, but the complexity of the USA healthcare system continues to serve as a barrier to healthcare access [4]. In the four largest states California, Florida, New York, and Texas, the rate of uninsured adults ages 19 to 64 varies from 12-30% [5].

Race is also a factor in access to healthcare. Studies have demonstrated that compared to Whites, Blacks do not receive similar treatment in the U.S. healthcare system. This is independent of the reduced access to healthcare facilities that Blacks often experience [6]. Black individuals are more likely to have poor sleep quality and greater risk factors for sleep apnea than White individuals. These differences persist despite adjusting for confounders such as medical comorbidities and socioeconomic status [7]. A Philadelphia-based cross-sectional study of 9,714 individuals assessed self-reported sleep quality in relation to socioeconomic factors including education level, employment status and level of poverty. African-Americans and Latinos reported poorer sleep quality in comparison with Whites. Participants with lower incomes were also found to have significantly poorer sleep quality. Post-college education is a protective factor against poor sleep. White subjects in lower poverty levels demonstrated the highest odds for poor sleep. This contrasts with other race/ethnic groups who did not have an increased likelihood of poor sleep after adjusting for the same covariates as above. These studies demonstrate that "sleep disparity" in the USA population evident in self-reported lower sleep quality is strongly associated with poverty and ethnicity [8].

A significant barrier to health care access in the rural USA is reluctance to seek health care in rural areas. This stems from cultural and financial limitations and is exacerbated when factoring in decreased range of services, availability of trained physicians willing to work in rural areas, limited public transport, and decreased availability of reliable internet service. Rural residents tend to have poorer health outcomes than urban individuals. Rural areas also have difficulty attracting and retaining physicians contributing to further inequity [9].

Health literacy impacts an individual's ability to access care. Patients who delay getting care and have difficulty finding providers generally have lower health literacy skills than individuals with adequate health literacy. This issue continues to persist even when controlling for employment, cognitive function, insurance status, poverty, and race/ethnicity. The probability that individuals seek medical care in a timely manner decreases in individuals with lower health literacy [10]. Over one-third of U.S. adults (~80 million) have limited health literacy which is defined as difficulty in reading, understanding and applying health information (*e.g.* written language on appointment reminders, discharge instructions, informed consent, medical forms, insurance applications, medical bills, medication instructions, and health education materials). This leads to poorer health outcomes, decreases patient safety, and reduces healthcare access and quality [11]. Universal health literacy precautions have been advocated by multiple professional organizations. These include providing literacy aimed at a lower educational level and accessible information in multiple formats including multiple languages. Eliminating medical jargon, providing information or instructions in a concise step wise fashion, limiting the focus of a visit to three key points or tasks, and assessing for comprehension after medical visits are all key to ensure higher health literacy. Visual aids in the form of diagrams, graphs and graphic illustrations may also increase patient understanding [12]. The use of mobile health applications (apps) to improve health literacy is a pioneering field to empower underserved patients and their caregivers in comprehending and applying medical information. There are several challenges associated to this approach including unequal, limited access to mobile technology, user error and limitations of adapting mobile health apps to different platforms, in addition to privacy and security concerns [13].

Barriers to providing the state of the care stem not only from the patient's perspective but also from the provider's perspective. This starts at the beginning of medical training. Medical schools across 12 countries (Australia, Canada, India, Indonesia, Japan, Malaysia, New Zealand, Singapore, South Korea, Thailand, United States, and Viet Nam) demonstrated that the average amount of time spent on sleep education is under 2.5 hours, with 27% of the 409 medical schools surveyed providing no sleep education. Schools in Australia, the United States and Canada report providing more than 3 hours of education. Schools in Southeast Asia including Indonesia, Malaysia, and Viet Nam provide no sleep education. Despite the high prevalence of sleep disorders, these findings demonstrate the lack of sleep education in medical training in proportion to patients affected by sleep disorders [14]. Analysis of sleep-related parameters from the 2005-2006 National Health and Nutrition Examination Survey in 6,139 individuals over the age of 16 demonstrated a lower prevalence of sleep disorders in the USA than previously reported in the literature. This suggests underdiagnosis of sleep disorders by primary care physicians [15]. Due to limited sleep education during their training, many providers may not recognize OSA symptoms, and fail to associate disease-associated comorbidities or behaviors with sleep quality impacted by sleep disorders. Although common, many PCPs do not routinely screen for sleep disorders. Many patients may present with OSA symptoms during a PCP visit and if not routinely screened referrals to a sleep specialist would be limited. Increased educational opportunities for PCPs on how to screen for OSA as well as long-term effects on cardiovascular morbidity and mortality can lead to earlier and more frequent identification of sleep disorders [16]. Currently, a little more than 6,000 physicians are boarded certified in sleep medicine. This board-certified workforce is insufficient in meeting the demands of a disproportionate population of patients who have a sleep disease, including an estimated 23.5 million adults with undiagnosed OSA [17]. The AASM is striving to reduce the number of patients with undiagnosed and untreated obstructive sleep apnea (OSA) by 10% by 2023 [18].

SPECIFIC SLEEP DISORDERS CHALLENGES

The STOP-Bang questionnaire has been demonstrated to have a strong positive predictive value to screen for moderate to severe OSA. Out of 187 participants in a primary care setting in Houston, Texas, 61% had scores of 3 and higher on the STOP-Bang questionnaire (OSA - Intermediate Risk). Only 39% (45 participants) agreed to undergo sleep studies. Of these 45 participants who underwent sleep studies, 67% were diagnosed with moderate to severe OSA and recommendations to initiate continuous positive airway pressure (CPAP) machine therapy. This study highlights the feasibility and effectiveness of routine screening and early identification of OSA in the primary care setting [19]. Screening and detection for OSA can be difficult in the elderly population. A retrospective study in US non-hospital and hospital-based clinics demonstrated a lower incidence of sleep apnea in individuals over 75 years of age compared to those between 65 and 74 years of age. It is important to take into consideration that individuals over 75 years of age have multiple comorbidities that take priority which may result in underreporting of sleep apnea symptoms. Elderly individuals may be reluctant to report their symptoms due to concerns and perceptions about sleep apnea testing and treatment [20].

The frequency of adult outpatient visits for obstructive sleep apnea was assessed using the U.S. National Hospital Ambulatory Medical Care Survey database from 1993-2010. The diagnosis of sleep apnea during outpatient visits in comparison to hospital-based and non-hospital-based practices was more frequent in 2010 in relation to 1993. Primary care providers (33%) pulmonologists (17%), and otolaryngologists (10%) were more likely to provide sleep apnea diagnoses. Neurologists (6%), cardiologists (5%) and psychiatrists (2%) were more likely to report sleep apnea during the study period than other specialties [21]. The distribution of regional geographic locations of sleep apnea visits from 1993-2010 was reported as Northeast (21%), West (21%), Midwest (22%), and South (35%). The prevalence of obesity and health insurance status partially contributes to these geographic differences [21].

The estimated cost for diagnosing and treating OSA in the United States in 2015 was estimated by Frost & Sullivan at approximately $12.4 billion. Physician office visits and testing are approximately 7% of these costs. Positive airway pressure (PAP) machines and related accessories provided by Durable Medical Equipment organizations and custom oral appliances account for another 50%. Multiple surgical treatments are available to treat OSA and comprise the remaining 43% of OSA treatment costs. It is estimated that 29.4 million U.S. adults have OSA however only 20% (5.9 million) individuals have been diagnosed. The cost per patient averages $2,105 with a denominator of 5.9 million patients diagnosed. When removing surgical costs, this average decreases to $1,190. The payor mix of insurers and employers has not adopted aggressive OSA diagnosis and treatment. Although there is initial investment cost, the overall cost of treating individuals with OSA is significantly less than leaving the condition untreated [20]. Other treatment options outside of PAP and surgery include OSA lifestyle changes consisting of weight management and/or nocturnal body positioning. If lifestyle modifications are not enough, 3% undergo surgery and 6% are fitted for custom oral appliances. The preferred treatment approach of PAP therapy consists of CPAP, AutoPAP, or Bilevel PAP and is utilized by approximately 85% of those diagnosed with OSA (approximately 5 million). Approximately 60% of patients (3 million) are compliant with their treatment [17].

The cost of treating sleep disorders in the US is estimated to be $16 billion [22]. Coverage policies to control these costs have been implemented by The Centers for Medicare and Medicaid Services (CMS) and other national and local payers. A focus on out-of-center sleep testing to diagnose OSA as well as the use of autoPAP in lieu of in-center PAP titration studies focuses on reducing the cost of testing and treatment. Primary care and independent diagnostic testing facilities have been diagnosing OSA instead of board-certified sleep physicians to reduce costs billed by specialists. Expanding national durable medical equipment chains instead of utilizing local durable medical equipment aims to decrease cost and nationalize supply chains [22].

Insurance status can delay care. Primary outcomes of insurance-related procedure cancellation rate, time from drug-induced sleep endoscopy (DISE) and upper airway stimulation (UAS) treatment recommendations were reviewed at Thomas Jefferson University, a single academic center. This was a retrospective chart review of Medicare and private insurance patients who underwent UAS from 2015-2018. In comparison to private insurance patients, Medicare patients who underwent UAS had less insurance-related treatment delays, shorter waiting periods, and fewer procedure cancellations. Private insurance patients faced prior authorization barriers. This resulted in the initial denial of almost half the patients. After the appeals process, 21.1% of patients continued to be denied for treatment. While only 6.4% of patients with Medicare coverage were denied [23].

Another common sleep disorder with multiple negative health impacts is insomnia. Direct and indirect healthcare costs related to insomnia have been estimated at $100 billion US dollars per year. Quality of life (QOL), impaired cognition, mood, and productivity can all be affected by insomnia [24].

The America Insomnia Survey (AIS) collected results from October 2008 to July 2009 and estimates the prevalence of insomnia at 23.2%. Insomnia resulted in lost work performance due to absenteeism. This insomnia to individual-level association was the equivalent of 11.3 days, accounting for $2280 of individual-level lost capital. These estimates generalized the total US workforce annualized at the population-level of 252.7 days and a loss of $63.2 billion in productivity secondary to insomnia [25].

Restless legs syndrome (RLS) and its economic impact have not been extensively investigated. A study from 2011 explored factors including expenditures, healthcare resource use, and lost productivity reported by patients. Patients with primary RLS reported a mean productivity loss of 1 day/week. As RLS symptom severity increased, RLS-related costs increased affecting work productivity, sleep disturbance, and health status. Moderately severe RLS results in 20 to 50% workplace productivity loss highlighting high personal and social costs. RLS is often underdiagnosed and treated. These study findings suggest improvements in RLS diagnosis and treatment should be a major public health priority given the high prevalence and social costs [26].

It is important to note that COVID-19 significantly impacted access to care and introduced new challenges.

CULTURAL, RACIAL AND AGE CHALLENGES

Strategies to reduce the discrepancies in health care of racial and ethnic minorities compared with Whites need to focus on culturally competent services. In order to break down linguistic and cultural barriers, a focus on understanding health-related attitudes, beliefs, and different cultural practices can improve services and close gaps in health status [27]. Racial and ethnic minorities in the United States are more likely to report short (≤6 hours) sleep durations, in comparison to non-Hispanic white. Short sleep duration is linked to cardiovascular disease, diabetes, obesity and overall, increased mortality. Poor health outcomes are also associated with poor sleep quality. Minority populations are at increased risk for poor sleep quality and sleep complaints are difficult to assess given linguistic barriers [28].

US adolescents routinely sleep more than the recommended 8 hours on school nights, as many as two-thirds do not achieve this recommendation. Compared to their white peers, racial and ethnic minority children and adolescents are more likely to have poorer sleep quality and shorter sleep duration. A review of 23 studies assessing sleep in American children and adolescents ages 6-19 years found that White youth regularly had greater sufficient sleep than minority youth and Hispanics had more than Blacks [29]. A two-arm randomized control trial to evaluate the effectiveness of a tailored intervention was assessed from 2010-2014 among black patients with metabolic syndrome at four community-based clinics in Brooklyn, New York. This intervention used culturally and linguistically tailored OSA health messages delivered by a trained health educator. These messages were based on patients' readiness to change and addressed unique barriers that prevented behavior change. The tailored intervention increased sleep consultations and evaluation of OSA among blacks. No significant difference was found between the two arms. The defined success of this tailored intervention was attributed to its focus on addressing sociocultural factors, primarily discontent with health-care providers and health-care services among black adolescents [30].

When assessing the adult population in the US, almost one-third get an inadequate amount of sleep. Among working American adults, the less educated, those living alone, and racial/ethnic minorities are at a greater risk for short sleep duration [31]. Long work hours, variable shift work, or working in high stress professions place an individual at increased risk for short sleep duration and subsequent physical, and mental health consequences.

The National Health Interview Survey (NHIS) from 2010-2018 assessed the prevalence of short sleep duration (< 7 hours) in working American adults on an annual basis. Short sleep duration risk factors included falling in the age bracket of 45-64 years, identifying as African American, holding less than a bachelor's degree, being separated, divorced, or widowed, and having a family structure of more than one child at home. Individuals living in the South had the highest prevalence of short sleep duration in any given year compared to their counterparts. Short sleep duration and poor sleep quality are associated with adverse health outcomes [31].

Racial/ethnic minorities are at increased risk for short sleep duration and poor sleep quality. Sleep quality of recent immigrants suggest that the acculturation process is linked to insufficient sleep among Asian, Black, and Latino immigrants and present as psychosomatic disorders, OSA, REM behavior disorder, and short sleep duration [28].

Patients with sleep-disordered breathing (SDB) have a high prevalence of comorbidities that increase their susceptibility to COVID-19. The traditional treatment with positive pressure devices (PAP) is challenging because of increased transmission risk due to PAP-induced droplets and aerosol. During the initial lockdown and mitigation period in 2020, the use of telemedicine rapidly emerged as an option to continue access to care and management of OSA in a safe manner [32]. Diagnostic testing was temporarily suspended as sleep centers closed over concerns of rising COVID-19 rates and risk of infection of staff and patients. Expansion of home sleep testing devices and placing patients on auto-CPAP allowed for continued diagnostic and management access for OSA patients [33]. Even before COVID-19, a retrospective study of sleep telemedicine at the Milwaukee VAMC demonstrated increased efficiency of sleep services and improved follow-ups [34]. Many sleep centers have continued to offer telemedicine services in addition to in-person scheduling after COVID-19 vaccination campaigns were enacted and medical staff members returned to the office and sleep laboratory.

CLINICAL AND RESEARCH KNOWLEDGE GAP

Sleep Medicine has evolved over the past 40 years due to new discoveries in the science of sleep and circadian rhythms, and the advancement in the knowledge of pathophysiology of sleep disorders [35].

The Centers for Disease Control and Prevention (CDC) has engaged the Sleep and Sleep Disorders team with a mission to raise awareness about the problem of sleep disorders, sleep insufficiency, and the influence of sleep in health and disease states. Approximately 70 million Americans identify with chronic sleep problems. Insufficient sleep is associated with chronic disease, decreased quality of life, injury, increased health care cost, psychiatric disorders, and reduced work productivity. Sleep problems are major contributors to depression and obesity but are rarely addressed. Public health research conducted by the Sleep and Sleep

Disorders team analyzes the relationships between insufficient sleep, chronic disease, and social outcomes [36]. The Sleep and Sleep Disorders Team has implemented new sleep questions for the Behavioral Risk Factor Surveillance System (BRFSS) which is part of the CDC's public health surveillance system. The BRFSS is the world's largest health survey system and tracks health conditions and risk behaviors in the United States *via* telephone annually since 1984.

The BRFSS provides critical information for monitoring national and state population health. A limitation of the BRFSS surveys is the lack of enough samples. This results in the inability to provide direct survey estimates for most counties or sub-county areas. To compensate, model multilevel regression and poststratification for small-area estimation of population health outcomes are used to estimate short sleep duration prevalence at different geographic levels [37]. These estimates are then used by communities, local policy makers, and program planners for public health program development and evaluation. In the past few years, the response rates for the BRFSS surveys have declined. It is prudent that new methods of weighting and cell phone sampling frames are reassessed. Question variations among surveys used and mode of data collection are some limitations of the BRFSS. Recognizing these challenges, revised methodologies and inclusion of cell phone data will be necessary to continue collecting population health data and the impact on sleep [38].

The National Healthy Sleep Awareness Project (NHSAP) was a collaboration between the CDC, the American Academy of Sleep Medicine and Sleep Research Society. NHSAP sought to improve surveillance of sleep health in the US by increasing scope of questions for the BRFSS.

As a result, the BRFSS has grown from approximately 100,000 telephone interviews to over 500,000 from 1993 to 2015. As the BRFSS continues to grow, this data should be utilized by sleep researchers in their published results regarding sleep health. The use of the data validates the utility of the information collected and that data are reviewed by policy makers and stakeholders working to improve the health and wellness of the US population [39].

Excessive daytime sleepiness and poor or unrefreshing sleep are frequent concerns in the primary care setting. Early detection of undiagnosed cases of sleep disorders is imperative to ensure timely intervention. Unfortunately, barriers to earlier diagnosis include the lack of education and training among non-sleep physicians regarding identification and treatment of sleep disorders. Screening tools in populations at high-risk for OSA in primary care could improve patient outcomes and reduce the complications of untreated OSA [40]. In an Australian study, PCPs were trained for 6 hours in the management of OSA. Patients who had moderate daytime sleepiness identified as Epworth Sleepiness Score ≥8 were randomly assigned to outpatient management by primary care physicians who had received training or a sleep specialist. After 6 months, primary care management was comparable to sleep specialist management which was measured by improvement in ESS, OSA symptoms and CPAP adherence [41].

The vast majority of PCPs are willing to assess for sleep disorders but very few will treat. This gap can be closed if PCPs were provided additional and adequate training in sleep medicine [42]. A provider survey demonstrates a large disparity between PCPs' prioritization of sleep disorders and reported low comfort levels with diagnosing and management. The use of screening questionnaires would aid PCPs in incorporating sleep disorder detection into their daily practice [43].

Teaching hospitals should encourage the growth of the field of sleep medicine. This focus should not only focus on physicians, but also on allied health staff, nurses, and technologists to support the diagnosis and treatment of common sleep disorders including OSA, insomnia, circadian rhythm disorders, restless legs syndrome, REM behavior disorder and others [17].

OSA is a common condition associated with cardiovascular outcomes based on the underlying pathophysiology (ie, endotypes) and its sequelae of disease (ie, phenotypes). Due to this variability, OSA is now being targeted as a disease responsive to precision medicine [44]. The care of these patients would take into account biomarker, genetic, pathophysiologic, phenotypic and treatment response characteristics of precision medicine methods [45].

Significant research advances regarding the pathophysiology and disease progression of OSA have been made. The next step should focus on targeting the molecular and cellular processes that link the circadian clock with multiple mechanisms seen in OSA (ie, autonomic dysregulation, inflammation, metabolic dysfunction). These links will help to identify the role of circadian dysregulation in the development of OSA. A proposed mechanism of multiple physio-pathological mechanisms is seen in Fig. (**1**) [46]. Hypoxia affects both clock dysregulation and sleep fragmentation. Sleep fragmentation can influence clock dysregulation by intrinsic or extrinsic mechanisms (ie, epigenetics), as well as the regulation of oxygenation. These intrinsic and extrinsic mechanisms lead to inflammation resulting in the progression of cardiopulmonary disease observed in untreated OSA.

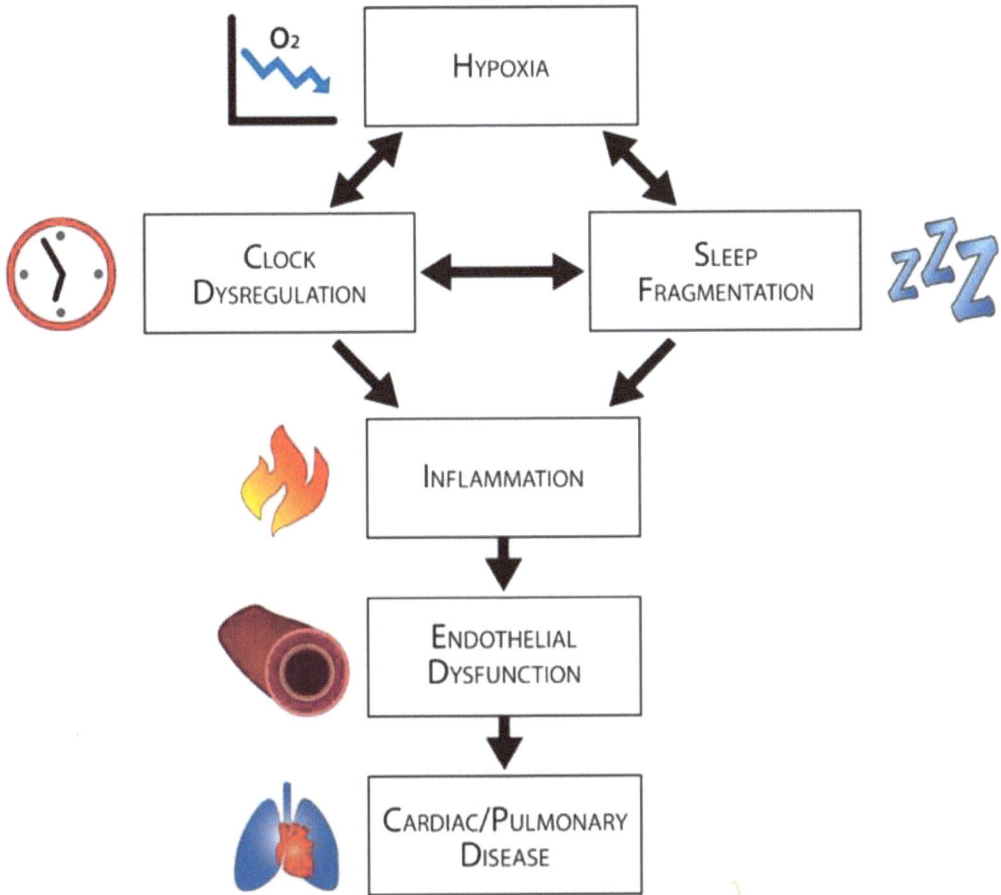

Fig. (1). A proposed mechanism for the role of circadian clock dysregulation, sleep fragmentation, and hypoxia in the pathophysiologic progression of cardiopulmonary disease seen in untreated obstructive sleep apnea with involvement of inflammation, endothelial dysfunction and cardiac/pulmonary diseases. Causes of hypoxia include sleep related hypoventilation, cheyne stokes breathing, central sleep apnea and obstructive sleep apnea. Figure was obtained from von Allmen *et al* [47].

In regard to cultural and racial gaps, the lack of sleep studies in ethnic minorities is one major research limitation in the field of sleep medicine. Sleep medicine research should also focus on reducing racial and ethnic disparities. For example, more research is needed on children, minority older adults and veterans. Sleep medicine providers should engage in cross-cultural education to enhance and provide more integrative care. There is a need to assess the inter-ethnic differences comparing US-born, foreign-born Caribbean blacks [28], Asians, and Hispanics living in urban and rural areas. African Americans have higher percentages of severe OSA compared to other racial groups, suggesting a delay in the initial diagnosis. This could explain at least in part the rate of suboptimal outcomes after OSA treatment. Among adults with OSA, adherence to CPAP is significantly lower in African Americans. The reasons for these disparities, especially in outcomes, are not very well understood. This is one reason why research on the minority population should be a priority [47]. Findings of these investigations will hopefully lead to targeted approaches to reduce racial and ethnic disparities.

CONCLUSION

Over the last 40 years, sleep medicine has continued to evolve due to new discoveries in the science of sleep and circadian rhythms, and the knowledge advances regarding pathophysiology of sleep disorders. There are significant clinical centers including over 2,500 AASM accredited sleep centers and 95 sleep medicine fellowship training programs and these numbers continue to grow.

The challenges to accessing and delivering optimal management for sleep medical conditions in the USA can be divided in 3 very well-connected major areas: patient, health care system, and health care providers. The main barriers in the patient setting include affordability, socioeconomic status, racial/ethnic inequities, poor health literacy, and restricted healthcare access during the COVID-19 pandemic.

The burden of chronic sleep problems affects approximately 70 million Americans. Specific sleep teams such as The Sleep and Sleep Disorders Team from the Centers for Disease Control and Prevention from the USA have continued to raise awareness about the problem of sleep insufficiency and sleep disorders and the importance of sleep health for the nation's overall health.

Much collaboration has been made for incorporating sleep health measures in the Behavioral Risk Factor Surveillance System and other CDC surveillance data. These findings are necessary to address the clinical and knowledge gaps as well as racial and health disparities impacting patients and their sleep disorders. Continued research and dissemination is key as policy makers and stakeholders work to improve the health and wellness of the US population.

CONSENT FOR PUBLICATION

Not applicable.

CONFLICT OF INTEREST

The authors declare no conflict of interest, financial or otherwise.

ACKNOWLEDGEMENT

Declared none.

REFERENCES

[1]   Loomis AL, Harvey EN, Hobart GA. Cerebral states during sleep, as studied by human brain potentials. J Exp Psychol 1937; 21(2): 127-44.
[http://dx.doi.org/10.1037/h0057431]

[2]   American Academy of Sleep Medicine. Accreditation Process and Policies 2020.

[3]   Dickman SL, Himmelstein DU, Woolhandler S. Inequality and the health-care system in the USA. Lancet 2017; 389(10077): 1431-41.
[http://dx.doi.org/10.1016/S0140-6736(17)30398-7] [PMID: 28402825]

[4]   Clarke JL, Bourn S, Skoufalos A, Beck EH, Castillo DJ. An Innovative Approach to Health Care Delivery for Patients with Chronic Conditions. Popul Health Manag 2017; 20(1): 23-30.
[http://dx.doi.org/10.1089/pop.2016.0076] [PMID: 27563751]

[5]   Rasmussen PW, Collins SR, Doty MM, Beutel S. Health care coverage and access in the nation's four largest states. Results from the Commonwealth Fund Biennial Health Insurance Survey, 2014. Issue Brief (Commonw Fund) 2015; 7: 1-12.
[PMID: 25890978]

[6]   Pandi-Perumal SR, Abumuamar AM, Spence DW, Chattu VK, Moscovitch A, BaHammam AS. Racial/Ethnic and Social Inequities in Sleep Medicine: The Tip of the Iceberg? J Natl Med Assoc 2017; 109(4): 279-86.
[http://dx.doi.org/10.1016/j.jnma.2017.04.005] [PMID: 29173935]

[7]   Petrov ME, Lichstein KL. Differences in sleep between black and white adults: an update and future directions. Sleep Med 2016; 18: 74-81.
[http://dx.doi.org/10.1016/j.sleep.2015.01.011] [PMID: 25754383]

[8]   Patel NP, Grandner MA, Xie D, Branas CC, Gooneratne N. "Sleep disparity" in the population: poor sleep quality is strongly associated with poverty and ethnicity. BMC Public Health 2010; 10(1): 475.
[http://dx.doi.org/10.1186/1471-2458-10-475] [PMID: 20701789]

[9]   Douthit N, Kiv S, Dwolatzky T, Biswas S. Exposing some important barriers to health care access in the rural USA. Public Health 2015; 129(6): 611-20.
[http://dx.doi.org/10.1016/j.puhe.2015.04.001] [PMID: 26025176]

[10]   Levy H, Janke A. 2016.

[11]   Berkman ND, Sheridan SL, Donahue KE, Halpern DJ, Crotty K. Low health literacy and health outcomes: an updated systematic review. Ann Intern Med 2011; 155(2): 97-107.
[http://dx.doi.org/10.7326/0003-4819-155-2-201107190-00005] [PMID: 21768583]

[12]   Hersh L, Salzman B, Snyderman D. Health Literacy in Primary Care Practice. Am Fam Physician 2015; 92(2): 118-24.
[PMID: 26176370]

[13]   Kim H, Goldsmith JV, Sengupta S, *et al.* Mobile Health Application and e-Health Literacy: Opportunities and Concerns for Cancer Patients and Caregivers. J Cancer Educ 2019; 34(1): 3-8.
[http://dx.doi.org/10.1007/s13187-017-1293-5] [PMID: 29139070]

[14]   Mindell JA, Bartle A, Wahab NA, *et al.* Sleep education in medical school curriculum: A glimpse across countries. Sleep Med 2011; 12(9): 928-31.
[http://dx.doi.org/10.1016/j.sleep.2011.07.001] [PMID: 21924951]

[15]   Ram S, Seirawan H, Kumar SKS, Clark GT. Prevalence and impact of sleep disorders and sleep habits in the United States. Sleep Breath 2010; 14(1): 63-70.

[http://dx.doi.org/10.1007/s11325-009-0281-3] [PMID: 19629554]

[16]   Miller JN, Berger AM. Screening and assessment for obstructive sleep apnea in primary care. Sleep Med Rev 2016; 29: 41-51.
[http://dx.doi.org/10.1016/j.smrv.2015.09.005] [PMID: 26606318]

[17]   Sullivan F. Hidden health crisis costing America billions: underdiagnosing and undertreating obstructive sleep apnea draining health care system. American Academy of Sleep Medicine 2018.

[18]   Rosen IM. Change is the Only Constant in Life (and in Sleep Medicine). J Clin Sleep Med 2018; 14(6): 1025-30.
[http://dx.doi.org/10.5664/jcsm.7174] [PMID: 29852896]

[19]   Ononye T, Nguyen K, Brewer E. Implementing protocol for obstructive sleep apnea screening in the primary care setting. Appl Nurs Res 2019; 46: 67-71.
[http://dx.doi.org/10.1016/j.apnr.2019.02.005] [PMID: 30853078]

[20]   Namen AM, Forest DJ, Huang KE, *et al.* Physicians Report Sleep Apnea Infrequently in Older and Older Vulnerable Adults. J Am Geriatr Soc 2017; 65(9): 2023-8.
[http://dx.doi.org/10.1111/jgs.14929] [PMID: 28470836]

[21]   Namen AM, Chatterjee A, Huang KE, Feldman SR, Haponik EF. Recognition of Sleep Apnea Is Increasing. Analysis of Trends in Two Large, Representative Databases of Outpatient Practice. Ann Am Thorac Soc 2016; 13(11): 2027-34.
[http://dx.doi.org/10.1513/AnnalsATS.201603-152OC] [PMID: 27585409]

[22]   El-Feky WH, Evans DA. Sleep Medicine Coding and Coverage Guidelines 2017.
[http://dx.doi.org/10.1212/CON.0000000000000494]

[23]   Patel J, Topf MC, Huntley C, Boon M. Does Insurance Status Impact Delivery of Care with Upper Airway Stimulation for OSA? Ann Otol Rhinol Laryngol 2020; 129(2): 128-34.
[http://dx.doi.org/10.1177/0003489419878454] [PMID: 31544468]

[24]   Taddei-Allen P. Economic burden and managed care considerations for the treatment of insomnia. Am J Manag Care 2020; 26(4) (Suppl.): S91-6.
[PMID: 32282179]

[25]   Kessler RC, Berglund PA, Coulouvrat C, *et al.* Insomnia and the performance of US workers: results from the America insomnia survey. Sleep 2011; 34(9): 1161-71.
[http://dx.doi.org/10.5665/SLEEP.1230] [PMID: 21886353]

[26]   Allen RP, Bharmal M, Calloway M. Prevalence and disease burden of primary restless legs syndrome: Results of a general population survey in the United States. Mov Disord 2011; 26(1): 114-20.
[http://dx.doi.org/10.1002/mds.23430] [PMID: 21322022]

[27]   Stephenson J. Cultural Barriers to Care. JAMA 1999; 282(23): 2201.
[http://dx.doi.org/10.1001/jama.282.23.2201-JHA90010-4-1] [PMID: 10605959]

[28]   Williams NJ, Grandner MA, Snipes SA, *et al.* Racial/ethnic disparities in sleep health and health care: importance of the sociocultural context. Sleep Health 2015; 1(1): 28-35.
[http://dx.doi.org/10.1016/j.sleh.2014.12.004] [PMID: 26229976]

[29]   Guglielmo D, Gazmararian JA, Chung J, Rogers AE, Hale L. Racial/ethnic sleep disparities in US school-aged children and adolescents: a review of the literature. Sleep Health 2018; 4(1): 68-80.
[http://dx.doi.org/10.1016/j.sleh.2017.09.005] [PMID: 29332684]

[30]   Jean-Louis G, Newsome V, Williams NJ, Zizi F, Ravenell J, Ogedegbe G. Tailored Behavioral Intervention Among Blacks With Metabolic Syndrome and Sleep Apnea: Results of the MetSO Trial. Sleep 2017; 40(1)
[http://dx.doi.org/10.1093/sleep/zsw008] [PMID: 28364475]

[31]   Khubchandani J, Price JH. Short Sleep Duration in Working American Adults, 2010–2018. J Community Health 2020; 45(2): 219-27.

[http://dx.doi.org/10.1007/s10900-019-00731-9] [PMID: 31489537]

[32]   Voulgaris A, Ferini-Strambi L, Steiropoulos P. Sleep medicine and COVID-19. Has a new era begun? Sleep Med 2020; 73: 170-6.
       [http://dx.doi.org/10.1016/j.sleep.2020.07.010] [PMID: 32836085]

[33]   Thorpy M, Figuera-Losada M, Ahmed I, *et al.* Management of sleep apnea in New York City during the COVID-19 pandemic. Sleep Med 2020; 74: 86-90.
       [http://dx.doi.org/10.1016/j.sleep.2020.07.013] [PMID: 32841850]

[34]   Baig MM, Antonescu-Turcu A, Ratarasarn K. Impact of Sleep Telemedicine Protocol in Management of Sleep Apnea: A 5-Year VA Experience. Telemed J E Health 2016; 22(5): 458-62.
       [http://dx.doi.org/10.1089/tmj.2015.0047] [PMID: 26974884]

[35]   Shepard JW Jr, Buysse DJ, Chesson AL Jr, *et al.* History of the development of sleep medicine in the United States. J Clin Sleep Med 2005; 1(1): 61-82.
       [http://dx.doi.org/10.5664/jcsm.26298] [PMID: 17561617]

[36]   Sleep and Sleep Disorders Tem tCfDCaPC. National Center for Chronic Disease Prevention and Health Promotion, Division of Population Health. 2017.

[37]   Zhang X, Holt JB, Lu H, *et al.* Multilevel regression and poststratification for small-area estimation of population health outcomes: a case study of chronic obstructive pulmonary disease prevalence using the behavioral risk factor surveillance system. Am J Epidemiol 2014; 179(8): 1025-33.
       [http://dx.doi.org/10.1093/aje/kwu018] [PMID: 24598867]

[38]   Pierannunzi C, Hu SS, Balluz L. A systematic review of publications assessing reliability and validity of the Behavioral Risk Factor Surveillance System (BRFSS), 2004–2011. BMC Med Res Methodol 2013; 13(1): 49.
       [http://dx.doi.org/10.1186/1471-2288-13-49] [PMID: 23522349]

[39]   Morgenthaler TI, Croft JB, Dort LC, Loeding LD, Mullington JM, Thomas SM. Development of the National Healthy Sleep Awareness Project Sleep Health Surveillance Questions. J Clin Sleep Med 2015; 11(9): 1057-62.
       [http://dx.doi.org/10.5664/jcsm.5026] [PMID: 26235156]

[40]   Aurora RN, Quan SF. Quality Measure for Screening for Adult Obstructive Sleep Apnea by Primary Care Physicians. J Clin Sleep Med 2016; 12(8): 1185-7.
       [http://dx.doi.org/10.5664/jcsm.6064] [PMID: 27397659]

[41]   Chai-Coetzer CL, Antic NA, Rowland LS, *et al.* Primary care vs specialist sleep center management of obstructive sleep apnea and daytime sleepiness and quality of life: a randomized trial. JAMA 2013; 309(10): 997-1004.
       [http://dx.doi.org/10.1001/jama.2013.1823] [PMID: 23483174]

[42]   Klingman KJ, Morse A, Williams N, Grandner M, Perlis ML. Sleep Disorders Screening in Primary Care: Prevalence of Diagnosis and Treatment in the EMR. Sleep (Basel) 2020; 43: A448-9.

[43]   Senthilvel E, Auckley D, Dasarathy J. Evaluation of sleep disorders in the primary care setting: history taking compared to questionnaires. J Clin Sleep Med 2011; 7(1): 41-8.
       [http://dx.doi.org/10.5664/jcsm.28040] [PMID: 21344054]

[44]   Light M, Owens RL, Schmickl CN, Malhotra A. Precision Medicine for Obstructive Sleep Apnea. Sleep Med Clin 2019; 14(3): 391-8.
       [http://dx.doi.org/10.1016/j.jsmc.2019.05.005] [PMID: 31375207]

[45]   Zinchuk A, Yaggi HK. Phenotypic Subtypes of OSA. Chest 2020; 157(2): 403-20.
       [http://dx.doi.org/10.1016/j.chest.2019.09.002] [PMID: 31539538]

[46]   Dudley KA, Patel SR. Disparities and genetic risk factors in obstructive sleep apnea. Sleep Med 2016; 18: 96-102.
       [http://dx.doi.org/10.1016/j.sleep.2015.01.015] [PMID: 26428843]

[47]   von Allmen DC, Francey LJ, Rogers GM, *et al.* Circadian Dysregulation: The Next Frontier in Obstructive Sleep Apnea Research. Otolaryngol Head Neck Surg 2018; 159(6): 948-55.
[http://dx.doi.org/10.1177/0194599818797311] [PMID: 30200807]

CHAPTER 2

Sleep Medicine in Canada

Zachary L. Adirim[1] and **Brian J. Murray**[1,*]

[1] *Division of Neurology, Department of Medicine, Sunnybrook Health Sciences Centre, University of Toronto, Toronto, Ontario, Canada*

Abstract: Canada has an expansive, challenging geography with diverse demographics. The country is an industrialized and democratic nation situated at the northern end of the Americas. Canada provides universal healthcare to all residents through a single-payer system administered by its provinces and territories. Data suggests common sleep disorders are present at similar rates in other industrialized nations, with the exception of a larger number of shift workers and arctic residents subject to circadian disruption. Canada has 'punched above its weight' in contributing to the field of sleep medicine, with numerous well-known pioneering specialists in areas ranging from pathophysiology and diagnostic development, to pharmacologic, therapeutic and device treatment. The practice of sleep medicine is provided by trained physicians in neurology, respirology, psychiatry, internal medicine, family practice, otolaryngology, pediatrics, as well as psychology and dentistry amongst other providers. Major challenges to Canadian sleep medicine include limited public healthcare funding, variable funding mechanisms across the nation's jurisdictions, limited access to diagnostic and therapeutics, and conflicts-of-interest with business. Certain demographic groups are particularly at-risk, including socioeconomically challenged communities, indigenous populations, and other diverse minority groups. Canada's characteristics and challenges provide it with substantial research opportunities and a chance to lead in such areas as epidemiology, sleep medicine genetics, ethnic and cultural aspects, circadian and shift work considerations, home polysomnography and post-COVID transitions to more virtual sleep medicine care.

Keywords: Apnea, Canada, Circadian, COVID-19, Hypersomnolence, Insomnia, Narcolepsy, Restless, REM, Sleep.

BACKGROUND

Canada is the northernmost country in North America, bordering the Pacific Ocean to the west, the Arctic Ocean to the North, and the Atlantic Ocean to the East boasting the longest coastline in the world [1]. Its territory expands over 9.94 million square kilometres, making it the world's second-largest country by total

---

* **Corresponding author Brian J. Murray:** Division of Neurology, Department of Medicine, Sunnybrook Health Sciences Centre, University of Toronto, Toronto, Ontario, Canada Tel: +1-416-480-6100 ext. 2461; Fax: +1-416-480-6092; E-mail: brian.murray@utoronto.ca

Hrayr P. Attarian, Marie-Louise M. Coussa-Koniski & Alain Michel Sabri (Eds.)

area [1]. It shares the world's longest bi-national border with its only land neighbour, the United States of America [1].

The northern extent of the country leads to reduced daylight in the winter and can contribute to problems of circadian rhythms.

Canada's climate ranges from arctic and subarctic in the north, to subarctic throughout the central regions, warm-summer humid continental in the south and southeast, and oceanic and warm-summer Mediterranean in the southwest. Thus, winter and summer temperatures vary greatly across the country, with temperate to relatively warm winters and mild summers on the southwest coast, cold winters and warm summers in the prairies, and cold, cold winters and humid summers in the Great Lakes regions, and cold winters and mild summers on the east coast.

Canada's geology and ecology are varied, with a permafrost and tundra region in the north, a mountainous western region dominated by boreal forests including the coast and Rocky Mountain ranges, prairies in the centre, and deciduous lowland forests in the east along the Great Lakes and Atlantic Ocean.

For millennia, the land of what is now Canada was home to numerous indigenous communities. European expeditions led chiefly by the United Kingdom (UK) and France gradually colonized the lands from the 16th to 19th centuries, with the British eventually gaining autonomous control of 'British North America', and thereafter ceding autonomy peacefully to self-government gradually culminating in the UK's recognition of Canadian independence with the Statue of Westminster in 1931.

Canada is a parliamentary democracy, formed as a confederacy of ten provinces and three territories, together consisting of a total population of nearly 38 million people [1]. One of the least densely populated countries in the world, Canada can have difficulties providing care in many remote communities. Canada's populace is highly urbanized, and located in close proximity to its southern border [1]. The six largest urban areas of Toronto, Montreal, Vancouver, Calgary, Edmonton and Ottawa together make up nearly half of the country's population. Most bulk of sleep medicine care is administered from larger urban centres.

Canada is one of the most ethnically and linguistically diverse countries in the world, driven by one of the highest per-capita immigration and refugee resettlement rates among nations. Nearly one-quarter of the population are first-generation immigrants, and belong to visible minorities [2]. Official languages are English and French, with the majority English-speaking in all provinces except Quebec, which retains a strong cultural distinctness in this regard. A sizeable indigenous community making up 4.9% of the population is present across all provinces, however, most highly concentrated in the Northern Territories of Yukon, Northwest Territories and Nunavut [2]. A fifth of the country's population speaks a non-official tongue, most commonly Punjabi, Italian, Spanish, German, Cantonese, Tagalog and Arabic in order of magnitude [1]. This makes the translation of patient materials challenging.

Canada's population, while aging alongside other industrialized countries around the world, has the second-lowest proportion of those aged 65 and older, and the largest distribution of working-age adults among G7 countries [3].

Canada is ranked in the top category of 'very high', ranking twelfth among nations according to the Human Development Index [4]. It ranks 34th in GDP per capita of $48,300 [5], and boasts a median household income of $70,336 [6]. A substantial 14.2% of the population is low-income [6], and 8.7% lives in poverty [7].

Canada mandates the provision of universal healthcare to all residents and citizens, which is administered provincially and territorially. According to this system, the federal government provides funding support to the provincial and territorial systems, according to their agreement to provide healthcare according to standards of universality, accessibility, portability, comprehensiveness and public administration. The federal mandate is oriented for medically necessary care, which does not permit private healthcare providers. Canada does not allow private hospitals. Moreover, it does not include provision of paramedical services such as psychology, dentistry, or prescription medications. While subsidization provisions exist for children, seniors and social assistance recipients, the general population pays out of pocket, or has private insurance plans supplied by their workplaces or privately purchased to cover these expenses.

Canadian citizens access routine healthcare through a primary care provider (PCP), most commonly a family physician for adults, and family physician or pediatrician for children. The PCP manages routine health issues *via* clinical assessment, the utilization of outpatient investigations such as laboratory testing or imaging, and the prescription of treatments. Referrals for more specialized medical care are made from PCPs. Canadians are unable to directly seek care from specialist providers such as sleep specialists, unless referred by their PCP or another specialist.

EPIDEMIOLOGICAL DATA OF SLEEP DISORDERS IN CANADA
Insomnia

An epidemiological survey of adults across Canada showed 40% cases describing at least one symptom of insomnia [8]. Nearly one-sixth of Canadians polled reported prior visits with healthcare providers for assessment of sleep disruption [8]. Sleep problems were more common in females, most common at ages 30-60yrs, and associated with lower educational level [8]. Interestingly, French-speaking Canadians reported less insomnia symptoms and fewer medical appointments for sleep-related concerns than English-speaking residents, while at the same time, utilizing increased amounts of prescribed medications [8]. Residents in prairie provinces self-treated with alcohol more than those in other regions [8].

Circadian Rhythm Disorders

While limited data is available regarding the epidemiology of circadian rhythms disorders in Canada, trends regarding the employment structure and arctic latitudes provide insights into unique Canadian circadian rhythm considerations.

According to Statistics of Canada, 28% of employed Canadians are engaged in shift work [9], an irregular work schedule which may involve predominant daytime, evening, or on-call work. This is higher than comparable industrialized economies including Europe at 21% [10] and the USA at 18-26% [11]. Shift work is associated with a doubling of the baseline risk of insomnia [12], increased risk of fatal occupational incidents [13], and a variety of other health-related concerns including cardiovascular diseases [14], metabolic syndrome [15], GI diseases [14], various cancers [16, 17] and mental health disorders [18].

Canada's provinces and territories observe daylight saving time changes biannually with the exception of the central prairie province of Saskatchewan, which has provided an important unique control for circadian shift research. Review of Ministry of Transportation data has shown statistically significant increased rates of traffic accidents in the week following the spring shift forward in which people lose one hour of sleep and decreased rates following the fall shift backward in which people gained one hour of sleep [19].

Seasonal variations in sunlight in the arctic create natural challenges for maintaining a normal circadian rhythm. Circadian drive is drastically altered for those living in artic environments, with as much as constant exposure to sunlight in summer months, and complete absence in winter months. Residence in arctic regions has been associated with insomnia in both summer and winter months [20, 21]. Additionally, increased melatonin production has been demonstrated in Arctic residents during the winter months [22 - 24], as well as reduced sleep efficiency, total sleep time and slow-wave sleep in Antarctic residents outside of Canada [25]. Recent studies on residents of the northernmost permanently inhabited community in the world - Alert, Canada found reductions in sleep during the summer months compared with the winter, and a trend towards increased melatonin production [26]. Canada's population living in such an extreme environment provides a unique opportunity for work in this area.

Restless Legs Syndrome

Restless Legs Syndrome (RLS) prevalence studies have demonstrated a wide distribution globally. A South Asian study found a rate of 2.9% [27], East Asian studies have shown rates of 0.9-8.35% [28 - 31], while European countries have measured between 3-15% [32]. Canada sits within this distribution at 10-15% [33] with a notably increased preponderance in French-speaking groups in Canada [33]. Notably, a multitude of historical studies have been conducted with variable clinical definitions, and a most recent Western study utilizing a formal diagnostic algorithm showed a rate of 6.2% [34].

Studies of the French Canadian population of Quebec have been illuminating in the study of the genetics of restless legs syndrome. Research in these groups have demonstrated the contribution of heritability, noting a positive family history in over three-quarters of cases [35]. Numerous genetic loci were discovered with whole exome sequencing studies, including a large-meta analysis identifying 19 loci associated with RLS [36]. Further studies however, have not been able to demonstrate evidence of causative agency of various of these genetic variants [37, 38]. A recent 2019 population-based genetic study looking at the 19 previously identified genetic loci [36] alongside clinical questionnaires, interestingly found the highest risk variant to be MEIS1, which is involved in ferritin expression in the iron homeostatic pathway thereby aligning with a known pathophysiological mechanism of RLS [39]. A further 2020 association study looking at 18 previously identified RLS-associated genetic variants identified five variants that were statistically significant, and that increased symptom cluster reported on questionnaire was associated with increased genetic findings [40].

Obstructive Sleep Apnea

Three percent of Canadian adults report having been diagnosed with OSA, while over 25% of Canadian adults reported clusters of symptoms and risk factors suggesting a high risk of having or developing OSA [41]. Of the 736,000 Canadians diagnosed, 77% of them report having been referred to a sleep laboratory, and of the 4.66 million at high-risk, only 5% have been referred [41]. This suggests that over 150,000 Canadians diagnosed with OSA were not diagnosed *via* sleep study, and over 4.4 million of those at high-risk have not been investigated. A 2014 study demonstrated predictors of sleep laboratory testing referral including male gender, middle age, overweight, chronic conditions, having a regular medical doctor, report of symptoms, and place of residence [42].

There are considerable provincial variations in prevalence rates. The most populous province of Ontario, has the highest rate of OSA diagnosis at 4.6%, the highest sleep laboratory testing referral rate of 7.7%, and hosts over three-quarters of the total Canadian Sleep Laboratory beds [42]. It is thought that less financial support for sleep assessment in other provinces has led to more problematic under-recognition of sleep disorders. For example, the second most populous province of Quebec, was found to have the lowest OSA prevalence of 1.9%, the lowest sleep laboratory testing referral rate of 2%, and just one tenth of the sleep laboratory bed capacity in the country [42]. The more sparsely populated provinces and territories of Prince Edward Island, Newfoundland and Labrador, Yukon, Nunavut and Northwest Territories do not have any testing capacity at all [42].

CURRENT PRACTICE OF SLEEP MEDICINE

Facilities

While Canada mandates single-payer universal healthcare provision to citizens administered provincially, there is significant interprovincial variability in the funding of sleep medicine. In terms of diagnostics, sleep studies are performed at either standalone private sleep laboratories which are the majority, or at public sleep laboratories located within hospitals. In the most populous province of Ontario, public funding is available for polysomnography at numerous sleep laboratories and there are a reasonably sufficient number of sleep specialists. In other provinces, there are significantly fewer sleep laboratories and sleep specialists available. This is associated with substantial wait-times and in some provinces a complete lack of availability, leading to increased reliance on at-home technologies for assessment. In many provinces, sleep laboratory diagnostics are either not funded by provincial universal healthcare, or only partially, leaving individuals to pay out of pocket with or without the contribution of their own private insurance coverage.

With regard to the treatment of suspected sleep-related disorders, there is large variability in provincial funding for CPAP treatment for OSA, and generally no coverage of dental devices for OSA, while surgical interventions are covered by public healthcare funding. Pharmaceuticals are subsidized according to provincial benefits plans with varying coverage, and there is limited availability of publicly-funded psychotherapeutic intervention such as cognitive behavioral therapy for insomnia (CBT-I), with private non-pharmacological resources concentrated in urban areas.

As of 2010, the number of sleep laboratory beds per capita in Canadian provinces in descending order, was Ontario 4.1, Quebec and Saskatchewan 1.0, Manitoba

0.8, British Columbia 0.7, Alberta and Nova Scotia 0.6, New Brunswick 0.5, followed by the other five provinces and territories which were without any sleep laboratory bed [42]. As discussed above, there is evidence suggesting that geographic location predicts diagnosis and severity of OSA in Canadian studies [42, 43].

PRACTITIONERS & TRAINING SYSTEMS

Physicians

Sleep medicine medical care in Canada is provided by physicians of a variety of specialties. A 2019 study in Ontario found CPAP most commonly prescribed by respirology, followed by psychiatry, internal medicine, family medicine, neurology and others with most practicing one-third of their clinical hours in sleep medicine [44].

Specialists in the fields of Pediatrics, General Internal Medicine, Neurology, Otalaryngology-Head and Neck Surgery, Psychiatry or Respirology have typically had several options for provincial recognition of sleep medicine expertise. An Accreditation Council for Graduate Medical Education (ACGME)-accredited fellowship program in the USA is one such pathway. Secondly, one may complete an academic unaccredited fellowship in sleep medicine in Canada which demonstrates equivalency in breadth to the aforementioned USA-training route. Thirdly, one may complete a non-academic, unaccredited personalized fellowship with numerous statutes set out for breadth of experience. Thus, Canada has provisioned guidelines largely in striving for equivalency with those of the American Association of Sleep Medicine (AASM) in the United States of America (USA).

Currently, the Royal College of Physicians and Surgeons of Canada does not recognize sleep as a specialty. The formal designation of sleep specialization is conferred on physicians registered as satisfying the competency training requirements for the area of focused competence (AFC) in Sleep Disorder Medicine as of a new program in 2018. This will formally facilitate high quality accredited sleep medicine speciality training programs with a mandate for multidisciplinary training.

Technologists

Sleep Technologists obtain credentials to work in sleep medicine laboratories by enrolling in College or University courses which provide theoretical and clinical instruction to students from a variety of backgrounds. Admission in such courses generally does not require a prior bachelor's level degree. Graduates are then eligible to write a standardized global licensing examination to gain standing as a Certified Polysomnographic Technician (CPSGT), allowing them to earn the Registered Polysomnographic Technologist (RPSGT) credential and register with the global Board of Registered Polysomnographic Technologists (BRPT). There are a few training programs in Canada, and much on-the-job experience.

Dentists

Dentists play an important role in the care of patients with sleep disordered breathing and obstructive sleep apnea (OSA). In Canada, following diagnosis of mild-moderate sleep disordered breathing or OSA by a physician, taking into account patient preference, patient's may be referred to dentists with expertise in sleep dentistry for the fitting with an oral appliance treatment. Additionally, dentists may provide oral devices for patients with bruxism identified by clinical examination or polysomnography. Canada's federally mandated universal healthcare does not provide the requirement for coverage of dentistry or orthodontics. Provinces and territories generally do not cover dental care, with most individuals thus obtaining dental care out of pocket, or *via* private insurance.

Psychologists

Psychologists play an integral role in the provision of non-pharmacological therapies for sleep disorders. In Canada, psychotherapy provided by physicians is covered under the single-payer Medicare program across all provinces and territories. Psychotherapy provided by other practitioners including psychologists however, is generally not covered, or covered in a time-limited or partially-refunded fashion. Thus, psychologists providing psychotherapeutic intervention for patients with sleep disorders are generally doing so independently, or as part of a private sleep laboratory in a fee-for-service manner. Additionally, despite the strong evidence for the effectiveness of Cognitive Behavioral Therapy for Insomnia (CBT-I), there appears to be limited training in this modality in general clinical psychology training in Canada. A 2009 study looking at training programs in Canada and the USA found that just 6% of programs provided formal training, and less than 5% offered internship options [45]. In practice, this is evident, with a general paucity of trained practitioners available and long waitlists being common.

Clinical psychologists in Canada obtain their credential after completing post-graduate training in psychology. The form of this post-graduate training may vary from M.A., M.Sc., or more commonly Ph.D.-level programs, which must include a supervised clinical component, and upon completion allow the practitioner to complete provincial-based licensing examinations and join the provincial and national psychologist associations.

Professional Societies, Regulatory Bodies and Guidelines

Professional Societies

The primary sleep medicine professional society in Canada is the Canadian Sleep Society (CSS). Formed in 1986, it is a multidisciplinary organization with membership including physicians, sleep technologists, psychologists, dentists and other allied health professionals. The CSS holds biannual conferences and intervening educational events for members.

Regulatory Bodies

The Royal College of Physicians and Surgeons of Canada (RCPSC) is the national regulatory college of Canadian physicians. The RCPSC mandates the training requirements and specialization options for physicians. Currently, the RCPSC categorizes sleep medicine under the title of 'Sleep Disorder Medicine' as an AFC diploma – a "highly specialized discipline of specialty medicine that addresses a legitimate societal need but does not meet the Royal College criteria for a specialty, foundation program or subspecialty" [46]. As mentioned above, Canadian physicians have recently obtain the opportunity to obtain this designation.

Provinces and territories generally have their own regulatory bodies for physicians which respect the national standards set by the RCPSC and are, usually named in a similar manner to their parent federal organization. For example, the largest province of Ontario is regulated by the College of Physicians and Surgeons of Ontario (CPSO). These regulatory bodies register all physicians in their jurisdiction, strive to uphold the utmost quality of care, manage investigations and disciplinary procedures for physicians, and guide standards for their professional conduct. Additionally, sleep laboratories are assessed or accredited by the provincial healthcare regulator to ensure operation according to clinical safety and care standards generally developed in conjunction with review of clinical guidelines and consultation with experts in the field.

Practice Guidelines

The Canadian Sleep Society (CSS) has published various position papers related to sleep, and the Canadian Thoracic Society (CTS) published guidelines on sleep disordered breathing in 2006 [47]. Provincial regulatory bodies, in addition to accrediting sleep laboratories may publish expert guidelines. The College of Physicians and Surgeons of Ontario (CPSO), published the Clinical Practice Parameters and Facility Standards most recently in 2016, under the leadership of a specialized sleep medicine task force of Ontario physicians in the field [48]. This guideline covered a range of sleep medicine care, from facility staffing, equipment maintenance and supply standards to diagnostic parameters and treatment suggestions in the treatment of sleep disorders [48].

Driving Regulations

Canada's national standards regarding the safety of individuals to operate motor vehicles are outlined by the Canadian Council of Motor Transport Administrators. Provinces and territories then establish legislation governing driver's licensing within their jurisdiction based upon this guideline. The regulation regarding driving in patients with medical disorders that may impact driving safety, including sleep disorders thus rests with provinces and territories. This leaves considerable variability across provinces. Ontario allows physicians discretionary authority to report individuals suffering from any medical condition that may endanger their driving ability [49], while Quebec specifically cites an apnea-hypopnea [42] index of 30 events/hour as an upper limit for patients with obstructive sleep apnea (OSA) [50]. British Columbia distinguishes between treated and untreated OSA and between private and commercial drivers, whereas Alberta leaves primary responsibility for informing motor transport authorities to the patient [50].

CHALLENGES TO THE PRACTICE OF SLEEP MEDICINE IN CANADA

Financial Coverage for Care

Canada's universal healthcare is administered by provinces, with great variability in provision of some aspects of healthcare including sleep medicine care. This lack of consistency in funding, leads to provinces relying on different funding models for sleep medicine care. Given the limited access to data regarding the breadth of sleep disorders, obstructive sleep apnea (OSA)-associated funding data will be looked at in depth as emblematic of sleep medicine as a whole.

Canada is regarded to have insufficient funding sources to allow for adequate diagnosis and treatment of obstructive sleep apnea (OSA) [42]. This is despite Canadian studies showing cost-effectiveness of treatment of moderate-severe OSA with incremental cost-utility ratios ranging from $7420-43,899 [51]. As noted above, the funding of sleep medicine diagnostics and treatment is variable across provinces. While provinces such as Ontario provide publicly-funded diagnostic polysomnography, others provide minimal public funding. Additionally, some provinces fund CPAP treatment, while others leave this to individuals or their private insurance policies. Oral devices are generally not funded across provinces, while surgical intervention is covered across provinces. The average cost for non-surgical treatments in British Columbia, a province that provides no co-payment or reimbursement is $800-$2500 for CPAP, and $400-2800 for oral devices [52].

Funding concerns may be prohibitive for a large segment of patients, and dissuasive for an even larger portion. A recent USA national population study found a statistically significant relationship between household income level and PAP adherence [53]. A 2016 study in Ontario, which boasts the second-most generous public funding for CPAP looked at addresses of patients to indirectly glimpse at financial capacity and CPAP adherence. While it did not find a statistically significant association between neighbourhood wealth and CPAP acceptance, living in higher-income neighbourhoods was associated with a 27% increased chance of accepting CPAP compared to the lowest-income neighbourhood [54].

Access to Care

As discussed above, Canada is an extraordinarily expansive, sparsely populated, highly urbanized nation. This presents healthcare challenges in traversing the large geographical distances to provide equitable care to smaller communities. Additionally, Canada's national college of physicians does not recognize sleep medicine as a distinct specialty nor subspecialty, and there are currently no formally accredited fellowships offered in the country. The combinations of these factors lends itself to a general lack of sleep medicine physicians and sleep laboratory facilities, which is unevenly distributed across the country.

Many provinces and territories were without any sleep laboratories [42]. On a more micro level, within such provinces rural residents are often required to travel to attend sleep specialty appointments or studies. Unsurprisingly then, there is Canadian research showing that geographic location predicts diagnosis and severity of OSA [42, 43]. In one such study, controlling for sex, age, obesity and education, travel remained a predictor of severity of OSA severity, with each ten minutes of travel associated with an AHI increase of 1.4 [43]. Even in Ontario, the province with the largest number of sleep laboratory beds per capita [42], less than half of the patients undergo polysomnographic testing within 6 months of initial primary care assessment for OSA, and almost half of the patients are started on CPAP empirically without titration [55].

Conflict of Interest

The lack of consistent funding of sleep medicine lends itself to thriving for-profit entities providing diagnostic sleep laboratory testing and treatments such as CPAP which are not covered by universal healthcare. In fact, an estimated 20-80% of Canadians outside of Ontario with suspected OSA are seen by private sleep providers [42]. Moreover, across all provinces and territories in Canada, there is a lack of reimbursement of costs associated with home sleep studies. This permits entities to charge patients with limited access to alternatives or who are subject to long waiting times for more convenient at-home assessment, which while shown to be non-inferior to level 1 polysomnography in simple OSA cases [56, 57], unfortunately is not standard of care in those with cardiopulmonary comorbidities or pre-test consideration of sleep comorbidities [58]. Similarly, lack of laboratory access makes it difficult to assess the breadth of sleep disorders medicine including narcolepsy, and parasomnias. Private diagnostic providers may have financial incentive to prescribe treatments such as CPAP given they are to be paid for directly by the customer, even if not necessarily indicated such as mild OSA which may be treated positionally or with an oral device. Moreover, providers may further be incentivized financially to recommend upgrades in equipment, which may be unnecessary and costly for consumers. Such conflict concerns may additionally arise for non-home-based diagnostic sleep testing in some provinces which do not accredit and license diagnostic providers.

Private sleep medicine providers currently play a pivotal role in ensuring that as many Canadians as possible are afforded with the resources of diagnostic testing of basic sleep disorders, and are provided with evidence-based treatments for such ailments. Considering the public healthcare funding limitations and geographic challenges in sleep medicine care in Canada, they are especially relied upon. With that in mind, when conflicts are present one must maintain adequate oversight to ensure the public is best served.

PATIENT GROUP CONSIDERATIONS

Socioeconomic

Socioeconomic factors are well-known contributors to healthcare outcomes. Low socioeconomic status is associated with increased all-cause mortality [59] and decreased life expectancy [60], and has been shown to increase the risk of avoidable or preventable hospitalizations in the USA [61], in Australia [62], in Europe [63, 64], and in Canada [65]. Given Canada's reliance on private provision of sleep medicine healthcare, socioeconomic status may affect an individual's sleep medicine care and outcomes.

In the USA, a population study has found a statistically significant relationship between household income level and PAP adherence [53]. In Ontario, which boasts the second-most generous public funding for CPAP, living in higher-income neighbourhoods was associated with a 27% increased chance of accepting CPAP compared to the lowest-income neighbourhood [54], and an association between household income and the purchase of a CPAP device [66]. In Alberta, a cohort study providing publically-funded CPAP and close follow-up demonstrated high CPAP compliance, and decreasing ESS scores [67]. Suggesting a more complex relationship however, a recent Ontario study found that receiving social assistance was associated with longer waiting time to the diagnosis of OSA, however living in a poor neighbourhood was associated with a shorter waiting time [55]. While there remains a paucity of data to clarify the picture of the link between socioeconomic status and sleep medicine outcomes, there appears an empiric trend towards decreased access to care and lack of evidence-based treatment uptake due to socioeconomic factors, which likely is associated with poorer outcomes.

Indigenous Populations

The Federal government classifies indigenous status according to their registration under the Indian Act, with those registering being classified as status Indians. Inuit people are classified separately, however are offered largely identical services. The designation of status-Indian or recognized Inuit provides specified access to government programs such as full Medicare benefits and extended healthcare benefits provided federally, as opposed to non-status Indians who are provided with benefits according to provincial legislation.

Canada's indigenous populations, when analyzed according to the Human Development Index (HDI) would rank as the 63rd most developed nation, as opposed to Canada's ranking within the top five as of 2007 [68]. Indigenous communities are overrepresented in poverty and low socioeconomic data, unemployment, lower educational attainment, and decreased access to healthcare [69]. Indigenous youth suffer disproportionately poor healthcare outcomes such as infant mortality, obesity, diabetes, tuberculosis, injuries and suicide [70], while a large summary of health data has shown that communities as a whole have lower life expectancy, higher rates of infectious disease, chronic disease, mental health conditions, substance use disorders, violent experiences, and suicide [71].

Studies of indigenous populations and sleep disorders have identified a higher prevalence of sleep disruption on polysomnography [72] and mild-mod, mod-severe OSA in the USA [73]. In Canada, indigenous populations have been found to have higher rates of insomnia, apnea symptoms, RLS symptoms [74], and lower sleep duration compared to other ethnicities [75]. New Zealand research has further shown Indigenous Maori ethnicity to be associated with more severe symptoms' burden, excessive sleepiness, and poor compliance with treatment [76 - 78]. Extrapolating non-Canadian data in combination with Canadian data, one may reasonably conclude a higher likely burden of sleep disorders in indigenous populations.

While indigenous Canadians are provided with publicly-funded extended health benefits federally unlike other ethnic groups, which theoretically may allow for increased access to costly diagnostic testing and OSA treatments, the limited access to public sleep facilities is a further barrier. A Saskatchewan study looking at indigenous pathways to care for OSA found that status Indians were subject to longer waiting times for polysomnography, and a more arduous logistical process to obtain publicly-funded CPAP machines [79]. The complexity of ensuring access to optimal sleep medicine care to indigenous populations is evident, and is a challenge which is ongoing.

Ethnicity

Canada is a highly multi-ethnic and multi-linguistic society with significant annual net migration.

Many ethnic and linguistic minority populations are at-risk due to difficulties accessing sleep medicine care in their language of understanding, or *via* translation, or due to challenges navigating the Canadian health system. To combat this impediment, in large Canadian cities, some Family Medicine and Specialty clinics provide dedicated care in numerous languages. With the limited supply of sleep medicine physicians in Canada however, such a solution is likely impractical, thereby relying on further systems assistance methodology.

Prior studies have shown differential sleep architecture patterns among various ethnicities [72, 75] including significantly decreased sleep time among non-white ethnicities [75], however there is limited available data suggesting different normative ranges based on such noted differences. Until such cross-ethnic data is further analyzed therefore, a more generalized approach taking into account such differences may be more suitable for the Canadian multicultural practice. A recent Canadian meta-analysis ventured to establish empirically-based polysomnography norms across ethnicities [80] which may aid in accurately scoring sleep studies in Canada, and other multiethnic societies.

CANADIAN SLEEP MEDICINE NEEDS & OPPORTUNITIES

Shift Work

Canada has a comparably larger population of shift workers compared with other industrialized nations which can contribute to sleep morbidity. While a most parsimonious fix would be prevention, the durability and economic necessity of such labor this may have limited applicability. Additionally, given the fixed causal factor, treatments have largely revolved around multifactorial attempts to minimize sequelae. These include symptomatic management for improving daytime sleep with sleep aids, melatonin and cognitive behavioral therapy for insomnia (CBT) and/or wakefulness with scheduled naps, caffeine and alertness agents. Increased research has focused on circadian adjustments with supplemental light treatment and non-pharmacological lifestyle changes, however evidence of effectiveness remains limited [81, 82]. Canadian sleep medicine requires further research into managing shift-work disorder (SWD), which is an underrecognized issue in the country.

Light and Circadian Problems

Seasonal variations in sunlight in arctic regions are associated with subjective and objective markers of sleep disruption. While a proportionally small population of Canadians live in arctic regions, arctic studies looking at morbidity associated with seasonal light variations are thought to be applicable to temperate urban environments which also experience significant seasonal shifts in daylight [22]. Early research at remedying sleep disruption in arctic regions looked at the use of hypnotic agents with some benefit [83]. More recent research has focussed on circadian adjustments including winter morning exposure to bright light, summer avoidance of evening exposure to sunlight and summer administration of melatonin to advance phase with some positive results. Moving forward, research is required to devise novel and widely easily implementable treatment regimes.

Data Repositories

One advantage of the single payer system is that information can be accessed to study health systems services in the form of a variety of epidemiological investigations. A number of standardized provincial and federal registries have contributed greatly to epidemiological research such as the Institute for Clinical Evaluative Sciences based in Ontario.

Genetic Diversity

Canada's multiethnic, multilingual and multicultural society translates well towards advancing research generalizable to regions across the world. A recent Ontario population study demonstrated ethnic differences noted in sleep-related symptoms, sleep duration, and comorbidities of depression, stroke and diabetes [75]. While such cross-sectional population-based studies must be interpreted with caution given confounding variables such as socioeconomic status differences among ethnicities in Canada, it represents an opportunity for Canadian sleep medicine to raise ethno-genetic differences that may be further studied across the world.

A recent study to establish normative values for polysomnography across ethnicities was performed in Toronto. Initial Rechtschaffen and Kales sleep scoring criteria [84] has yielded to the 2007 American Association of Sleep Medicine (AASM) criteria [85]. The published meta-analysis incorporates global data towards developing a unified standard for laboratory normative value reference ranges world-wide [80].

Genetic studies in the French-majority province of Quebec have yielded considerable dividends in developing an understanding of the genetics of restless legs syndrome (RLS) and other neurological diseases. In substantial part, such genetic research has been made possible by the collaborative CARTaGENE biobank program – a population-based cohort biobank project in Quebec. A recent 2020 Quebec review of genetic loci of RLS demonstrates the increasing recognition of genetic loci and their association with severity of questionnaire-reported symptoms [40]. Moving forward, Canada is well-placed to further identify genetic links to sleep disorders with the CARTaGENE biobank program in Quebec, and across the country with the nationally-associated Canadian Partnership for Tomorrow Project (CPTP) which is likely to allow further genetic investigation of health conditions including sleep disorders.

Home Polysomnography

A confluence of factors including geographic, policy-related, financial and ethnocultural contribute to Canada's challenges in providing sleep medicine care to its population. A promising development which may allow increased reach is home diagnostic sleep testing. Such technology, could allow for increased testing capacity, and significantly increased reach to the many regions without any sleep laboratories in Canada. There remain such challenges as provincial healthcare policy on whether to provide co-payments or full coverage of such diagnostic testing, and providing access to sleep medicine physicians for follow-up which may require increased recruitment and/or training pathways.

Currently, the utility of home sleep testing is largely confined to sleep disordered breathing and obstructive sleep apnea (OSA) and thus named home sleep apnea tests (HSATs). HSATs often do not utilize EEG, EOG, or EMG sensors, rather, level 3 HSATs are generally reliant on pulse oximeters to monitor oxygen and heart rate, belts to measure respiratory movement and cannulas to measure airflow. HSATs relying on these four signals have been found to be able to diagnose sleep disordered breathing and OSA [56, 57, 86, 87]. Given their more limited view of a person's sleep, HSATs have been shown to be less sensitive, and may underestimate the severity of sleep disordered breathing and/or OSA in comparison with the gold standard of polysomnography [88]. The Canadian

Agency for Drugs and Technologies in Health (CADTH) reviewed research in the field, and concluded that HSATs may be useful in the diagnosis for patients with high suspicion of moderate-severe OSA with no comorbidities [88]. The American Academy of Sleep Medicine (AASM) recently published a position statement supporting the use of HSAT devices at physician's discretion to diagnose OSA or evaluate treatment efficacy if a sleep physician may review and interpret HSAT device data [89].

Further research looking at the validity and reliability of HSATs for OSA diagnostic testing and treatment follow-up could provide further possibility of increased access for Canadians with undiagnosed or under-treated OSA. While current provincial healthcare plans do not provide funding for such diagnostics, with increasing evidence and cost-effectiveness data this may present a possible future avenue for change in the financial coverage for sleep medicine in Canada.

THE COVID-19 ERA & TELE-SLEEP MEDICINE

The Coronavirus 2019 (COVID-19) pandemic remains ongoing at the time of this writing, and as such will be discussed under conditions that limit the certainty which may surface in the coming months and years.

The first COVID-19 diagnosis in Canada occurred on January 27th 2020, with community transmission then recognized on March 5th 2020. Subsequently, the nation's number of presumed and confirmed cases and fatalities quickly accelerated prompting the country to implement a physical distancing campaign and provinces to close all non-essential services to curb the spread of the pandemic. As the nation acclimated to this 'new normal' from March 2020 onwards, the medical system shifted alongside. Elective procedures, non-emergent medical care, and outpatient practices were largely curtailed or rapidly tasked to shift to telemedicine or virtual healthcare including sleep medicine. Laboratories have reopened in a cautious fashion.

The transition of a significant proportion of the Canadian healthcare industry to telemedicine was a paramount change. While provinces differed in the nuts and bolts of implementing such care, the shift did occur across the country. In Ontario, the health authorities had invested in a proprietary videoconference software Ontario Telemedicine Network (OTN) which practitioners were encouraged to employ for video-consultations, while in other provinces, clinicians utilized various enterprise software services, and across the country telephone was employed as a resource if no others were possible. Fortunately, numerous software companies, and OTN were already certified compliant with Canada's privacy legislation to facilitate this.

In sleep medicine, sleep laboratories were closed across the nation, and clinics that continued operating generally did so *via* telemedicine. For complex patients with severe sleep apnea and comorbidities this meant challenging management decisions. For those awaiting titrations or diagnostic testing it naturally led to increased consideration of utilization of HSATs and auto-titrating CPAP treatment. While we remain in the 'fog of war' with respect to COVID19, this may present a penultimate adjustment of Canadian sleep medicine practice towards increasing consideration of remote diagnostic tools, and empiric auto-titrating CPAP treatment given the lack of access to care in the country, and long waiting times. Canadian sleep medicine, as with numerous specialties may resurrect from the pandemic with permanently altered patient-centred care.

CONCLUSION

Healthcare in Canada is federally mandated to be universal and accessible to all citizens, which is administered provincially with some variation in the extent of coverage of non-essential services including sleep medicine. Across the country however, there are long waiting times for clinical testing and specialist appointments, which has led to the burgeoning of a private sleep medicine clinic industry, which allows private charging of patients given the lack of public funding, which is rare in Canadian healthcare. A Royal College of Physicians and Surgeons of Canada recognition of the area of 'focused competence' should help ensure quality training experiences. The rapid transition to remote care across specialties, with ongoing disruptions to in-person polysomnography provides both challenges and opportunities for Canada to increasingly uptake home polysomnography, and to the provision of sleep medicine specialty care *via* teleconference tools to ensure access.

CONSENT FOR PUBLICATION

Not applicable.

CONFLICT OF INTEREST

The authors declare no conflict of interest, financial or otherwise.

ACKNOWLEDGEMENT

Declared none.

REFERENCES

[1]   Central Intelligence Agency. The World Factbook - Canada 2020 Available from:. https://www.cia.gov/library/publications/the-world-factbook/geos/ca.html

[2]   Statistics Canada. Immigration and ethnocultural diversity 2016 Available from:. https://www150.statcan.gc.ca/n1/en/subjects/immigration_and_ethnocultural_diversity

[3]   Statistics Canada. Analysis: Population by age and sex 2019 Available from:. https://www150.statcan.gc.ca/n1/pub/91-215-x/2018002/sec2-eng.htm

[4]   Programme UND. Programme UND. Human Development Index and its components 2018 Available from:. http://hdr.undp.org/en/composite/HDI

[5]   Central Intelligence Agency. The World Factbook - Country Comparison GDP per capita 2019 [Available from:. https://www.cia.gov/library/publications/the-worl--factbook/rankorder/2004rank.html

[6]   Statistics Canada. 2016 Census topic: Income 2019 Available from:. https://www12.statcan.gc.ca/census-recensement/2016/rt-td/inc-rev-eng.cfm

[7]   Statistics Canada. Canada's Official Poverty Dashboard 2020 Available from:. https://www150.statcan.gc.ca/n1/pub/11-627-m/11-627-m2020018-eng.htm

[8]   Morin CM, LeBlanc M, Bélanger L, Ivers H, Mérette C, Savard J. Prevalence of insomnia and its treatment in Canada. Can J Psychiatry 2011; 56(9): 540-8.
[http://dx.doi.org/10.1177/070674371105600905] [PMID: 21959029]

[9]   Williams C. Work-life balance of shift workers.Perspectives. 2008.

[10]   Eurofound. Sixth European Working Conditions Survey - Overview report (2017 update). Publications Office of the European Union. 2017.

[11]   Drake C. Shift work, shift-work disorder, and jet lag Principles and practice of sleep medicine. 5th ed. St. Louis, MO: Elsevier Saunders 2011; pp. 784-98.

[12]   Drake CL, Roehrs T, Richardson G, Walsh JK, Roth T. Shift work sleep disorder: prevalence and consequences beyond that of symptomatic day workers. Sleep 2004; 27(8): 1453-62.
[http://dx.doi.org/10.1093/sleep/27.8.1453] [PMID: 15683134]

[13]   Akerstedt T, Fredlund P, Gillberg M, Jansson B. A prospective study of fatal occupational accidents - relationship to sleeping difficulties and occupational factors. J Sleep Res 2002; 11(1): 69-71.
[http://dx.doi.org/10.1046/j.1365-2869.2002.00287.x] [PMID: 11869429]

[14]   Knutsson A. Health disorders of shift workers. Occup Med (Lond) 2003; 53(2): 103-8.
[http://dx.doi.org/10.1093/occmed/kqg048] [PMID: 12637594]

[15]   Biggi N, Consonni D, Galluzzo V, Sogliani M, Costa G. Metabolic syndrome in permanent night workers. Chronobiol Int 2008; 25(2-3): 443-54.
[http://dx.doi.org/10.1080/07420520802114193] [PMID: 18484373]

[16]   Davis S, Mirick DK. Circadian disruption, shift work and the risk of cancer: a summary of the evidence and studies in Seattle. Cancer Causes Control 2006; 17(4): 539-45.
[http://dx.doi.org/10.1007/s10552-005-9010-9] [PMID: 16596308]

[17]   Schernhammer ES, Kroenke CH, Laden F, Hankinson SE. Night work and risk of breast cancer. Epidemiology 2006; 17(1): 108-11.
[http://dx.doi.org/10.1097/01.ede.0000190539.03500.c1] [PMID: 16357603]

[18]   Shields M. Shift work and health. Health Rep 2002; 13(4): 11-33.
[PMID: 15069802]

[19]   Coren S. Daylight savings time and traffic accidents. N Engl J Med 1996; 334(14): 924-5.
[http://dx.doi.org/10.1056/NEJM199604043341416] [PMID: 8596592]

[20]   Pallesen S, Nordhus IH, Nielsen GH, *et al.* Prevalence of insomnia in the adult Norwegian population. Sleep 2001; 24(7): 771-9.
[PMID: 11683480]

[21]   Nilssen O, Lipton R, Brenn T, Höyer G, Boiko E, Tkatchev A. Sleeping problems at 78 degrees north: the Svalbard Study. Acta Psychiatr Scand 1997; 95(1): 44-8.
       [http://dx.doi.org/10.1111/j.1600-0447.1997.tb00372.x] [PMID: 9051160]

[22]   Arendt J. Biological rhythms during residence in polar regions. Chronobiol Int 2012; 29(4): 379-94.
       [http://dx.doi.org/10.3109/07420528.2012.668997] [PMID: 22497433]

[23]   Kauppila A, Kivelä A, Pakarinen A, Vakkuri O. Inverse seasonal relationship between melatonin and ovarian activity in humans in a region with a strong seasonal contrast in luminosity. J Clin Endocrinol Metab 1987; 65(5): 823-8.
       [http://dx.doi.org/10.1210/jcem-65-5-823] [PMID: 3667880]

[24]   Adamsson M, Laike T, Morita T. Annual variation in daily light exposure and circadian change of melatonin and cortisol concentrations at a northern latitude with large seasonal differences in photoperiod length. J Physiol Anthropol 2017; 36(1): 6.
       [http://dx.doi.org/10.1186/s40101-016-0103-9] [PMID: 27435153]

[25]   Bhattacharyya M, Pal MS, Sharma YK, Majumdar D. Changes in sleep patterns during prolonged stays in Antarctica. Int J Biometeorol 2008; 52(8): 869-79.
       [http://dx.doi.org/10.1007/s00484-008-0183-2] [PMID: 18807075]

[26]   Paul MA, Love RJ, Hawton A, Arendt J. Sleep and the endogenous melatonin rhythm of high arctic residents during the summer and winter. Physiol Behav 2015; 141: 199-206.
       [http://dx.doi.org/10.1016/j.physbeh.2015.01.021] [PMID: 25615594]

[27]   Panda S, Taly A, Sinha S, Gururaj G, Girish N, Nagaraja D. Sleep-related disorders among a healthy population in South India. Neurol India 2012; 60(1): 68-74.
       [http://dx.doi.org/10.4103/0028-3886.93601] [PMID: 22406784]

[28]   Cho SJ, Hong JP, Hahm BJ, *et al.* Restless legs syndrome in a community sample of Korean adults: prevalence, impact on quality of life, and association with DSM-IV psychiatric disorders. Sleep 2009; 32(8): 1069-76.
       [PMID: 19725258]

[29]   Tsuboi Y, Imamura A, Sugimura M, Nakano S, Shirakawa S, Yamada T. Prevalence of restless legs syndrome in a Japanese elderly population. Parkinsonism Relat Disord 2009; 15(8): 598-601.
       [http://dx.doi.org/10.1016/j.parkreldis.2009.02.014] [PMID: 19346151]

[30]   Chen NH, Chuang LP, Yang CT, *et al.* The prevalence of restless legs syndrome in Taiwanese adults. Psychiatry Clin Neurosci 2010; 64(2): 170-8.
       [http://dx.doi.org/10.1111/j.1440-1819.2010.02067.x] [PMID: 20447013]

[31]   Shi Y, Yu H, Ding D, Yu P, Wu D, Hong Z. Prevalence and risk factors of restless legs syndrome among Chinese adults in a rural community of Shanghai in China. PLoS One 2015; 10(3)e0121215
       [http://dx.doi.org/10.1371/journal.pone.0121215] [PMID: 25803876]

[32]   Ohayon MM, Roth T. Prevalence of restless legs syndrome and periodic limb movement disorder in the general population. J Psychosom Res 2002; 53(1): 547-54.
       [http://dx.doi.org/10.1016/S0022-3999(02)00443-9] [PMID: 12127170]

[33]   Lavigne GJ, Montplaisir JY. Restless legs syndrome and sleep bruxism: prevalence and association among Canadians. Sleep 1994; 17(8): 739-43.
       [PMID: 7701186]

[34]   Allen RP, Walters AS, Montplaisir J, *et al.* Restless legs syndrome prevalence and impact: REST general population study. Arch Intern Med 2005; 165(11): 1286-92.
       [http://dx.doi.org/10.1001/archinte.165.11.1286] [PMID: 15956009]

[35]   Xiong L, Montplaisir J, Desautels A, *et al.* Family study of restless legs syndrome in Quebec, Canada: clinical characterization of 671 familial cases. Arch Neurol 2010; 67(5): 617-22.
       [http://dx.doi.org/10.1001/archneurol.2010.67] [PMID: 20457962]

[36] Schormair B, Zhao C, Bell S, *et al.* Identification of novel risk loci for restless legs syndrome in genome-wide association studies in individuals of European ancestry: a meta-analysis. Lancet Neurol 2017; 16(11): 898-907.
[http://dx.doi.org/10.1016/S1474-4422(17)30327-7] [PMID: 29029846]

[37] Gan-Or Z, Zhou S, Ambalavanan A, *et al.* Analysis of functional GLO1 variants in the BTBD9 locus and restless legs syndrome. Sleep Med 2015; 16(9): 1151-5.
[http://dx.doi.org/10.1016/j.sleep.2015.06.002] [PMID: 26298793]

[38] Akçimen F, Spiegelman D, Dionne-Laporte A, Gan-Or Z, Dion PA, Rouleau GA. Screening of novel restless legs syndrome–associated genes in French-Canadian families. Neurol Genet 2018; 4(6)e296
[http://dx.doi.org/10.1212/NXG.0000000000000296] [PMID: 30637332]

[39] Akcimen F, Ross JP, Sarayloo F, Liao C, De Barros Oliveira R, Ruskey JA, *et al.* Genetic and epidemiological characterization of restless legs syndrome in Quebec. Sleep (Basel) 2019.

[40] Akçimen F, Ross JP, Sarayloo F, *et al.* Genetic and epidemiological characterization of restless legs syndrome in Québec. Sleep 2020; 43(4)zsz265
[http://dx.doi.org/10.1093/sleep/zsz265] [PMID: 31665514]

[41] The Canadian Community Health Survey 2009. www.statcan.gc.ca/cgi-bin/ imdb/p2SV.pl?Function =getSurvey&SDDS=3226&lang=en&db=imdb&adm=8&dis=2

[42] Evans J, Skomro R, Driver H, *et al.* Sleep laboratory test referrals in Canada: sleep apnea rapid response survey. Can Respir J 2014; 21(1): e4-e10.
[http://dx.doi.org/10.1155/2014/592947] [PMID: 24288698]

[43] Allen AJMH, Amram O, Tavakoli H, Almeida FR, Hamoda M, Ayas NT. Relationship between Travel Time from Home to a Regional Sleep Apnea Clinic in British Columbia, Canada, and the Severity of Obstructive Sleep. Ann Am Thorac Soc 2016; 13(5): 719-23.
[http://dx.doi.org/10.1513/AnnalsATS.201509-613BC] [PMID: 26814425]

[44] Grant-Orser A, Bray-Jenkyn K, Allen B, George CF, Shariff SZ, Povitz M. Profile of CPAP-prescribing physicians in Ontario, Canada: A secular trend analysis. Canadian Journal of Respiratory, Critical Care, and Sleep Medicine 2019; 3(1): 50-5.
[http://dx.doi.org/10.1080/24745332.2018.1507616]

[45] Meltzer LJ, Phillips C, Mindell JA. Clinical psychology training in sleep and sleep disorders. J Clin Psychol 2009; 65(3): 305-18.
[http://dx.doi.org/10.1002/jclp.20545] [PMID: 19132641]

[46] Canada RCoPaSo. Area of Focused Competence (Diploma) 2020 [Available from:. http://www.royalcollege.ca/rcsite/credentials-exams/exam-eligibility/areas-focussed-competence-afc-d iploma-e

[47] Fleetham J, Ayas N, Bradley D, *et al.* Canadian Thoracic Society guidelines: diagnosis and treatment of sleep disordered breathing in adults. Can Respir J 2006; 13(7): 387-92.
[http://dx.doi.org/10.1155/2006/627096] [PMID: 17036094]

[48] Ontario TCoPaSo. Clinical Practice Parameters and Standards — Sleep Medicine 4th Edition 2016 [Available from: . https://www.cpso.on.ca/admin/CPSO/media/Documents/physician/your-practice/quality-in-practice/cpgs-other-guidelines/ihf-standards-sleep-medicine.pdf

[49] Ontario Ministry of Transportation Report a medically unfit driver: healthcare practitioners. http://www.mto.gov.on.ca/english/safety/medically-unfit-driver-physicians.shtml#law

[50] Ayas N, Skomro R, Blackman A, *et al.* Obstructive sleep apnea and driving: A Canadian Thoracic Society and Canadian Sleep Society position paper. Can Respir J 2014; 21(2): 114-23.
[http://dx.doi.org/10.1155/2014/357327] [PMID: 24724150]

[51] Interventions for the treatment of obstructive sleep apnea in adults: a health technology assessment 2017.

[52]   Pendharkar SR, Povitz M, Bansback N, George CFP, Morrison D, Ayas NT. Testing and treatment for obstructive sleep apnea in Canada: funding models must change. CMAJ 2017; 189(49): E1524-8.
[http://dx.doi.org/10.1503/cmaj.170393] [PMID: 29229714]

[53]   Pandey A, Mereddy S, Combs D, *et al.* Socioeconomic Inequities in Adherence to Positive Airway Pressure Therapy in Population-Level Analysis. J Clin Med 2020; 9(2): 442.
[http://dx.doi.org/10.3390/jcm9020442] [PMID: 32041146]

[54]   Kendzerska T, Gershon AS, Tomlinson G, Leung RS. The Effect of Patient Neighborhood Income Level on the Purchase of Continuous Positive Airway Pressure Treatment among Patients with Sleep Apnea. Ann Am Thorac Soc 2016; 13(1): 93-100.
[http://dx.doi.org/10.1513/AnnalsATS.201505-294OC] [PMID: 26473580]

[55]   Povitz M, Bray Jenkyn K, Kendzerska T, *et al.* Clinical pathways and wait times for OSA care in Ontario, Canada: A population cohort study. Canadian Journal of Respiratory, Critical Care, and Sleep Medicine 2019; 3(2): 91-9.
[http://dx.doi.org/10.1080/24745332.2018.1512841]

[56]   Kuna ST, Gurubhagavatula I, Maislin G, *et al.* Noninferiority of functional outcome in ambulatory management of obstructive sleep apnea. Am J Respir Crit Care Med 2011; 183(9): 1238-44.
[http://dx.doi.org/10.1164/rccm.201011-1770OC] [PMID: 21471093]

[57]   Corral J, Sánchez-Quiroga MÁ, Carmona-Bernal C, *et al.* Conventional Polysomnography Is Not Necessary for the Management of Most Patients with Suspected Obstructive Sleep Apnea. Noninferiority, Randomized Controlled Trial. Am J Respir Crit Care Med 2017; 196(9): 1181-90.
[http://dx.doi.org/10.1164/rccm.201612-2497OC] [PMID: 28636405]

[58]   El Shayeb M, Topfer LA, Stafinski T, Pawluk L, Menon D. Diagnostic accuracy of level 3 portable sleep tests *versus* level 1 polysomnography for sleep-disordered breathing: a systematic review and meta-analysis. CMAJ 2014; 186(1): E25-51.
[http://dx.doi.org/10.1503/cmaj.130952] [PMID: 24218531]

[59]   Katikireddi SV, Niedzwiedz CL, Dundas R, Kondo N, Leyland AH, Rostila M. Inequalities in all-cause and cause-specific mortality across the life course by wealth and income in Sweden: a register-based cohort study. Int J Epidemiol 2020; 49(3): 917-25.
[http://dx.doi.org/10.1093/ije/dyaa053] [PMID: 32380544]

[60]   Chetty R, Stepner M, Abraham S, *et al.* The Association Between Income and Life Expectancy in the United States, 2001-2014. JAMA 2016; 315(16): 1750-66.
[http://dx.doi.org/10.1001/jama.2016.4226] [PMID: 27063997]

[61]   Moy E, Chang E, Barrett M. Potentially preventable hospitalizations - United States, 2001-2009. MMWR Suppl 2013; 62(3): 139-43.
[PMID: 24264504]

[62]   Page AAS, Glover J, Hetzel D. Atlas of avoidable Hospitalisations in Australia: ambulatory care-sensitive conditions. Adelaide 2007.

[63]   Dimitrovová K, Costa C, Santana P, Perelman J. "Evolution and financial cost of socioeconomic inequalities in ambulatory care sensitive conditions: an ecological study for Portugal, 2000–2014". Int J Equity Health 2017; 16(1): 145.
[http://dx.doi.org/10.1186/s12939-017-0642-7] [PMID: 28810869]

[64]   Weeks WB, Ventelou B, Paraponaris A. Rates of admission for ambulatory care sensitive conditions in France in 2009–2010: trends, geographic variation, costs, and an international comparison. Eur J Health Econ 2016; 17(4): 453-70.
[http://dx.doi.org/10.1007/s10198-015-0692-y] [PMID: 25951924]

[65]   Information CIfH Hospitalization disparities by socio-economic status for males and females Canadian Institute for Health Information. CIHI 2010.

[66]   Simon-Tuval T, Reuveni H, Greenberg-Dotan S, Oksenberg A, Tal A, Tarasiuk A. Low

socioeconomic status is a risk factor for CPAP acceptance among adult OSAS patients requiring treatment. Sleep 2009; 32(4): 545-52.
[http://dx.doi.org/10.1093/sleep/32.4.545] [PMID: 19413149]

[67]   Sin DD, Mayers I, Man GCW, Pawluk L. Long-term compliance rates to continuous positive airway pressure in obstructive sleep apnea: a population-based study. Chest 2002; 121(2): 430-5.
[http://dx.doi.org/10.1378/chest.121.2.430] [PMID: 11834653]

[68]   Reading JL. 2007.

[69]   Bougie E, Kelly-Scott K, Arriagada P. The education and employment experiences of First Nations people living off reserve, Inuit, and Metis: selected findings from the 2012 Aboriginal Peoples Survey. Statistics Canada 2013.

[70]   Greenwood ML, de Leeuw SN. Social determinants of health and the future well-being of Aboriginal children in Canada. Paediatr Child Health 2012; 17(7): 381-4.
[PMID: 23904782]

[71]   Adelson N. The embodiment of inequity: health disparities in aboriginal Canada. Can J Public Health 2005; 96(S2) (Suppl. 2): S45-61.
[http://dx.doi.org/10.1007/BF03403702] [PMID: 16078555]

[72]   Redline S, Kirchner HL, Quan SF, Gottlieb DJ, Kapur V, Newman A. The effects of age, sex, ethnicity, and sleep-disordered breathing on sleep architecture. Arch Intern Med 2004; 164(4): 406-18.
[http://dx.doi.org/10.1001/archinte.164.4.406] [PMID: 14980992]

[73]   Young T, Peppard PE, Gottlieb DJ. Epidemiology of obstructive sleep apnea: a population health perspective. Am J Respir Crit Care Med 2002; 165(9): 1217-39.
[http://dx.doi.org/10.1164/rccm.2109080] [PMID: 11991871]

[74]   Froese CL, Butt A, Mulgrew A, *et al.* Depression and sleep-related symptoms in an adult, indigenous, North American population. J Clin Sleep Med 2008; 4(4): 356-61.
[http://dx.doi.org/10.5664/jcsm.27237] [PMID: 18763428]

[75]   Singh M, Hall KA, Reynolds A, Palmer LJ, Mukherjee S. The Relationship of Sleep Duration with Ethnicity and Chronic Disease in a Canadian General Population Cohort. Nat Sci Sleep 2020; 12: 239-51.
[http://dx.doi.org/10.2147/NSS.S226834] [PMID: 32346318]

[76]   Mihaere KM, Harris R, Gander PH, *et al.* Obstructive sleep apnea in New Zealand adults: prevalence and risk factors among Māori and non-Māori. Sleep 2009; 32(7): 949-56.
[http://dx.doi.org/10.1093/sleep/32.7.949] [PMID: 19639758]

[77]   Gander PH, Marshall NS, Harris R, Reid P. The Epworth Sleepiness Scale: influence of age, ethnicity, and socioeconomic deprivation. Epworth Sleepiness scores of adults in New Zealand. Sleep 2005; 28(2): 249-54.
[http://dx.doi.org/10.1093/sleep/28.2.249] [PMID: 16171250]

[78]   Baldwin DR, Kolbe J, Troy K, *et al.* Comparative clinical and physiological features of Maori, Pacific Islanders and Europeans with sleep related breathing disorders. Respirology 1998; 3(4): 253-60.
[http://dx.doi.org/10.1111/j.1440-1843.1998.tb00131.x] [PMID: 10201052]

[79]   Marchildon GP, Katapally TR, Beck CA, *et al.* Exploring policy driven systemic inequities leading to differential access to care among Indigenous populations with obstructive sleep apnea in Canada. Int J Equity Health 2015; 14(1): 148.
[http://dx.doi.org/10.1186/s12939-015-0279-3] [PMID: 26683058]

[80]   Boulos MI, Jairam T, Kendzerska T, Im J, Mekhael A, Murray BJ. Normal polysomnography parameters in healthy adults: a systematic review and meta-analysis. Lancet Respir Med 2019; 7(6): 533-43.
[http://dx.doi.org/10.1016/S2213-2600(19)30057-8] [PMID: 31006560]

[81]   Slanger TE, Gross JV, Pinger A, *et al.* Person-directed, non-pharmacological interventions for

sleepiness at work and sleep disturbances caused by shift work. Cochrane Libr 2016; 2016(8)CD010641
[http://dx.doi.org/10.1002/14651858.CD010641.pub2] [PMID: 27549931]

[82]   Lowden A, Öztürk G, Reynolds A, Bjorvatn B. Working Time Society consensus statements: Evidence based interventions using light to improve circadian adaptation to working hours. Ind Health 2019; 57(2): 213-27.
[http://dx.doi.org/10.2486/indhealth.SW-9] [PMID: 30700675]

[83]   Lingjærde O, Bratlid T, Westby OC, Gordeladze JO. Effect of midazolam, flunitrazepam, and placebo against midwinter insomnia in northern Norway. Acta Psychiatr Scand 1983; 67(2): 118-29.
[http://dx.doi.org/10.1111/j.1600-0447.1983.tb06731.x] [PMID: 6133412]

[84]   Rechtschaffen A, Kales A. A manual of standardized terminology, techniques and scoring system for sleep staging of human subjects. Los Angeles, CA: Brain Information Service, Brain Research Institute, UCLA 1968.

[85]   Iber C, Ancoli-Israel S, Chesson A, Quan SF. The AASM manual for the scoring of sleep and associated events: rules, terminology and technical specifications. 2007.

[86]   Skomro RP, Gjevre J, Reid J, *et al.* Outcomes of home-based diagnosis and treatment of obstructive sleep apnea. Chest 2010; 138(2): 257-63.
[http://dx.doi.org/10.1378/chest.09-0577] [PMID: 20173052]

[87]   Berry RB, Sriram P. Auto-adjusting positive airway pressure treatment for sleep apnea diagnosed by home sleep testing. J Clin Sleep Med 2014; 10(12): 1269-75.
[http://dx.doi.org/10.5664/jcsm.4272] [PMID: 25348244]

[88]   Portable monitoring devices for diagnosis of obstructive sleep apnea at home: review of accuracy, cost-effectiveness, guidelines, and coverage in Canada. CADTH Technol Overv 2010; 1(4)e0123
[PMID: 22977413]

[89]   Rosen IM, Kirsch DB, Chervin RD, *et al.* Clinical Use of a Home Sleep Apnea Test: An American Academy of Sleep Medicine Position Statement. J Clin Sleep Med 2017; 13(10): 1205-7.
[http://dx.doi.org/10.5664/jcsm.6774] [PMID: 28942762]

CHAPTER 3

Sleep Medicine in Mexico

Ulises Jiménez Correa[1,*] and **Horacio Balám Álvarez García**[1]

[1] *Sleep Disorder Clinic, Faculty of Medicine, Research Division, National Autonomous University of Mexico, 04510 Ciudad de México, CDMX, Mexico*

Abstract: Sleep medicine is a fascinating and still growing field in Mexico. We describe some historical background as well as some clinical and basic research topics that have been studied more recently. We also describe the main characteristics of the clinical practice of sleep medicine, some clinical practice guides for sleep disorders, regulatory bodies for the certification of physicians who practice sleep medicine, and the main types of professional positions in the care of patients with sleep disorders in Mexico. We also detail some of the challenges facing sleep medicine in Mexico, including the limited availability of professional training and human resource specialized in sleep medicine, and the need to implement governmental and public health actions to address sleep disorders in the Mexican population. Finally, we mention the implications of the COVID-19 pandemic in the operation of sleep clinics and the changes that have been implemented in the patient care model.

Keywords: Sleep Medicine, Current Practice, Insomnia, Mexico, Sleep Apnea.

INTRODUCTION

The beginning of basic sleep research is attributed to researchers such as Dr. Raúl Hernández Peón, Dr. Augusto Fernández Guardiola, Dr. René Raúl Drucker Colín [1] and Dr. Fructuoso Ayala Guerrero, all of whom have been researchers at the National Autonomous University of Mexico (UNAM). One of the first courses on sleep science offered in Mexico was "The Psychophysiology of Sleep", which has been taught since 1971 in the Faculty of Psychology at UNAM. One of the first books on sleep science in Mexico was called "Psicofisiología del sueño," published in 1983 [2]. Sleep medicine is a relatively recent area of the health sciences in Mexico, whose roots can be traced back to the 1980s in some sleep laboratories located in the National Institute of Neurology and Neurosurgery, in the Mexican Institute of Psychiatry (today the National Institute of Psychiatry)

[*] **Corresponding author Ulises Jiménez Correa:** Sleep Disorder Clinic, Faculty of Medicine, Research Division, National Autonomous University of Mexico. 04510 Ciudad de Mexico, CDMX, Mexico; Tel: 52+55 56232690; E-mail: ulisesjc@yahoo.com

Hrayr P. Attarian, Marie-Louise M. Coussa-Koniski & Alain Michel Sabri (Eds.)

and different areas of the UNAM (such as the Faculties of Psychology and Medicine; as well as the Institute of Biomedical Research).

CLINICAL AND BASIC RESEARCH TOPICS

Some Mexican contributions to clinical sleep medicine have been in the topics of restless legs syndrome [3], psychology and sleep [4], sleep-disordered breathing [5], parasomnias [6] and neurodevelopment and sleep [7]. These lines of research have mainly been pursued in sleep disorder clinics at national institutes of health or public universities. Basic sleep research has mainly addressed sleep phylogeny [8, 9], psychopharmacology and sleep [10, 11] and sleep restriction [12]. These studies have been published by research groups based at public universities.

Over the last 40 years, sleep medicine has developed gradually in Mexico, fighting against two main obstacles: a) budget constraints in the federal health system, and b) little or no inclusion of sleep science or sleep medicine in the curricula of professionals in key fields such as medicine, psychology, dentistry, and physical therapy.

Sleep Medicine and Education

Over the years, specific courses and even degree programs have emerged, such as the Masters in Sleep Disorders at the Faculty of Psychology at UNAM, as well as postgraduate courses and medical specialties in sleep medicine in areas such as psychiatric disorders and sleep, sleep breathing disorders, and comprehensive sleep medicine [13]. Currently, however, there are no technical training programs or bachelor's or doctorate level degrees in sleep medicine in Mexico.

Scientific Societies Studying Sleep

There are three existing sleep-related scientific societies in Mexico. The Mexican Society for Sleep Medicine and Research was established in 1998, the Mexican Academy of Sleep Medicine in 2011, and the Mexican Association of Oral Sleep Medicine in 2019. These civil associations aim mainly to research sleep and sleep disorders, as well as provide training through courses, annual meetings and diploma courses. They also participate in health promotion activities such as the annual celebration of World Sleep Day.

Current Practice of Sleep Medicine

Sleep medicine is practiced in a public medicine setting at some university health facilities, such as the UNAM Sleep Disorders Clinic at Eduardo Liceaga General Hospital of Mexico. National Health Institutes also have some sleep clinic facilities, for example at the Ramón de la Fuente Muñiz National Institute of

Psychiatry, Ismael Cossío Villegas National Institute of Respiratory Diseases, or the Salvador Zubirán National Institute of Medical Sciences and Nutrition. All of these centers have limited infrastructure and personnel, leading to long waiting lists, however, patients benefit from low costs for consultations and polysomnographic diagnosis. In Mexico, sleep medicine is also available in private practice at sleep labs, sleep disorder centers and medical, dental or psychological consultations.

There are specialized sleep disorder centers for specific patient groups. For example, the Ismael Cossío Villegas National Institute of Respiratory Diseases cares mainly for patients with sleep-disordered breathing, while the Ramón de la Fuente Muñiz National Institute of Psychiatry cares for patients with mental disorders. There are also sleep disorder clinics that serve patients of any age (from premature neonates with central sleep apnea risk to elderly with symptoms of REM Sleep Behavior Disorder; RBD) and have the ability to diagnose most sleep disorders.

Sleep medicine is practiced mainly by physicians such as neurologists, psychiatrists, internists, geriatricians, pediatricians, and pulmonologists, as well as by psychologists and dentists. In Mexico, physicians can be certified in sleep medicine through the councils of pulmonology, neurology, psychiatry, neurophysiology and otolaryngology. However, there are currently no specific organizations to certify other health professionals (such as psychologists or dentists) in sleep medicine or as polysomnography technicians.

Clinical practice guidelines related to sleep medicine have mostly been prepared by task forces comprising physicians, dentists and psychologists. These include the clinical guides for the diagnosis and treatment of sleep disorders [14]; detection, diagnosis and treatment of obstructive sleep apnea syndrome in adults [15]; and for diagnosis and treatment of insomnia in the elderly [16]; as well as the international multicentric consensus [5]. These publications have the academic endorsement of national government agencies such as the Mexican Institute of Social Security (IMSS) and the Ministry of Health.

Patients have access to diagnostic services such as polysomnographic records or multiple sleep latencies tests (though actigraphy is not yet available as a diagnostic tool), CPAP device titration, cognitive behavioral therapy for insomnia [17], dental treatment for sleep-disordered breathing, and pharmacological treatment. With respect to pharmacological treatment, government health agencies offer free drug therapy for insomnia, but this is limited to some benzodiazepines (mainly clonazepam, lorazepam or diazepam), anti-histamines (such as hydroxyzine or diphenhydramine), antidepressants (*i.e.* amitriptyline, fluoxetine, paroxetine), antipsychotics (quetiapine and olanzapine), or anticonvulsants (pregabaline, gabapentine or valproic acid) [18, 19]. Government health services such as IMSS or the Institute of Security and Social Services for government employees (ISSSTE) can provide treatment for patients with sleep apnea with CPAP devices through subrogation to private companies.

In Mexico, there are four main payment systems for services in sleep disorder clinics: 1) through social security, which is free to the patient but have highly limited availability and are mostly located in Mexico City, Monterrey, and Guadalajara; 2) public health services subrogated to private companies; 3) private practice, which is more widely available but is more expensive and mainly address specific for sleep disorders related to psychiatric, neurological, and breathing morbidities; and 4) through insurance companies, though very few companies currently cover sleep medicine consultation and Polysomnography records (PSGr).

It is important to mention that the consultation services of the sleep medicine specialist, PSGr and CPAP devices are very expensive for the majority of the population, making sleep medicine still difficult to access in Mexico for the average patient. There are few sleep clinics in the country, and indirect costs such as transportation, food and lodging expenses must be considered in addition to direct medical costs.

Cultural Factors Affecting Sleep Medicine

One of the main cultural factors impacting sleep medicine is self-medication or misuse of medications. According to clinical experience, approximately 90% of insomnia incidences are patients who use over-the-counter medicine (without guidance on the dosage) or consume hypnotics without following a specialist's indications (*i.e.* dose, duration of consumption or combination with other medical drugs, alcohol or illegal drugs).

CHALLENGES IN SLEEP MEDICINE AND FUTURE DIRECTIONS

In terms of education on sleep medicine, it is necessary to incorporate knowledge about sleep medicine especially in recently created health areas, such as physical therapy. The number of health professionals trained in sleep medicine also needs to increase if sleep medicine is to be made available outside the three largest cities in the country. It is also important to make available training courses for technicians in polysomnography as well as sleep medicine at the bachelor's and postgraduate levels. This would help improve care by reducing waiting times for consultation and could also make clinical services more affordable.

Although there are few epidemiological studies on sleep disorders in Mexico [20, 21], there have been some studies on the symptoms of insomnia and sleep apnea, which could indicate that health authorities are beginning to consider sleep disorders a health priority. In Mexico, public health campaigns have not yet integrated sleep and its disorders, for example by bringing awareness to the role of drowsiness in vehicular accidents or the importance of sleep in preventing metabolic diseases.

CONCLUSION

Finally, the covid-19 pandemic has caused sleep clinics to close for at least half a year across the country and the world, making it necessary to perform consultations *via* telemedicine platforms and clinical training of physicians *via* distance education [17]. This has had the advantage of improving access to consultation throughout the country, significantly increasing access to clinical services, at least in the case of patients with insomnia. However, social distancing measures and, above all, the conversion of hospitals to COVID-19 wards, have limited the availability of in-person sleep clinics located within hospitals. This, in turn, has caused an increase in the number of PSG type 2 records instead of type 1 polysomnography.

It is possible that in the immediate future, the services of sleep clinics will have to be restricted to patients with critical illnesses, and most polysomnograms will be carried out on an outpatient basis.

CONSENT FOR PUBLICATION

Not applicable.

CONFLICT OF INTEREST

The authors declare no conflict of interest, financial or otherwise.

ACKNOWLEDGEMENT

The authors wish to thank to Sergio Aguilar, Fructuoso Ayala, Romel Gutiérrez, Elizabeth Luna, Humberto Medina, Miguel Otero, Alejandra Sainos and Carlos Toledo for providing important information for the preparation of the manuscript.

REFERENCES

[1]   Pedemonte M, Brockmann PE, DelRosso LM, Andersen ML. Past, present, and future of sleep medicine research in Latin America. J Clin Sleep Med 2021; 17(5): 1133-9.
[http://dx.doi.org/10.5664/jcsm.9152] [PMID: 33583492]

[2]   Corsi-Cabrera M. Psicofisiología del sueño. First Edition. México: Trillas. 1983.

[3]   Osses-Rodríguez L, Urrea-Rodríguez A, Jiménez-Genchi A. Improvement of restless legs syndrome with a plantar pressure device. Neurologia (Engl Ed). 2020; S0213-4853: pp. (20)30421-7.
[http://dx.doi.org/10.1016/j.nrl.2020.11.003]

[4]   Fernández-Cruz KA, Jiménez-Correa U, Marín-Agudelo HA, Castro-López C, Poblano A. Proposing the Clinical Inventory of Sleep Quality. Sleep Sci 2016; 9(3): 216-20.
[http://dx.doi.org/10.1016/j.slsci.2016.10.002] [PMID: 28123664]

[5]   Mediano O, González Mangado N, Montserrat JM, *et al.* Spanish Sleep Network. International Consensus Document on Obstructive Sleep Apnea. Arch Bronconeumol (Engl Ed). 2021; S0300-2896: p. (21)00115-0.
[http://dx.doi.org/10.1016/j.arbres.2021.03.017]

[6]   Jiménez-Correa U, Santana-Miranda R, Barrera-Medina A, *et al.* Parasomnias in patients with addictions-a systematic review. CNS Spectr 2020; 1-8.
[http://dx.doi.org/10.1017/S1092852920001911] [PMID: 33092679]

[7]   Santana-Miranda R, Murata C, Bruni O, *et al.* Cyclic alternating pattern in infants with congenital hypothyroidism Brain Dev 41(1): 66-71.
[http://dx.doi.org/10.1016/j.braindev.2018.07.002]

[8]   Cruz-Aguilar MA, Ayala-Guerrero F, Jiménez-Anguiano A, Santillán-Doherty AM, García-Orduña F, Velázquez-Moctezuma J. Sleep in the spider monkey (*Ateles geoffroyi*): A semi-restrictive, non-invasive, polysomnographic study. Am J Primatol 2015; 77(2): 200-10.
[http://dx.doi.org/10.1002/ajp.22322] [PMID: 25231936]

[9]   Mexicano G, Montoya-Loaiza B, Ayala-Guerrero F. Sleep characteristics in the quail Coturnix coturnix. Physiol Behav 2014; 129: 167-72.
[http://dx.doi.org/10.1016/j.physbeh.2014.02.041] [PMID: 24582668]

[10]   Rojas-Zamorano JA, Esqueda-Leon E, Jimenez-Anguiano A, Cintra-McGlone L, Mendoza Melendez MA, Velazquez Moctezuma J. The H1 histamine receptor blocker, chlorpheniramine, completely prevents the increase in REM sleep induced by immobilization stress in rats. Pharmacol Biochem Behav 2009; 91(3): 291-4.
[http://dx.doi.org/10.1016/j.pbb.2008.07.011] [PMID: 18700151]

[11]   Ayala-Guerrero F, Mexicano G, Gutiérrez-Chávez CA, Lazo LA, Mateos EL. Effect of gabapentin on sleep patterns disturbed by epilepsy. Epilepsy Behav 2019; 92: 290-6.
[http://dx.doi.org/10.1016/j.yebeh.2018.12.012] [PMID: 30731295]

[12]   García-García F, Priego-Fernández S, López-Muciño LA, Acosta-Hernández ME, Peña-Escudero C. Increased alcohol consumption in sleep-restricted rats is mediated by delta FosB induction. Alcohol 2021; 93: 63-70.
[http://dx.doi.org/10.1016/j.alcohol.2021.02.004] [PMID: 33662520]

[13]   Vizcarra-Escobar D, Fabián-Quillama RJ, Fernández-Gonzáles YS. Sleep societies and sleep training programs in Latin America. J Clin Sleep Med 2020; 16(6): 983-8.
[http://dx.doi.org/10.5664/jcsm.8422] [PMID: 32118575]

[14]   Instituto Mexicano del Seguro Social. Diagnóstico y Tratamiento de los Trastornos del Sueño 2010. http://www.imss.gob.mx/profesionales/guiasclinicas/gpc.htm.

[15]   Secretaría de salud. Detección, diagnóstico y tratamiento del síndrome de apnea obstructiva del sueño en los tres niveles de atención. México. [Date of Access July 23, 2021}. Disponible en:. https://cenetec-difusion.com/gpc-sns/?p=867.

[16]   Instituto Mexicano del Seguro Social. Diagnóstico y Tratamiento del Insomnio en el Anciano http://www.imss.gob.mx/profesionales/guiasclinicas/Pages/guias.aspx.

[17]   Álvarez-García HB, Jiménez-Correa U, de Almondes KM. Effectiveness of a brief behavioral intervention for insomnia (BBII) during the COVID-19 pandemic: Mexican case report. Sleep Sci 2020; 13(3): 210-3.

[http://dx.doi.org/10.5935/1984-0063.20200055] [PMID: 33381289]

[18]   PML Latinoamérica. Catálogo de medicamentos. México. [Date of Access June 24, 2021]. Disponible en:. https://www.medicamentosplm.com/Home/Medicamento/a/1

[19]   Consejo de Salubridad General. Cuadro Básico y Catalogo de Medicamentos. Edición 2016. México. Consultado 24 junio 2021]. Disponible en:. http://www.csg.gob.mx /contenidos/priorizacion/ cuadro-basico/med/catalogos.html

[20]   Instituto Nacional de Salud Pública (INSP). Encuesta Nacional de Salud y Nutrición de Medio Camino. Informe Final de Resultados. México, [Consultado 23 julio 2021] Disponible en: . https://www.gob.mx/cms/uploads/attachment/file/209093/ENSANUT.pdf

[21]   Guerrero-Zúñiga S, Gaona-Pineda EB, Cuevas-Nasu L, *et al.* Prevalencia de síntomas de sueño y riesgo de apnea obstructiva del sueño en México. Salud Publica Mex 2018; 60(3, may-jun): 347-55. [http://dx.doi.org/10.21149/9280] [PMID: 29746752]

CHAPTER 4

Sleep Medicine in Australia

Nicole Grivell[1,2], **Alexander Sweetman**[1,2], **Nicole Lovato**[1,2], **Andrew Vakulin**[1,2] and **Ching Li Chai-Coetzer**[1,2,3,*]

[1] *National Centre for Sleep Health Services Research, Bedford Park, South Australia, Australia*

[2] *Adelaide Institute for Sleep Health/FHMRI Sleep Health, College of Medicine and Public Health, Flinders University, Bedford Park, South Australia, Australia*

[3] *Southern Adelaide Local Health Network, SA Health, Bedford Park, South Australia, Australia*

Abstract: This chapter explores the current context of sleep medicine in Australia. Detailed descriptions of the providers involved in sleep health care, the services available for the assessment and management of sleep disorders, the professional organisations supporting and advocating for sleep medicine, Australian clinical guidelines, and the barriers limiting the provision of best practice sleep health care are presented within this chapter. Sleep medicine is available within Australia by means of publicly funded specialist-led sleep services such as public hospital outpatient clinics and sleep laboratories, and private referral options including specialist sleep physicians, sleep psychologists and private sleep laboratories. Access to publicly funded sleep services are often limited by long wait times for assessment and management, insufficient numbers of sleep-trained providers and long distances to travel for those individuals located in rural and remote areas. Private sleep services offer shorter waiting times than public sleep services, however the associated costs of accessing private treatment mean that it is limited to those with the financial means to afford it. Subsidies for many treatments for sleep disorders, such as continuous positive airway pressure and mandibular advancement splints, are also restricted to those on government benefits and/or those who hold private health insurance coverage. Research exploring new models of care for sleep health care within the primary care setting is currently being conducted in an effort to improve access to care for the many Australians living with sleep disorders.

Keywords: Australia, Barriers to care, Healthcare delivery, Insomnia, Obstructive sleep apnea, Sleep medicine.

* **Corresponding author Ching Li Chai-Coetzer:** Adelaide Institute for Sleep Health, Flinders University, Mark Oliphant Building, Level 3, 5 Laffer Drive, Bedford Park SA 5042, Australia; Tel: +61 8 7221 8313; Fax: +61 8 8490 3253; Email: chingli.chai-coetzer@sa.gov.au

Hrayr P. Attarian, Marie-Louise M. Coussa-Koniski & Alain Michel Sabri (Eds.)

THE AUSTRALIAN HEALTHCARE SYSTEM

The Australian healthcare system is composed of a complex mix of services that include public and private hospitals, primary health care (*e.g.* general practitioners [GPs], allied health, dental, community and public health) and specialist medical services which are funded by the government (state/territory or federal) and non-government sources (*e.g.* not-for-profit organisations, private health insurers, and individual out-of-pocket payments). In 2017-18, more than two-thirds (AUD$126.7 billion; 68.3%) of total health expenditure in Australia was funded by governments [1]. The Australian health system utilises a hybrid model of financing with healthcare funded through either taxation or privately *via* a voluntary private health insurance system. A universal, taxpayer-funded public health insurance scheme known as Medicare was introduced in Australia in 1984 and currently provides free or subsidised access to public hospital services as well as consultations, investigations and treatment by health professionals. Medicare consists of three main parts – hospital, medical and pharmaceutical. Government subsidised medical services and prescription medications are set out in the Medicare Benefits Schedule (MBS) and Pharmaceutical Benefits Schedule (PBS), respectively [2, 3]. Government-funded healthcare and support services are also provided by the Department of Veterans' Affairs (DVA) to war veterans, serving and former members of the Australian Defence Force, Australian Federal Police and their families [4].

CURRENT PRACTICE OF SLEEP MEDICINE IN AUSTRALIA

Sleep Medicine Practitioners

In Australia, the first point of contact for patients with a suspected sleep disorder is typically within primary health care *via* a GP who may then refer patients to specialist sleep services for sleep physician review and/or polysomnography (PSG) testing. PSGs can be conducted overnight at home or in a sleep laboratory, and are provided by specialist sleep services within public hospitals or privately-operated sleep centres. Specialist sleep centres are overseen by qualified sleep medicine physicians and typically employ sleep technicians, scientists and/or nurses. Many sleep centres have affiliations with, or refer patients to see, Ear, Nose and Throat (ENT) surgeons, dentists, sleep-trained or general psychologists, other specialist physicians, such as neurologists and psychiatrists who may have a special interest in sleep disorders management, and allied health practitioners (*e.g.* dieticians, exercise physiologists and pharmacists).

Sleep Medicine Training in Australia

The typical pathway for qualification as a sleep medicine physician in Australia is through completion of specialist Respiratory Medicine training (minimum of two core years following completion of Basic Physician Training), and one year of specialist Sleep Medicine training *via* the Royal Australasian College of Physicians [5, 6]. Thus, almost all physicians practising within the sleep field in Australia are dually certified in Respiratory and Sleep Medicine. Unlike medical practitioners, nurses are not required to complete formal sleep-related education to work in sleep health. There are also no formal educational requirements to become a sleep technologist, although sleep technologists commonly have degrees in science, nursing or psychology and a graduate certificate in sleep science is available for those individuals interested in pursuing a career as a sleep technologist. For dentists wishing to practice dental sleep medicine, there is currently no formal certification available, however a Fellowship in Dental Sleep Medicine has recently been introduced by the Australasian Sleep Association. For psychologists, the Australian Psychological Society offers a 'Foundations in Sleep Psychology' online course that provides an overview of insomnia, sleep apnoea, and circadian rhythm disorders but there is currently no formal program for accreditation to administer Cognitive Behavioural Therapy for Insomnia (CBTi) that is recognised throughout Australia. Additional training programs are being developed to increase the amount of sleep health education in post-graduate psychology university programs [7, 8], and CBTi training-and-accreditation programs are offered through Australian professional sleep and psychology bodies.

Sleep Study Testing and Obstructive Sleep Apnea Management

The cost of sleep physician consultations is covered in part by the MBS if patients are referred by a GP to see the specialist. There are several MBS items available for the investigation of sleep disorders in adults and children, including in-laboratory (level 1) or at-home (level 2) diagnostic polysomnography (PSG), treatment initiation and treatment effectiveness PSG studies, as well as daytime hypersomnolence testing (*i.e.* Multiple Sleep Latency Tests [MSLT] and Maintenance Of Wakefulness Tests [MWT]) [9, 10]. Limited-channel (*i.e.* level 3 and 4) sleep studies are not currently subsidised in Australia. Medicare criteria mandate that GPs who wish to directly refer patients for diagnostic laboratory or home PSG must confirm that patients have a high pre-test probability of symptomatic, moderate-severe obstructive sleep apnea (OSA) by meeting the following criteria [1]: an OSA50 score ≥5, STOP-BANG score ≥3 or high-risk score on Berlin Questionnaire; plus [2] an Epworth Sleepiness Scale score ≥8 [11 - 14]. Otherwise, patients must have professional attendance with a qualified sleep medicine or respiratory physician prior to PSG testing. These criteria were introduced by Medicare in November 2019 following concerns about the rapid rise in claims for publicly funded laboratory and home-based sleep study item numbers [15 - 17].

Treatments available in Australia for the management of OSA include continuous positive airway pressure (CPAP) therapy, mandibular advancement splints (MAS), posture control devices and upper airway surgery. Patients who are confirmed to have a diagnosis of OSA in whom CPAP therapy is recommended may have their CPAP equipment provided by a public hospital if eligibility criteria for government-subsidised equipment are fulfilled. Eligibility criteria vary across states/territories and local health networks, and are often based on OSA severity, symptoms (*e.g.* excessive daytime sleepiness) and medical co-morbidities in patients who meet specified welfare entitlements (*e.g.* Health Care Card or Pensioner Concession Card holders). Patients who are not eligible for government-subsidised equipment are required to purchase their own device from a private CPAP provider (*e.g.* CPAP retailer or pharmacy). There is little to no government funding available to cover the cost of MAS, which needs to be custom-made and fitted by appropriately trained dentists. The cost of CPAP or MAS (and related dental costs) may be partially reimbursed by private health insurers, but the rebate amount can vary considerably, depending on the type and level of health insurance purchased.

The Bettering the Evaluation And Care of Health (BEACH) program is a cross-sectional survey that includes 1,000 new and randomly sampled general practitioners per year to identify rates of identification and management of health conditions in Australia [18]. Data from the BEACH program showed that the management rate of new cases of OSA in primary care had risen steadily from 35 to 118 per 100,000 patient encounters between 2000 to 2014, and previously diagnosed obstructive sleep apnea (OSA) problems from 94 to 296 per 100,000 encounters. Interestingly, the gender ratio of patients being managed for OSA had changed from 4:1 (male:female) to approximately 2:1 during this time. The referral rate for OSA by GPs was 59% (medical referral to a respiratory or sleep clinic in 90% of all referrals; surgical [*e.g.* ear, nose and throat surgeon] referral in 3%; and "other" specialist referral in 7%) [19].

Insomnia Management

Psychologists are central to the provision of psychological services, including insomnia management, within Australia. Insomnia is well-recognised to be dominated by psychological causes. These causes require strategic behavioural modifications to break the cycle of poor sleep habits and self-fulfilling worry about chronic poor sleep. The best evidence-based care is Cognitive Behavioural Therapy for Insomnia (CBTi) [20], administered by a psychologist, which produces robust and durable therapeutic improvements, extending well beyond the period of therapy [21, 22].

General practitioners in Australia can refer patients with insomnia to a psychologist, with a Better Access Initiative GP Mental Health Care Treatment Plan (MHTP) [23 - 25]. GPs can claim reimbursement through the public healthcare system for the development of a MHTP in consultation with the patient. This treatment plan allows patients to access up to 10 sessions with a psychologist (increased to 20 sessions during the COVID-19 pandemic), subsidised by the public health system. These visits can be provided by telehealth, with funding for telehealth available for those in rural and remote areas, and more recently for the entire Australian population in light of the COVID-19 pandemic [23]. Depending on the fees charged by the psychologist, this subsidy can be sufficient to cover a substantial proportion of treatment costs for the patient however, at present GPs rarely consider referral to a psychologist, with GPs instead commonly providing sleep hygiene information and/or a prescription for medications to manage insomnia [26 - 28]. This is a sub-optimal practice with evidence that sleep hygiene is not an effective stand-alone treatment for insomnia and recommendations that non-drug interventions such as CBTi and brief behavioural therapy for insomnia should be used as first-line treatment for the management of chronic insomnia [29, 30].

Australian adults seek advice and treatment for insomnia in a range of settings. In 2019, Reynolds and colleagues [31] reported the results of a population-based survey in Australia that investigated the most common help-seeking approaches used to manage insomnia symptoms. This report found that 30% of adults had discussed sleep with a doctor or healthcare professional in the past year. Of those with chronic insomnia (14.8% of the sample), less than half had discussed sleep with a healthcare professional over the past year. A small proportion of the adult population reported using herbal supplements (4-5%), prescription medicines (8-12%), or CBTi approaches (3-4%) to manage sleep problems.

The BEACH program also investigated changes in general practitioner management of insomnia between 2000 and 2015 [27]. They found that insomnia was managed in approximately 1.5% of all general practice encounters, and that 90% of these appointments resulted in a sedative-hypnotic medicine prescription. There was a gradual reduction in the prescription of temazepam, and an increase in the prescriptions of melatonin, mirtazapine and quetiapine over time. Most of these medications are associated with adverse side effects, and dependence and withdrawal effects [32 - 34]. Non-pharmacological management advice was provided in about 20% of encounters.

Online information and 'apps' claiming to treat insomnia symptoms are prolific throughout the world, but do not always provide evidence-based information or advice. Although digital CBTi programs that provide tailored therapy recommendations have been developed and studied extensively in North America and Europe, there are currently no interactive self-guided digital CBTi programs available in Australia [35, 36]. This Way Up, an Australian Government subsidised service that offers online services based on cognitive behavioural therapy, however, does provide a freely available eBook "Managing Insomnia", alongside a suite of other digital mental health services [37].

PROFESSIONAL ORGANISATIONS WITHIN AUSTRALIAN SLEEP MEDICINE

Australasian Sleep Association

The Australasian Sleep Association (ASA) (www.sleep.org.au) is the peak professional and scientific organisation representing sleep clinicians and researchers working across all areas of sleep health and medicine in Australia and New Zealand [38]. The primary role of the ASA is to lead and promote sleep health and sleep science, provide professional development for members, foster research and establish clinical standards. It also supports community engagement, education and consultation including broader advocacy activities to promote sleep health and research. The ASA has over 900 members across Australia and organises a range of activities throughout the year including workshops, webinars and seminars, local state branch conferences along with the Australia and New Zealand Sleep Science Association (ANZSSA) and the flagship Australasian sleep medicine annual scientific meeting, the Sleep DownUnder Conference. This annual 3-day conference showcases the latest clinical and basic research and practice with a strong emphasis on showcasing and nurturing early career clinicians and scientists. The ASA provides a range of awards to support higher degree research and clinical students and early career researchers, including travel awards, the prestigious new investigator award, seed grants, travel scholarships and leadership awards.

Alongside the ANZSSA and the National Association of Testing Authorities (NATA), the ASA co-runs the Sleep Disorders Services Accreditation program, providing input into the development, training and accreditation of sleep laboratories in Australia and New Zealand to maintain sleep disorders services accreditation. NATA administers and conducts the accreditation program, with sleep services who wish to be accredited required to meet the necessary requirements of the program and undergo reaccreditation every four years.

The ASA is also involved in advocacy activities at the community level working with the Sleep Health Foundation, and at the government level promoting sleep health as a priority area for health and wellbeing. This work is essential towards increasing government investment into sleep health research and health professions education in sleep health management, including primary care providers.

Thoracic Society of Australia and New Zealand

The Thoracic Society of Australia and New Zealand (TSANZ) (www.thoracic.org.au/) is a professional body representing a diverse range of health professions including medical specialists, researchers, academics, nurses, physiotherapists and other health professionals working in the field of respiratory and sleep medicine. It is a health promotion charity committed to improving knowledge, understanding and prevention of lung disease through research and health promotion. The TSANZ plays a key role in setting and implementing the highest quality standards for the diagnosis and management of patients with respiratory and sleep disorders.

Australia and New Zealand Sleep Science Association

The Australia and New Zealand Sleep Science Association (ANZSSA) (www.anzsleepscience.org/) is the professional body for sleep technologists, physiologists, nurses and scientists in Australia. As with the ASA, it is a Company Limited by Guarantee and is governed by its constitution [39]. ANZSSA advocates for Sleep Technology as a health profession, contributes to the best practice and optimal patient sleep healthcare, and provides resources and support to members.

Sleep Health Foundation

The Sleep Health Foundation (SHF) (www.sleephealthfoundation.org.au/) is a not-for-profit health promotion charity organisation and the peak advocacy body for healthy sleep in Australia. The SHF aims to increase community knowledge about the importance of healthy sleep and sleep disorders, and to improve public health, safety and well-being. The SHF produces educational materials in conjunction with sleep experts for distribution to the public and commissions reports about the impacts of poor sleep health, safety and productivity to improve public awareness and understanding of sleep health. Recent publications by the

SHF include reports on the costs of poor sleep health [40], chronic insomnia disorder [31] and the impacts of inadequate sleep [41].

Australian Practice Guidelines

The ASA develops clinical standards which describe the minimum standards required for the provision of high-quality sleep disorders services in both private and public sectors. The ASA works with its members, and other professional groups including the TSANZ, to publish position statements and clinical guidelines on best-practice management of clinical sleep disorders. The ASA have released position statements on sleep studies in children [42] and adults [43], management of sleep disordered breathing with CPAP therapy [44], oral appliance devices [45], and surgery [46], management of narcolepsy [47], and non-pharmacological strategies to manage insomnia [48].

A suite of community-facing online resources [49] are produced by the SHF to provide information on a range of areas including; paediatric sleep problems, sleep apnoea, CPAP therapy and other non-CPAP treatments for OSA, relationships between sleep and other mental and physical health disorders, circadian rhythm disorders, chronic insomnia, CBTi, and healthy sleep/lifestyle advice.

In 2015, the Royal Australian College of General Practitioners (RACGP) produced a guideline for general practitioners on insomnia and anxiety management with prescription and non-pharmacological approaches (revised in 2019) [29]. This guideline strongly encourages CBTi as the 'first line' treatment for insomnia in general practice patients.

The National Centre for Sleep Health Services Research (NCSHSR) [50] is a multi-disciplinary and multi-institutional group of sleep and respiratory researchers, clinicians, health economists, implementation experts, industry partners and professional society representatives that was established in 2018 and funded by a National Health and Medical Research Council Centres of Research Excellence grant. The aim of the NCSHSR is to improve the management of sleep disorders within primary care and translate new evidence into Australian general practice. This group is preparing evidence-based guidelines, education and management pathways for OSA [51, 52] and chronic insomnia [53] to improve sleep service access and sleep disorders care within Australian general practice. Interactive OSA and insomnia management resources will be hosted online through the ASA website. The group have also worked with the RACGP to develop insomnia and OSA education resources for the CPD-accredited "CHECK" program, the official RACGP journal (Australian Journal of General Practice), and the online GP education system (gpLearning) [54, 55].

FACTORS INFLUENCING ACCESS TO SLEEP HEALTH CARE

Barriers to OSA Management

With OSA traditionally managed as a specialist-led condition in Australia, the increasing prevalence of OSA has culminated in long wait times for access to public, specialist-led outpatient services that offer assessment and management of OSA and other sleep disorders [56]. It was reported in a 2019 Australian Parliamentary Inquiry into sleep health awareness that an 18 month wait for an initial appointment in a public sleep outpatient clinic is common, with an additional 12 months for a PSG occurring at times [57]. Research by Grivell *et al.* [58] concurs, with Australian GPs reporting challenges accessing public sleep services within a reasonable timeframe for their patients. These significant wait times are largely limited to public services and can be avoided by a referral to a private sleep physician, however, this pathway can incur significant costs. Patients are almost always required to pay a gap fee above the scheduled Medicare subsidy when seeing private medical specialists in Australia and there are commonly fees above the scheduled Medicare subsidy and private health insurance rebates when undergoing a PSG at a private sleep laboratory [59]. These out-of-pocket costs mean that a private approach to sleep disorder management is limited to those with the financial means to afford it. OSA assessment and management can also be more challenging for individuals living in rural and remote areas of Australia. Australia is geographically large, making access to both public and private sleep services, which are more commonly located in metropolitan areas, difficult and can mean that patients are required to travel long distances to access services [57, 58, 60]. This is of particular concern for indigenous Australians with research by Woods *et al.* [60] finding that remoteness was one of the factors influencing access to sleep disorder management for Aboriginal and Torres Strait Islander people, with this population more likely to reside in remote areas.

Another option available for OSA assessment is for individuals to attend commercial CPAP retailers that offer Medicare subsidised level 2 home-based PSGs. Whilst this type of service offers shorter wait times for PSG testing, there is concern about a potential conflict of interest with many providers offering both diagnostic services and the sale of treatment devices such as CPAP masks and machines [61]. This may result in an incentive for private retailers to recommend CPAP therapy to patients with mild, asymptomatic OSA when it may not be clinically indicated and there is concern by the Australasian Sleep Association that this potential conflict of interest could limit the provision of impartial advice about treatment options and influence a patient's choice to explore treatments other than CPAP [44, 57].

One approach being considered by sleep researchers to address the access issues inherent in OSA care in Australia is the transition of management of less complex cases of OSA from specialist centres into the general practice setting [52]. This was explored in a randomised controlled trial by Chai-Coetzer *et al.* [62] who found that the management of uncomplicated OSA by GPs and general practice nurses was non-inferior to specialist-led care. Whilst this model would enable access to OSA management within an individual's local community with reduced wait times, limiting this model from the widespread translation at present is due to the lack of knowledge about the management of OSA and CPAP in both GPs and practice nurses, with GPs instead frequently referring patients on to specialist sleep services, and a funding model that does not currently support OSA diagnosis and CPAP initiation within general practice [58].

Barriers to Insomnia Care

Chronic insomnia is commonly managed within general practice with the management of sleep difficulties being one of the most common reasons for presentation within Australian general practice [27, 63]. GPs consider insomnia management to be within their scope of practice and frequently provide sleep hygiene and medication [26, 27]. This is despite GP guidelines recommending CBTi as the 'first line' treatment for chronic insomnia [29]. It is important to note that many sedatives and hypnotics are subsidised for patients in Australia by the PBS, so despite RACGP guidelines recommending short term or intermittent use, the minimal cost of these medications makes pharmaceutical management of insomnia a cost-effective option for individuals [29, 64].

For the management of complex cases of insomnia, a referral to a health professional trained in the delivery of CBTi is an option [48, 65], with Medicare funding available by means of a MHTP [25]. Whilst it is appropriate for a MHTP to be used for the treatment of chronic insomnia, until recent times the use of MHTPs for insomnia management has been limited by a lack of awareness of the eligibility of the plan to be used to address sleep difficulties by GPs, thus limiting access to subsidised visits for patients [24, 26]. Costs for the provision of CBTi by Australian psychologists is also not standardised and varies between providers, with many charging gap fees beyond the Medicare rebate making meeting the cost of CBTi difficult for some individuals, particularly without Medicare support [65]. Limited access to psychologists is compounded by a lack of tertiary specialist insomnia services and insufficient numbers of psychologists trained to administer CBTi, making an onward referral for insomnia management challenging for GPs [7]. Solutions that have been proposed to address the challenges of accessing CBTi in Australia involve increased participation by general practice. Ideas include the provision of brief behavioural therapy for insomnia (BBTi) or CBTi by GPs and/or practice nurses for patients with less complex insomnia as part of a stepped care approach, and provision of online CBTi through general practice [54]. Whilst these approaches potentially offer improved access for individuals with insomnia, particularly those who are financially disadvantaged and/or residing in remote or rural areas, they are currently under research investigation and are yet to be integrated into routine clinical practice [66, 67].

Cost of Treatments

Cost of specific treatments and devices can also be a factor influencing access to sleep health care [26, 58, 68]. CPAP equipment can cost in excess of $1200AUD and is not universally funded in Australia [57, 69]. Public CPAP provision is managed by individual states and territories or local health networks within Australia. In most states CPAP is provided at low or no cost to those individuals in receipt of a pensioner concession card or a low income or disability health care card, but access varies between regions in Australia, and even in areas within capital cities, with some areas having no access to publicly funded CPAP [57]. Additionally, in order to access publicly funded CPAP, patients must be seen within public outpatient clinics and contend with the associated lengthy wait times. For those not eligible for publicly funded CPAP, some private health insurance funds offer partial reimbursement for CPAP devices but there is no consistency in the amount of reimbursement. For patients that are unable to tolerate or choose not to use CPAP, there is no government funding for mandibular advancement splints (MAS) and rebates vary between private health insurance funds. With MAS devices costing approximately $1400-2000AUD and minimal/no public funding, access to MAS is limited to those who either hold private health insurance that provides a rebate for MAS or can afford the device outright [57].

The Australian government provides subsidies for the majority of pharmaceutical items for Australian citizens and residents by means of the Pharmaceutical Benefits Scheme (PBS), however exceptions exist that can mean considerable out-of-pocket costs for individuals [3]. For example, PBS-subsidised therapy for narcolepsy in Australia remains limited to dexamphetamine and modafinil/armodafinil in patients who meet specified criteria. The American Academy of Sleep Medicine and the Australasian Sleep Association both support the use of sodium oxybate for the management of narcolepsy, however it is not currently subsidised by the Australian Government *via* the PBS nor is it easily accessible [47, 70]. To obtain sodium oxybate in Australia, an application must be made to the Australian Government Special Access Scheme to import the medicine from overseas, and the annual out-of-pocket cost of treatment for patients is between $15,000 and $20,000AUD, a cost that is understandably prohibitive for many individuals [57, 71]. Furthermore, medications such as solriamfetol and pitolisant, which are recommended in current international guidelines as first-line treatments for narcolepsy are not currently available in Australia [72, 73].

Sleep Health Care for Indigenous Australians

Aboriginal and Torres Strait Islander people accounted for 3.3% of the Australian population in 2016 [74]. They have been shown to experience disease at a rate that is 2.3 times greater than non-Indigenous Australians, with chronic diseases contributing to 63% of this gap in health status [74, 75]. While recent research has found that Aboriginal and Torres Strait Islander (ATSI) people have higher rates of OSA than non-ATSI Australians [76], there remains a paucity of research exploring the prevalence and impact of sleep disorders on ATSI people. This is concerning given that work by Woods and colleagues [60] found that ATSI individuals are more likely to live remotely, thus limiting their access to sleep services, and they were less likely to attend follow up care for their sleep disorder. They attributed this reduced follow up care to factors including a lack of familiarity with sleep disorders, the complexity of CPAP treatment, environmental issues influencing sleep hygiene and a need for electricity. This potentially represents a system of care provision that does not meet the cultural needs of this population. Further research and investigation into culturally appropriate sleep health care for ATSI people is required, with input from representative leaders from ATSI communities needed to inform the development of appropriate research and clinical programs. An example of research of this kind is work by Benn and colleagues [77] who recently engaged Indigenous representatives and researchers experienced in Indigenous health to inform the development of a new, culturally appropriate assessment tool for the ATSI population, the Top End Sleepiness Scale, as an alternative to the Epworth Sleepiness Scale.

CONCLUSION

This chapter provides an overview of the current services and challenges to the delivery of adult sleep health services in Australia. Sleep disorder management is provided by a range of healthcare professionals within both public and private funding models. The increasing prevalence of common sleep disorders, significant demand for specialist sleep services and insufficient numbers of sleep-trained healthcare professionals have prompted the exploration of new models of care, including general practice settings. It is clear that disparities exist in accessing sleep medicine services and treatments in Australia, particularly for those unable to afford the out-of-pocket costs associated with the assessment and treatment of sleep disorders and for those located geographically distant from metropolitan sleep services. Despite having a universal health care system, access to sleep medicine services and treatments in Australia remains influenced by socio-economic status and geographical location, with those individuals with the means to follow the private referral process, hold private health insurance or purchase devices able to avoid the lengthy waits associated with the public sleep medicine system in Australia. By improving access to sleep health care, for example within primary care, it is expected that more Australians will have access to timely sleep disorder assessment and management within their local communities.

CONSENT FOR PUBLICATION

Not applicable.

CONFLICT OF INTEREST

The authors declare no conflict of interest, financial or otherwise.

ACKNOWLEDGEMENT

Declared none.

REFERENCES

[1]   Australian Institute of Health and Welfare. Australia's health. 2020.

[2]   Australian Government Services Australia. https://www.servicesaustralia.gov.au/individuals/medicare

[3]   Australian Government Department of Health. About the PBS 2021.https://www.pbs.gov.au/info/about-the-pbs

[4]   Australian Government Department of Veteran Affairs. Department of Veteran Affairs nd https://www.dva.gov.au/

[5]   Royal Australasian College of Physicians. Sleep Medicine Advanced Training Curriculum. Royal Australasian College of Physicians 2013.

[6]   Royal Australasian College of Physicians. Paediatric Sleep Medicine Advanced Training Curriculum. Royal Australasian College of Physicians 2013.

[7]   Meaklim H, Jackson ML, Bartlett D, *et al.* Sleep education for healthcare providers: Addressing deficient sleep in Australia and New Zealand. Sleep Health 2020; 6(5): 636-50.
[http://dx.doi.org/10.1016/j.sleh.2020.01.012] [PMID: 32423774]

[8]   Meaklim H, Rehm IC, Monfries M, Junge M, Meltzer LJ, Jackson ML. Wake up psychology! Postgraduate psychology students need more sleep and insomnia education. Aust Psychol 2021; 56(6): 485-98.
[http://dx.doi.org/10.1080/00050067.2021.1955614]

[9]   Australian Government Department of Health. http://www9.health.gov.au/ mbs/fullDisplay.cfm? type=note&q=DN.1.17& qt=noteID&criteria=sleep

[10]   Australian Government Department of Health. http://www9.health.gov.au/ mbs/fullDisplay.cfm?type =note&q=DN.1.23& qt=noteID&criteria=multiple%20sleep%20latency

[11]   Chai-Coetzer CL, Antic NA, Rowland LS, *et al.* A simplified model of screening questionnaire and home monitoring for obstructive sleep apnoea in primary care. Thorax 2011; 66(3): 213-9.
[http://dx.doi.org/10.1136/thx.2010.152801] [PMID: 21252389]

[12]   Chung F, Abdullah HR, Liao P. STOP-Bang Questionnaire. Chest 2016; 149(3): 631-8.
[http://dx.doi.org/10.1378/chest.15-0903] [PMID: 26378880]

[13]   Netzer NC, Stoohs RA, Netzer CM, Clark K, Strohl KP. Using the Berlin Questionnaire to identify patients at risk for the sleep apnea syndrome. Ann Intern Med 1999; 131(7): 485-91.
[http://dx.doi.org/10.7326/0003-4819-131-7-199910050-00002] [PMID: 10507956]

[14]   Johns MW. A new method for measuring daytime sleepiness: the Epworth sleepiness scale. Sleep 1991; 14(6): 540-5.
[http://dx.doi.org/10.1093/sleep/14.6.540] [PMID: 1798888]

[15]   Woods CE, Usher KJ, Jersmann H, Maguire GP. Sleep disordered breathing and polysomnography in Australia: trends in provision from 2005 to 2012 and the impact of home-based diagnosis. J Clin Sleep Med 2014; 10(7): 767-72.
[http://dx.doi.org/10.5664/jcsm.3868] [PMID: 25024654]

[16]   Marshall NS, Wilsmore BR, McEvoy RD, Wheatley JR, Dodd MJ, Grunstein RR. Polysomnography in Australia--trends in provision. J Clin Sleep Med 2007; 3(3): 281-4.
[http://dx.doi.org/10.5664/jcsm.26799] [PMID: 17561597]

[17]   Australian Government Department of Health. Changes to Diagnostic Services for Sleep Disorders 2019. http://www.mbsonline.gov.au/internet/mbsonline /publishing.nsf/Content/Factsheet-Sleep Disorders

[18]   The University of Sydney. https://www.sydney.edu.au/medicine-health/our-research/research-centres/bettering-the-evaluation-and-care-of-health.html n.d.

[19]   Cross NE, Harrison CM, Yee BJ, *et al.* Management of Snoring and Sleep Apnea in Australian Primary Care: The BEACH Study (2000–2014). J Clin Sleep Med 2016; 12(8): 1167-73.
[http://dx.doi.org/10.5664/jcsm.6060] [PMID: 27397666]

[20]   Morin CM. Cognitive-behavioral approaches to the treatment of insomnia. J Clin Psychiatry 2004; 65 (Suppl. 16): 33-40.
[PMID: 15575803]

[21]   Morin AK, Jarvis CI, Lynch AM. Therapeutic options for sleep-maintenance and sleep-onset insomnia. Pharmacotherapy 2007; 27(1): 89-110.
[http://dx.doi.org/10.1592/phco.27.1.89] [PMID: 17192164]

[22]   Jacobs GD, Pace-Schott EF, Stickgold R, Otto MW. Cognitive behavior therapy and pharmacotherapy for insomnia: a randomized controlled trial and direct comparison. Arch Intern Med 2004; 164(17): 1888-96.
[http://dx.doi.org/10.1001/archinte.164.17.1888] [PMID: 15451764]

[23]   Australian   Government   Department   of   Health.   Better   Access   Initiative 2021.https://www.health.gov.au/initiatives-and-programs/better-acc-ss-initiative?utm_source=health.gov.au&utm_medium=callout-au-o-custom&utm_campaign=digital_transformation

[24]   Liotta M. Does insomnia fall under mental health treatment plans? newsGP: Royal Australian College of General Practitioners; 2021 [Available from:. https://www1.racgp.org.au/newsgp/clinical/does-insomnia-fall-under-mental-health-treatment-p

[25]   Australian Government Department of Health. Medicare Benefits Schedule - Item 2715 n.d. Available from:. http://www9.health.gov.au/mbs/fullDisplay.cfm?type=item&q=2715

[26]   Haycock J, Grivell N, Redman A, *et al.* Primary care management of chronic insomnia: a qualitative analysis of the attitudes and experiences of Australian general practitioners. BMC Fam Pract 2021;

22(1): 158.
[http://dx.doi.org/10.1186/s12875-021-01510-z] [PMID: 34294049]

[27]　Miller CB, Valenti L, Harrison CM, *et al.* Time Trends in the Family Physician Management of Insomnia: The Australian Experience (2000–2015). J Clin Sleep Med 2017; 13(6): 785-90.
[http://dx.doi.org/10.5664/jcsm.6616] [PMID: 28454597]

[28]　Begum M, Gonzalez-Chica D, Bernardo C, Woods A, Stocks N. Trends in the prescription of drugs used for insomnia: an open-cohort study in Australian general practice, 2011–2018. Br J Gen Pract 2021; 71(712): e877-86.
[http://dx.doi.org/10.3399/BJGP.2021.0054] [PMID: 33950853]

[29]　Prescribing drugs of dependence in general practice Part B - Benzodiazepines. Royal Australian College of General Practitioners 2015.

[30]　Edinger JD, Arnedt JT, Bertisch SM, *et al.* Behavioral and psychological treatments for chronic insomnia disorder in adults: an American Academy of Sleep Medicine clinical practice guideline. J Clin Sleep Med 2021; 17(2): 255-62.
[http://dx.doi.org/10.5664/jcsm.8986] [PMID: 33164742]

[31]　Reynolds A, Appleton S, Gill T, Adams R. Chronic insomnia disorder in Australia: A report to the Sleep Health Foundation. Sleep Health Foundation 2019.

[32]　Qaseem A, Kansagara D, Forciea MA, Cooke M, Denberg TD. Management of Chronic Insomnia Disorder in Adults: A Clinical Practice Guideline From the American College of Physicians. Ann Intern Med 2016; 165(2): 125-33.
[http://dx.doi.org/10.7326/M15-2175] [PMID: 27136449]

[33]　Sweetman A, Putland S, Lack L, *et al.* The effect of cognitive behavioural therapy for insomnia on sedative-hypnotic use: A narrative review. Sleep Med Rev 2021; 56: 101404.
[http://dx.doi.org/10.1016/j.smrv.2020.101404] [PMID: 33370637]

[34]　Glass J, Lanctôt KL, Herrmann N, Sproule BA, Busto UE. Sedative hypnotics in older people with insomnia: meta-analysis of risks and benefits. BMJ 2005; 331(7526): 1169.
[http://dx.doi.org/10.1136/bmj.38623.768588.47] [PMID: 16284208]

[35]　Soh HL, Ho RC, Ho CS, Tam WW. Efficacy of digital cognitive behavioural therapy for insomnia: a meta-analysis of randomised controlled trials. Sleep Med 2020; 75: 315-25.
[http://dx.doi.org/10.1016/j.sleep.2020.08.020] [PMID: 32950013]

[36]　Zachariae R, Lyby MS, Ritterband LM, O'Toole MS. Efficacy of internet-delivered cognitive-behavioral therapy for insomnia – A systematic review and meta-analysis of randomized controlled trials. Sleep Med Rev 2016; 30: 1-10.
[http://dx.doi.org/10.1016/j.smrv.2015.10.004] [PMID: 26615572]

[37]　Grierson AB, Hobbs MJ, Mason EC. Self-guided online cognitive behavioural therapy for insomnia: A naturalistic evaluation in patients with potential psychiatric comorbidities. J Affect Disord 2020; 266: 305-10.
[http://dx.doi.org/10.1016/j.jad.2020.01.143] [PMID: 32056892]

[38]　Constitution. Australasian Sleep Association 2017.

[39]　Consitution of Australia and New Zealand Sleep Science Association Ltd 2019.

[40]　Rise and try to shine: The social and economic cost of sleep disorders in Australia. Sleep Health Foundation 2021.

[41]　Asleep on the job - costs of inadequate sleep in Australia. Sleep Health Foundation 2017.

[42]　Pamula Y, Nixon GM, Edwards E, *et al.* Australasian Sleep Association clinical practice guidelines for performing sleep studies in children. Sleep Med 2017; 36 (Suppl. 1): S23-42.
[http://dx.doi.org/10.1016/j.sleep.2017.03.020] [PMID: 28648225]

[43]　Douglas JA, Chai-Coetzer CL, McEvoy D, *et al.* Guidelines for sleep studies in adults – a position

statement of the Australasian Sleep Association. Sleep Med 2017; 36 (Suppl. 1): S2-S22.
[http://dx.doi.org/10.1016/j.sleep.2017.03.019] [PMID: 28648224]

[44]   ASA. Position Paper: Best Practice Guidelines for Provision of CPAP Therapy 2009 Available from:.
https://sleep.org.au/common/Uploaded%20files/Public%20Files/Professional%20resources/Sleep%20
Documents/Best%20Practice%20Guidelines%20for%20Provision%20of%20CPAP%20therapy.pdf

[45]   ASA. The use of oral appliances in the treatment of snoring and obstructive sleep apnoea: A position
Paper   of   the   Australasian   Sleep   Association   Available   from:.
https://sleep.org.au/common/Uploaded%20files/Public%20Files/ASA%20Membership/Guidelines/OA
%20Position%20paper.pdf

[46]   MacKay SG, Lewis R, McEvoy D, Joosten S, Holt NR. Surgical management of obstructive sleep
apnoea: A position statement of the Australasian Sleep Association *. Respirology 2020; 25(12): 1292-
308.
[http://dx.doi.org/10.1111/resp.13967] [PMID: 33190389]

[47]   Swieca J, Teng A, Davey M, Djavadkhani Y, Grunstein R, Banerjee D, *et al.* Australasian Sleep
Association position statement and guidelines, regarding the use of sodium oxybate in the treatment of
narcolepsy
2013.
https://sleep.org.au/common/Uploaded%20files/Public%20Files/Professional%20resources/Sleep%20
Documents/sodium%20oxybate.pdf

[48]   Ree M, Junge M, Cunnington D. Australasian Sleep Association position statement regarding the use
of psychological/behavioral treatments in the management of insomnia in adults. Sleep Med 2017; 36
(Suppl. 1): S43-7.
[http://dx.doi.org/10.1016/j.sleep.2017.03.017] [PMID: 28648226]

[49]   Sleep Health Foundation. Sleep Health Foundation Factsheets 2021 Available from:.
https://www.sleephealthfoundation.org.au/fact-sheets.html

[50]   NCSHSR. National Centre for Sleep Health Services Research: Positioning Primary Care at the centre
of Sleep Health Management 2018 Available from:. https://www.ncshsr.com/

[51]   Zwar N, Soenen S. Obstructive Sleep Apnoea Primary Care Resource, a National Centre for Sleep
Health Services Research Guideline 2021.

[52]   Sweetman A, Chai-Coetzer CL, Ryswyk EV, Vakulin A, Lovato N, Zwar N, *et al.* Assessment and
management of obstructive sleep apnoea in Australian general practice. Med Today in press

[53]   Sweetman A, Lovato N, Haycock J, Lack L. Improved access to effective non-drug treatment options
for insomnia in Australian general practice. Med Today 2020; 21(11): 14-21.

[54]   Sweetman A, Zwar NA, Grivell N, Lovato N, Lack L. A step-by-step model for a brief behavioural
treatment for insomnia in Australian general practice. Aust J Gen Pract 2021; 50(5): 287-93.
[http://dx.doi.org/10.31128/AJGP-04-20-5391] [PMID: 33928277]

[55]   Sweetman A, Chai-Coetzer CL. Royal Australian College of General Practitioners CHECK program:
Insomnia case study; Carmen has trouble falling asleep. Royal Australian College of General
Practitioners 2020.

[56]   Peppard PE, Young T, Barnet JH, Palta M, Hagen EW, Hla KM. Increased prevalence of sleep-
disordered breathing in adults. Am J Epidemiol 2013; 177(9): 1006-14.
[http://dx.doi.org/10.1093/aje/kws342] [PMID: 23589584]

[57]   Parliament of the Commonwealth of Australia. Bedtime Reading - Inquiry into Sleep Health
Awareness in Australia. House of Representatives Standing Committee on Health Aged Care and
Sport; . 2019.

[58]   Grivell N, Haycock J, Redman A, *et al.* Assessment, referral and management of obstructive sleep
apnea by Australian general practitioners: a qualitative analysis. BMC Health Serv Res 2021; 21(1):
1248.

[http://dx.doi.org/10.1186/s12913-021-07274-7] [PMID: 34794444]

[59]   Australian Government Department of Health. Annual Medicare statistics – 2009-10 onwards.. 2021.

[60]   Woods CE, McPherson K, Tikoft E, *et al.* Sleep Disorders in Aboriginal and Torres Strait Islander People and Residents of Regional and Remote Australia. J Clin Sleep Med 2015; 11(11): 1263-71.
[http://dx.doi.org/10.5664/jcsm.5182] [PMID: 26094934]

[61]   Hanes CA, Wong KKH, Saini B. Diagnostic pathways for obstructive sleep apnoea in the Australian community: observations from pharmacy-based CPAP providers. Sleep Breath 2015; 19(4): 1241-8.
[http://dx.doi.org/10.1007/s11325-015-1151-9] [PMID: 25801279]

[62]   Chai-Coetzer CL, Antic NA, Rowland LS, *et al.* Primary care vs specialist sleep center management of obstructive sleep apnea and daytime sleepiness and quality of life: a randomized trial. JAMA 2013; 309(10): 997-1004.
[http://dx.doi.org/10.1001/jama.2013.1823] [PMID: 23483174]

[63]   General Practice Health of the Nation 2020.

[64]   Australian Government Department of Health. N05C hypnotics and sedatives n.d. Available from:.
https://www.pbs.gov.au/browse/body-system?depth=3&codes=n05c

[65]   Cunnington D, Junge MF, Fernando AT. Insomnia: prevalence, consequences and effective treatment. Med J Aust 2013; 199(8): S36-40.
[PMID: 24138364]

[66]   Bartlett D, Galgut Y, Lobsey J, *et al.* 0393 Cognitive behavior therapy for insomnia administered by practice nurses in rural new south wales australia. Sleep (New York, NY). 2017;40(suppl_1):A146-A..

[67]   Sweetman A, Knieriemen A, Hoon E, *et al.* Implementation of a digital cognitive behavioral therapy for insomnia pathway in primary care. Contemp Clin Trials 2021; 107: 106484.
[http://dx.doi.org/10.1016/j.cct.2021.106484] [PMID: 34129952]

[68]   Hanes CA, Wong KKH, Saini B. Clinical services for obstructive sleep apnea patients in pharmacies: the Australian experience. Int J Clin Pharm 2014; 36(2): 460-8.
[http://dx.doi.org/10.1007/s11096-014-9926-9] [PMID: 24562977]

[69]   Streatfeild J, Hillman D, Adams R, Mitchell S, Pezzullo L. Cost-effectiveness of continuous positive airway pressure therapy for obstructive sleep apnea: health care system and societal perspectives. Sleep 2019; 42(12): zsz181.
[http://dx.doi.org/10.1093/sleep/zsz181] [PMID: 31403163]

[70]   Maski K, Trotti LM, Kotagal S, *et al.* Treatment of central disorders of hypersomnolence: an American Academy of Sleep Medicine clinical practice guideline. J Clin Sleep Med 2021; 17(9): 1881-93.
[http://dx.doi.org/10.5664/jcsm.9328] [PMID: 34743789]

[71]   Australian Government Department of Health. Special Access Scheme 2021 Available from: 2021.
https://www.tga.gov.au/form/special-access-scheme

[72]   Bassetti CLA, Kallweit U, Vignatelli L, *et al.* European guideline and expert statements on the management of narcolepsy in adults and children. Eur J Neurol 2021; 28(9): 2815-30.
[http://dx.doi.org/10.1111/ene.14888] [PMID: 34173695]

[73]   Sivam S, Chamula K, Swieca J, Frenkel S, Saini B. Narcolepsy management in Australia: time to wake up. Med J Aust 2021; 215(2): 62-63.e1.
[http://dx.doi.org/10.5694/mja2.51150] [PMID: 34145573]

[74]   Australian Bureau of Statistics. Estimates and Projections, Aboriginal and Torres Strait Islander Australians 2019 Available from:. https://www.abs.gov.au/statistics/people/aboriginal-and-torr-s-strait-islander-peoples/estimates-and-projections-aboriginal-and-torres-strai--islander-australians/latest-release

[75]   Australian Institute of Health and Welfare. Australian Burden of Disease Study: impact and causes of

illness and death in Aboriginal and Torres Strait Islander people 2011. Canberra: AIHW 2016.

[76] Heraganahally SS, Kruavit A, Oguoma VM, *et al.* Sleep apnoea among Australian Aboriginal and non-Aboriginal patients in the Northern Territory of Australia—a comparative study. Sleep 2020; 43(3): zsz248.
[http://dx.doi.org/10.1093/sleep/zsz248] [PMID: 31608397]

[77] Benn E, Wirth H, Short T, Howarth T, Heraganahally SS. The Top End Sleepiness Scale (TESS): A New Tool to Assess Subjective Daytime Sleepiness Among Indigenous Australian Adults. Nat Sci Sleep 2021; 13: 315-28.
[http://dx.doi.org/10.2147/NSS.S298409] [PMID: 33707978]

CHAPTER 5

Sleep Medicine Practice and Training in Saudi Arabia

Shaden O. Qasrawi[1] and **Ahmed S. BaHammam**[2,3,*]

[1] *Sleep Disorders Unit, Kingdom Hospital, Riyadh, Saudi Arabia*

[2] *Department of Medicine, University Sleep Disorders Center, King Saud University, Riyadh, Saudi Arabia*

[3] *The Strategic Technologies Program of the National Plan for Sciences and Technology and Innovation in the Kingdom of Saudi Arabia (08 MED511 02), Riyadh, Saudi Arabia*

Abstract: Sleep medicine as an independent medical specialty is relatively new in Saudi Arabia. Since its foundation, there has been significant growth and an increase in the number of sleep medicine physicians and technologists to meet the continuous increase in demand among the Saudi population. In response to the expansion of sleep medicine in Saudi Arabia, the Saudi Commission for Health Specialties (SCHS) established clear guidelines for the accreditation of sleep medicine physicians and technologists in 2012. Currently, there are two training programs providing structured training and certification in sleep medicine in Saudi Arabia. Despite this progress, there are still many difficulties hindering sleep medicine growth in Saudi Arabia, including the shortage of trained technicians, and specialists, the lack of financial support, and awareness of sleep disorders and their profound effects on healthcare workers and healthcare authorities. In the future, it is essential to introduce sleep medicine in the medical educational system at all levels to show the importance of early recognition and management of sleep disorders, in addition to developing research that is necessary to build knowledge about the prevalence of many sleep disorders in order to help to plan the number of sleep specialists and sleep facilities needed to meet the increasing demands. This chapter discusses the current practice of sleep medicine, and the challenges it faces in Saudi Arabia, in addition to the available data and research about common sleep disorders among the Saudi population.

Keywords: Barriers, Developing countries, Education, Polysomnography, Prevalence, Sleep disorders.

* **Corresponding author Ahmed S. BaHammam:** Department of Medicine, University Sleep Disorders Center, King Saud University, Riyadh, Saudi Arabia; Fax: +966 11 467 9495; E-mails: ashammam2@gmail.com; ashammam@ksu.edu.sa

Hrayr P. Attarian, Marie-Louise M. Coussa-Koniski & Alain Michel Sabri (Eds.)

INTRODUCTION

Saudi Arabia is the fifth largest country in Asia, with an estimated land area of 2,150,000 km^2 (830,000 miles^2). In the official census from 2019, Saudi Arabia's population was estimated to be 34.2 million people, with nearly two-thirds of its population under the age of 30 years and one-third under the age of 15 years old [1]. Although Arabs and Muslims have always expressed special interest in sleep as it is repeatedly cited in the Holy Qu'ran as one of God's signs, "And among His signs is your sleep by night and by day" (Sūrah 30, Ar-rūm, verse 23) [2], sleep medicine is considered a novel medical specialty in Saudi Arabia [3].

HEALTHCARE SERVICES IN SAUDI ARABIA

In Saudi Arabia, the Ministry of Health is the primary governmental healthcare provider (79% of the provided health services) [1, 4]. All Saudis as well as government workers have the right to free health care services supported by the government. The private sector also provides healthcare services (21%), particularly in cities and large towns, the expenses of which are usually covered by insurance companies or by the patients [5].

In 2010, the ratio of doctors and nurses per 10,000 residents in SAUDI ARABIA was 16 and 36, respectively; those numbers are less than those from countries of the developed world [4].

CURRENT PRACTICE OF SLEEP MEDICINE

Early and up to the mid1990s, pulmonologists in Saudi Arabia were relying on overnight pulse oximetry to establish the diagnosis of obstructive sleep apnea (OSA) and used to empirically initiate continuous positive airway pressure (CPAP) therapy and titrate the pressure to treat oxygen desaturation [6]. At that time, the lack of specialized sleep disorders clinics and facilities designated resulted in the occupation of hospital beds by patients with sleep disorders [7]. However, after the increase in the awareness of sleep medicine recently, several sleep disorders centers were opened [5].

In a survey in 2013, sleep disorders centers for diagnosing and treating sleep-related disorders were found in the three main cities in Saudi Arabia: Riyadh (six sleep facilities), Jeddah (seven sleep facilities), and Dammam (five sleep facilities) [8].

According to the national survey conducted in 2013, the number of beds/100,000 individuals, and the number of studies/100,000 individuals were 0.11 and 18.0, respectively [8]. The number of sleep medicine specialists (doctors who completed a minimum of 6 months of formal full-time fellowship training in sleep medicine) was 37, translating to 0.012/100,000 people [8]. The current members of the Saudi Sleep Medicine Group are 55 sleep medicine physicians and surgeons. Of all sleep studies conducted, 80% were performed for sleep-disordered breathing, 7% for movement disorders, 5% for narcolepsy, 7% addressed insomnia, and 1% investigated other conditions [8].

Almost 90% of sleep disorders facilities are run by Respiratory Medicine Physicians [8], the majority of whom were trained in North America. All sleep disorders facilities in Saudi Arabia observe the American Academy of Sleep Medicine (AASM) regulations for diagnosing and treating sleep disorders [5]. In addition to pulmonologists, there are many otolaryngologists in Saudi Arabia with a special interest in surgical interventions for OSA [5]. There are also dentists and maxillofacial surgeons in Saudi Arabia who provide treatment for OSA using mandibular advancement devices [5]. There is still a significant shortage of psychologists specializing in sleep medicine; therefore, sleep medicine physicians tend to offer cognitive behavioral therapy for insomnia [5].

SLEEP MEDICINE TRAINING AND ACCREDITATION

In response to the continuous increase in the demand for sleep medicine services in Saudi Arabia [3], the accreditation of sleep medicine physicians and technologists was vital to patient care.

Numerous studies have shown that accrediting sleep centers and certifying physicians were associated with better outcomes and better compliance and adherence to management plans in patients with sleep disorders [9, 10]. Additionally, the accreditation of sleep medicine as a unique self-governing medical specialty will pave the way to establishing a Saudi national fellowship training program in sleep medicine.

In planning for this assignment, the Saudi Commission for Health Specialties (SCFHS) established the National Committee for the Accreditation of Sleep Medicine Practice of Physicians and Technologists in 2011 [11], aiming at developing: 1) accreditation regulations for physicians to be classified as sleep medicine specialists; and 2) accreditation regulations for technicians to be classified as sleep medicine technologists [11].

A physician is accredited as a sleep physician if he/she is a medical doctor (MD) and is qualified in the subspecialty of sleep medicine and has competency in the clinical evaluation, physiological assessment, diagnosis, treatment, and prevention of sleep and circadian rhythm problems [5, 11]. The national committee used two routes to approve specializing in sleep medicine. The first route included physicians with board certification in sleep medicine from a University or medical commission recognized by the SCFHS, like the American Board of Health Specialties or a SCFHS-approved local training program [5, 11]. The second route included physicians with a certificate demonstrating the completion of at least 12 months of full-time, structured, hands-on clinical training with direct patient care in an organization recognized by the SCFHS [5, 11].

On the other hand, a sleep medicine technologist is accredited by the SCFHS if he/she has a bachelor's degree in respiratory care, nursing, electroneurodiagnostics, medicine (MD), dentistry, physical therapy or applied medical sciences and:

1) Has had at least 12 months of applied hands-on training (experience) under the observation of a sleep disorders physician and a full-time sleep technologist recognized by the SCFHC

2) or if the candidate finished at least 6 months of the above experience and is certified by the RPSGT (Board of Registered Polysomnographic Technologists), The American Board of Sleep Medicine's (ABSM) Sleep Technologist Registry or The Sleep Disorders Specialty Examination of the National Board for Respiratory Care [11].

Unfortunately, there is a shortage in the number of trained sleep medicine specialists and technologists [12]. In view of this shortage in Saudi Arabia, two academic centers have started sleep medicine fellowship programs. King Saud University (KSU) in Riyadh established a sleep medicine fellowship program in 2009, which is the first structured program, focusing on the clinical aspects of sleep medicine and building the research expertise desired for sleep medicine to grow [5]. Subsequently, a sleep medicine diploma program was also introduced in 2016 at King Abdulaziz University (KAU) in Jeddah [5]. In 2021, the SCFHS mandated a new National Committee to found a Training Program for the Saudi Fellowship in Adult Sleep Medicine and accreditations regulations for training centers, which was approved in the fourth quarter of 2021, and is expected to recruit applicants for 2023 [12].

Nevertheless, there is still no structured sleep technologists training program. To overcome the lack of trained sleep technologists, many intensive courses and workshops are being prepared to train additional sleep technologists, this is on top of 3 and 6 months structured sleep technologists training programs at KSU and KAU [5].

In 2009, and under the umbrella of the Saudi Thoracic Society, the Saudi Sleep Medicine Group was established [5]. This group, which comprises sleep medicine specialists from all over Saudi Arabia, holds yearly meetings that are well-joined by active physicians and technologists in the area [5].

Major Challenges Facing Sleep Medicine in Saudi Arabia

There are numerous challenges facing sleep medicine and sleep medicine practitioners in the country. The low number of qualified sleep doctors and technologists continues to be a major problem for the practice in Saudi Arabia [8]. The lack of qualified sleep technologists is considered the main hindrance in establishing sleep disorders centers in Saudi Arabia [8]. In two national surveys, more than 80% of hospitals attributed not having a specialized sleep disorders center to a lack of trained sleep technologists [8]. Fig. (**1**) demonstrates a summary the challenges facing sleep medicine in Saudi Arabia.

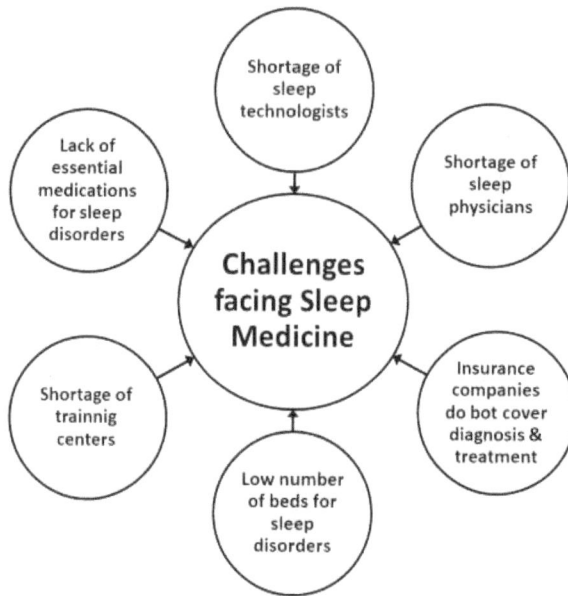

Fig. (1). An illustration of some of the challenges facing sleep medicine in Saudi Arabia.

There is generally a lack of awareness and limited knowledge of healthcare personnel about sleep problems [5]. Unfortunately, sleep medicine is not part of the medical schools' syllabi in Saudi Arabia [13]. Likewise, postgraduate doctors do not receive enough training or education on sleep medicine during their residency program [3]. This probably explains the limited knowledge about sleep disorders among practicing general physicians, which has been demonstrated in several studies [14 - 17]. This deficiency in sleep medicine knowledge and education is possibly responsible for the under-recognition and diagnosis of sleep disorders leading to delays in treatment [5]. There is also a lack of awareness of sleep problems and their serious consequences among the Saudi public [5].

Sadly, diagnosing and treating sleep disorders are not a priority for some decision-makers [5]. A national survey showed that "unconvinced administration" was one of the most important obstacles facing establishing sleep disorder facilities in about 50% of the hospitals in the Kingdom [8]. Another major hurdle to the expansion of sleep medicine in private hospitals is that some insurance policies do not include services provided for diagnosing OSA and treating the disorder with positive airway pressure therapy (PAP) or mandibular advancement devices. Even if the PAP therapy device is approved, the insurance companies will not approve the regular replacement of masks, tubings, and filters. Moreover, most insurance companies will not pay for the diagnostic procedures needed for other sleep disorders like narcolepsy [5].

Nearly all sleep disorders services in Saudi Arabia are hospital-based with no freestanding/outpatient sleep laboratories; this obviously limits patients' access to sleep service facilities [5]. Like many developing countries, the limited technical assistance of diagnostic machinery, the lack of after-sales service, and the poor training of the end-users is still an important problem facing sleep medicine practitioners in Saudi Arabia [18]. It is also very difficult to find the frequently used controlled medications for insomnia or narcolepsy (*e.g.*, modafinil, sodium oxybate, pitolisant, and others) since these medications' producers do not have a local distributor and are not approved by the Saudi Food and Drug Administration (Saudi FDA) [5]. Therefore, to obtain these medications, a distinct application through the hospital is needed, which causes patients with sleep disorders to go through extended intervals without medications [5].

Clinical and Research Knowledge Gap

Over the last three decades, there has been substantial development and progress in sleep medicine research all over the world; however, sleep research is still relatively underdeveloped in Arab countries, reflecting the underdevelopment of clinical service in general. In the area, Saudi Arabia was placed fourth after Turkey, Israel, and Iran in sleep medicine publications [19].

There is some research addressing the prevalence of different sleep disorders in Saudi Arabia. Sleep disorders are common among Saudi people [8]. A couple of studies that used the Berlin questionnaire to evaluate the prevalence of OSA risk factors and symptoms amongst middle-aged Saudi men and women revealed that

3 out of 10 Saudi men and 4 out of 10 Saudi women are at increased risk for OSA [20, 21].

Another study assessed OSA using polysomnography (PSG) in a randomly chosen group of 346 Saudi school employees aged 30-60 years. It showed that the rates of OSA (an apnea-hypopnea index ≥ 5) were 11.2% in men and 4.0% in women [22]. The prevalence of apnea-hypopnea index ≥ 5 plus daytime sleepiness was 2.8% (4.0% in men and 1.8% in women) [22]. Parent-reported snoring occurred in 17.9% of Saudi elementary school children [23]. The prevalence of narcolepsy with cataplexy in Saudis is 40/100,000 people [24, 25], which is similar to the range described in other studies that revealed the prevalence of narcolepsy type 1 (with cataplexy) to range from 25 to 50 per 100,000 individuals [26]. Another study showed the prevalence of restless legs syndrome (RLS) amongst Saudis to be 5% [27]. This prevalence falls within the described ranges of RLS (i.e., 3% to 12%) in other nations [27, 28]. Insufficient sleep and disturbances of biological sleep rhythms are major problems in Saudi adults and children [29, 30]. Excessive sleepiness among city drivers in Saudi Arabia was the subject of a 2014 study. Over the study period of 6 months, 12% of motor vehicle accidents were caused by sleepiness, and 25% of drivers reported falling asleep at least once during the monitoring period [8]. Among truck drivers, almost 95% reported accidentally falling asleep at least once while driving over the study period [31]. In a more recent study of commercial aircraft pilots in the Arabian Gulf region, 34% of the pilots had an Epworth Sleep Scale (ESS) score of > 10 (signifying excessive daytime sleepiness), and 45% stated falling asleep at the controls at least once without their copilot's knowledge [32]. In both studies, most participants recognized sleep deprivation as the cause of their excessive daytime sleepiness [5]. It is apparent that more studies are still required to build the necessary knowledge about the prevalence of sleep disorders in Saudi Arabia. Such work is important to teach healthcare service providers and decision-makers about the extent of the problem to help plan the number of sleep specialists and sleep services required to encounter those needs [5]. It is essential as well to expand postgraduate research programs for clinical and bench sleep research in all academic centers. Moreover, it is crucial to create a partnership among local centers, develop registries both at the national and the regional levels to record sleep disorders, and establish connections with prominent worldwide research centers, which will be reflected positively on the size and value of published work [5].

CONCLUSION

Despite the steady growth in sleep medicine practice and training in Saudi Arabia, there are still many obstacles hindering its development, including the shortage of trained sleep physicians and technologists in addition to the poor knowledge about sleep conditions and their effects amongst healthcare workers, healthcare authorities, and insurance companies. It is essential to introduce sleep medicine in training for medical students and physicians to raise awareness about the commonness and the grave consequences of sleep disorders. Population and strategic-planning research are also required to aid in planning the needed facilities and services for the increasing demands.

CONSENT FOR PUBLICATION

Not applicable.

CONFLICT OF INTEREST

The authors declare no conflict of interest, financial or otherwise.

ACKNOWLEDGEMENT

Declared none.

REFERENCES

[1]   Statistics GAf. The total population in 2019. https://www.stats.gov.sa/en/43. Accessed Jan 2021. 2019.

[2]   BaHammam A, Gozal D. Qur'anic insights into sleep. Nat Sci Sleep 2012; 4: 81-7.
       [http://dx.doi.org/10.2147/NSS.S34630] [PMID: 23620681]

[3]   BaHammam A. Sleep medicine in Saudi Arabia: Current problems and future challenges. Ann Thorac Med 2011; 6(1): 3-10.
       [http://dx.doi.org/10.4103/1817-1737.74269] [PMID: 21264164]

[4]   Almalki M, Fitzgerald G, Clark M. Health care system in Saudi Arabia: an overview. East Mediterr Health J 2011; 17(10): 784-93.
       [http://dx.doi.org/10.26719/2011.17.10.784] [PMID: 22256414]

[5]   Almeneessier AS, BaHammam AS. Sleep Medicine in Saudi Arabia. J Clin Sleep Med 2017; 13(4): 641-5.
       [http://dx.doi.org/10.5664/jcsm.6566] [PMID: 28212693]

[6]   Al-Mobeireek AF, Al-Kassimi FA, Al-Majed SA, Al-Hajjaj MS, Bahammam AS, Sultan I. Clinical profile of sleep apnea syndrome. A study at a university hospital. Saudi Med J 2000; 21(2): 180-3.
       [PMID: 11533778]

[7]   Bahammam A, Rahman AA. Hospital nights utilized for CPAP titration in obstructive sleep apnea syndrome patients in the absence of a proper sleep disorders center. Ann Saudi Med 2000; 20(1): 83-5.
       [http://dx.doi.org/10.5144/0256-4947.2000.83] [PMID: 17322756]

[8]   Bahammam A, Alsaeed M, AlAhmari M, AlBalawi I, Sharif M. Sleep medicine services in Saudi Arabia: The 2013 national survey. Ann Thorac Med 2014; 9(1): 45-7.
       [http://dx.doi.org/10.4103/1817-1737.124444] [PMID: 24551019]

[9]   Parthasarathy S, Haynes PL, Budhiraja R, Habib MP, Quan SF. A national survey of the effect of sleep medicine specialists and American Academy of Sleep Medicine Accreditation on management of obstructive sleep apnea. J Clin Sleep Med 2006; 2(2): 133-42.
[http://dx.doi.org/10.5664/jcsm.26506] [PMID: 17557485]

[10]   Pamidi S, Knutson KL, Ghods F, Mokhlesi B. The impact of sleep consultation prior to a diagnostic polysomnogram on continuous positive airway pressure adherence. Chest 2012; 141(1): 51-7.
[http://dx.doi.org/10.1378/chest.11-0709] [PMID: 21700685]

[11]   BaHammam A, Al-Jahdali H, AlHarbi A, AlOtaibi G, Asiri S, AlSayegh A. Saudi regulations for the accreditation of sleep medicine physicians and technologists. Ann Thorac Med 2013; 8(1): 3-7.
[http://dx.doi.org/10.4103/1817-1737.105710] [PMID: 23440260]

[12]   BaHammam AS, Al-Jahdali HH, Alenazi MH, Aleissi SA, Wali SO. Curriculum development for the Saudi sleep medicine fellowship program. J Taibah Univ Med Sci 2022; 17(5): 782-93.
[http://dx.doi.org/10.1016/j.jtumed.2021.12.014] [PMID: 36050948]

[13]   Almohaya A, Qrmli A, Almagal N, *et al.* Sleep medicine education and knowledge among medical students in selected Saudi Medical Schools. BMC Med Educ 2013; 13(1): 133.
[http://dx.doi.org/10.1186/1472-6920-13-133] [PMID: 24070217]

[14]   Alotair H, BaHammam A. Gender differences in Saudi patients with obstructive sleep apnea. Sleep Breath 2008; 12(4): 323-9.
[http://dx.doi.org/10.1007/s11325-008-0184-8] [PMID: 18369671]

[15]   Saleem AH, Al Rashed FA, Alkharboush GA, *et al.* Primary care physicians' knowledge of sleep medicine and barriers to transfer of patients with sleep disorders. Saudi Med J 2017; 38(5): 553-9.
[http://dx.doi.org/10.15537/smj.2017.5.17936] [PMID: 28439609]

[16]   BaHammam AS. Knowledge and attitude of primary health care physicians towards sleep disorders. Saudi Med J 2000; 21(12): 1164-7.
[PMID: 11360092]

[17]   BaHammam A. Polysomnographic characteristics of patients with chronic insomnia. Sleep Hypnosis 6. 2004; 6: 163-8.

[18]   Gitanjali B. Establishing a polysomnography laboratory in India: problems and pitfalls. Sleep 1998; 21(4): 331-2.
[http://dx.doi.org/10.1093/sleep/21.4.331] [PMID: 9646376]

[19]   Robert C, Wilson CS, Gaudy J-F, Arreto C-D. The evolution of the sleep science literature over 30 years: A bibliometric analysis. Scientometrics 2007; 73(2): 231-56.
[http://dx.doi.org/10.1007/s11192-007-1780-2]

[20]   Bahammam AS, Al-Rajeh MS, Al-Ibrahim FS, Arafah MA, Sharif MM. Prevalence of symptoms and risk of sleep apnea in middle-aged Saudi women in primary care. Saudi Med J 2009; 30(12): 1572-6.
[PMID: 19936423]

[21]   BaHammam AS, Alrajeh MS, Al-Jahdali HH, BinSaeed AA. Prevalence of symptoms and risk of sleep apnea in middle-aged Saudi males in primary care. Saudi Med J 2008; 29(3): 423-6.
[PMID: 18327372]

[22]   Wali S, Abalkhail B, Krayem A. Prevalence and risk factors of obstructive sleep apnea syndrome in a Saudi Arabian population. Ann Thorac Med 2017; 12(2): 88-94.
[http://dx.doi.org/10.4103/1817-1737.203746] [PMID: 28469718]

[23]   BaHammam A, AlFaris E, Shaikh S, Saeed AB. Prevalence of sleep problems and habits in a sample of Saudi primary school children. Ann Saudi Med 2006; 26(1): 7-13.
[http://dx.doi.org/10.5144/0256-4947.2006.7] [PMID: 16521868]

[24]   BaHammam AS, Alenezi AM. Narcolepsy in Saudi Arabia. Demographic and clinical perspective of an under-recognized disorder. Saudi Med J 2006; 27(9): 1352-7.

[PMID: 16951772]

[25] Al Rajeh S, Bademosi O, Ismail H, *et al.* A community survey of neurological disorders in Saudi Arabia: the Thugbah study. Neuroepidemiology 1993; 12(3): 164-78.
[http://dx.doi.org/10.1159/000110316] [PMID: 8272177]

[26] Longstreth WT Jr, Koepsell TD, Ton TG, Hendrickson AF, van Belle G. The epidemiology of narcolepsy. Sleep 2007; 30(1): 13-26.
[http://dx.doi.org/10.1093/sleep/30.1.13] [PMID: 17310860]

[27] BaHammam A, Al-sharani K, Al-zahrani S, Al-shammari A, Al-amri N, Sharif M. The prevalence of restless legs syndrome in adult Saudis attending primary health care. Gen Hosp Psychiatry 2011; 33(2): 102-6.
[http://dx.doi.org/10.1016/j.genhosppsych.2011.01.005] [PMID: 21596202]

[28] Ohayon MM, O'Hara R, Vitiello MV. Epidemiology of restless legs syndrome: A synthesis of the literature. Sleep Med Rev 2012; 16(4): 283-95.
[http://dx.doi.org/10.1016/j.smrv.2011.05.002] [PMID: 21795081]

[29] BaHammam A, Bin Saeed A, Al-Faris E, Shaikh S. Sleep duration and its correlates in a sample of Saudi elementary school children. Singapore Med J 2006; 47(10): 875-81.
[PMID: 16990963]

[30] Al-Hazzaa H, Abahussain NA, Musaiger AO, Al-Sobayel H, Qahwaji D. Prevalence of short sleep duration and its association with obesity among adolescents 15- to 19-year olds: A cross-sectional study from three major cities in Saudi Arabia. Ann Thorac Med 2012; 7(3): 133-9.
[http://dx.doi.org/10.4103/1817-1737.98845] [PMID: 22924070]

[31] Alahmari MD, Alanazi TM, Batawi AA, *et al.* Sleepy driving and risk of obstructive sleep apnea among truck drivers in Saudi Arabia. Traffic Inj Prev 2019; 20(5): 498-503.
[http://dx.doi.org/10.1080/15389588.2019.1608975] [PMID: 31120335]

[32] Aljurf TM, Olaish AH, BaHammam AS. Assessment of sleepiness, fatigue, and depression among Gulf Cooperation Council commercial airline pilots. Sleep Breath 2018; 22(2): 411-9.
[http://dx.doi.org/10.1007/s11325-017-1565-7] [PMID: 28884322]

CHAPTER 6

Sleep Medicine in the United Arab Emirates

Preeti Devnani[1,*], Sobia Farooq[2], Kelly L Huffman[1], Ayesha Ahmed[1] and Hadie Rifai[3]

[1] *Neurological Institute, Cleveland Clinic Abu Dhabi, Abu Dhabi, United Arab Emirates*

[2] *Respiratory Institute, Cleveland Clinic Abu Dhabi, Abu Dhabi, United Arab Emirates*

[3] *Surgical Subspecialities Institute, Cleveland Clinic Abu Dhabi, Abu Dhabi, United Arab Emirates*

Abstract: Sleep disorders are increasingly being recognized as a major health problem in the UAE. The rising prevalence, potentially modifiable risk factors, and impact on global health outcomes have prompted the growth of sleep medicine. The burden of under-recognized disease has encouraged patient and physician-centric education. Supported by nationalized health insurance plans, the medical fraternity has adopted a multi-disciplinary approach to optimize resources and outcomes, while recognizing that these measures are initial steps in the unique challenges posed.

Keywords: Cultural influence, CPAP compliance, Insomnia, Obstructive sleep apnea, Regulatory body.

INTRODUCTION

The United Arab Emirates (UAE) is on the Arabian Peninsula bordering Saudi Arabia and Oman, occupying a land mass of approximately 83,600 sq km. The UAE consists of a federation of seven different constitutional monarchies, Abu Dhabi (the capital), Ajman, Dubai, Fujairah, Ras Al Khaimah, and Umm Al Quwain. The UAE is a member of the Gulf Cooperation Council (GCC), which includes the countries of Bahrain, Kuwait, Oman, Qatar and Saudi Arabia) and part of the Middle East North Africa (MENA) region. UAE nationals are referred to as Emiratis, and while sharing close cultural ties with GCC countries, they retain their own cultural identity. The total population of the UAE is approximately 10 million people; 11.6% are Emiratis and the remaining 88.4% of the population consist of expatriates [1]. The majority of the UAE's population (85%) resides in the emirates of Dubai, Abu Dhabi and Sharjah [1]. The UAE is a

---

* **Corresponding author Preeti Devnani:** Neurological Institute, Cleveland Clinic Abu Dhabi, Abu Dhabi, United Arab Emirates; Tel: +1 216 444 2165; Fax- +1 216 636 0090; E-mail: devnanp@ccf.org

Hrayr P. Attarian, Marie-Louise M. Coussa-Koniski & Alain Michel Sabri (Eds.)
All rights reserved-© 2023 Bentham Science Publishers

Muslim country and 76% percent of UAE residents (including both citizens and non-citizens) are Muslim.

HEALTHCARE INFRASTRUCTURE

The UAE has a far-reaching comprehensive, government-funded health service, and a burgeoning private health sector that both deliver a high standard of care. Healthcare is regulated at both the Federal and Emirate level. To date, health care in the UAE has been funded mainly by the government. Public healthcare services are administered by different regulatory authorities in the UAE including the Ministry of Health and Prevention, the Health Authority-Abu Dhabi (HAAD), the Dubai Health Authority (DHA) and the Emirates Health Authority (EHA). Under the 'Thiqa' national insurance program, the Abu Dhabi Government provides full medical coverage for all UAE nationals living in Abu Dhabi. Citizens receive a Thiqa card, through which they have comprehensive access to a large number of private and public healthcare providers.

MEDICAL COVERAGE

Medical coverage for continuous positive airway pressure (CPAP) and Bi-level positive airway pressure (BiPAP) devices has to meet eligibility criteria, determined by the Health Authority of Abu Dhabi (HAAD) including central sleep apnea, obesity hypoventilation syndrome (OHVS) with BMI greater than 30, obstructive sleep apnea (OSAS). Similarly non-invasive positive pressure ventilation, BiPAP device is covered for chronic obstructive pulmonary disease, OHVS, end-stage lung diseases with respiratory failure in patients awaiting lung transplant (*e.g.*, chronic obstructive pulmonary disease, cystic fibrosis, idiopathic pulmonary fibrosis, and sarcoidosis), respiratory insufficiency/failure with kyphoscoliosis of the thoracic spine or other chest wall deformity, neuromuscular disease (*e.g.*, amyotrophic lateral sclerosis, myasthenia gravis, and polio). Requirements for coverage devices require prior authorization along with ICD and CPT codes with the highest level of specificity (Thiqa insurer). ENT and Dental sleep medicine services are readily available to help pursue alternative treatments.

Sleep Disorders in the UAE

The available empirical literature suggests that the prevalence of poor sleep and sleep disorders is high in the UAE. A recent study of a non-clinical population of 100 female Emirati university students found that 75% reported poor sleep quality and an average sleep duration of 6.1 hours (± 1.9) [2]. In UAE healthcare settings, 34% of patients with type II diabetes mellitus reported poor sleep quality. In culturally similar KSA, a cross-sectional study of 2,095 adults showed that 33.8%

of participants reported a sleep duration of less than 7 hours/night [2], 78.3% reported poor sleep quality [3], and 20.5% reported excessive daytime sleepiness [4]. Poor sleep is strongly correlated with smart-device overuse, and has increased considerably in Middle Eastern countries [1]. 47.5% of the population surveyed in three cities in UAE reported being heavy users of smart-devices, 74.5% of the participants used their smart-device at bedtime [5]. 81% of heavy smart device users were reported to be poor sleepers [5].

Sleep Disordered Breathing

Obstructive sleep apnea (OSA) is a common disease worldwide, primarily due to the obesity epidemic. In the UAE, the 2016 prevalence of obesity was estimated to be 29.9% of the adult population. The prevalence and major risk factors for sleep-disordered breathing within the UAE are similar to those in other countries. A study of 1,214 consecutive patients presenting to a primary healthcare clinic in Dubai, found that 20.9% were at high risk of OSA [6]. A higher risk was seen in Saudi Arabia, with 31.9% of the population presenting as high risk for OSA based on the Berlin Questionnaire (BQ) [7], a self-report measure demonstrated to reliably identify OSA [10]. A recent UAE-based study [8] examining sleep-disordered breathing based on self-report of snoring) showed 34.2% of participants reported snoring. Of these participants, 43.2% were at risk of OSA [8], as measured by the BQ [7]. Males, older adults (50–60 years) and obese participants were more likely to snore than their counterparts [8], and smoking, hypertension, and nasal septal deviation were all significantly correlated with snoring (p < .01) [8].

Restless Legs Syndrome

Restless legs syndrome (RLS) is estimated to impact 7 to 10% of young to middle aged people and 10 to 20% in those older than 60 years. In the Middle East region, in Saudi Arabia, 8.4% prevalence of RLS was observed in a study of 2682 participants [9]. Pregnancy, iron deficiency anemia (26.9%) and gastritis were the most frequent causes of RLS among females, whereas genetics, hypertension, and related neurological diseases were the main risk factors for RLS among men [10]. However, unlike findings of most studies, RLS significantly affects males more than females. Restless legs syndrome (RLS) affects the quality of life and survival in patients on hemodialysis with a smoking history contributing to a poor outcome. UAE-specific data is limited. Accurate diagnosis, access to tertiary clinics and time to diagnosis as well as pharmacotherapeutic options are showing a positive trend.

NARCOLEPSY

Narcolepsy is an under-recognized, often misdiagnosed sleep disorder. In a study by Almeneessier *et al.* from Saudi Arabia [11], the mean diagnostic delay was 9.1 ± 8.4 years, EDS was the main symptom that prompted patients to seek medical consultation. 82% of the patients were misdiagnosed or deemed to be suffering from cultural superstitions such as "evil eye," or "black magic" prior to obtaining appropriate care. UAE data specific are lacking; however, a recognized challenge includes limited pharmacotherapy with the non-availability of sodium oxybate. Appropriate tertiary clinic referrals for advanced diagnostics including multiple sleep latency tests are challenging. Strict regulation measures in relation to dispensing controlled substance stimulants and antidepressants are in place, with a centralized computerized database for state-led facilities to limit abuse and overprescriptions. Spreading awareness amongst primary care physicians and providing community support are essential measures.

Sleep Medicine in the UAE

There are no national guidelines for sleep medicine or the treatment of insomnia and other sleep disorders in the UAE. UAE health regulatory bodies endorse international sleep medicine guidelines provided by the American Academy of Sleep Medicine, American Thoracic Society, American College of Chest Physicians, and European Respiratory Society. There is little research in the field of sleep medicine focused specifically on the UAE. For this reason, we include in our review research from culturally similar countries in the GCC and MENA region. The majority of available research stems from Saudi Arabia, as the country has made significant advances in the field of sleep medicine in a relatively short period of time. For example, in 2000, BaHammam *et al.* noted that 40% of primary care physicians in Saudi Arabia did not consider sleep disorders to be a distinct specialty and only 15% had attended related lectures or training [12]. By 2013, the country had produced its own guidelines for the accreditation of sleep medicine physicians and technologists [13].

The UAE has 11 hospital-based and 2 private sleep laboratories. Most sleep programs lack a multidisciplinary approach with the exception of a few larger programs that start with a screening or basic evaluation by primary care providers followed by a formal detailed sleep evaluation in a sleep clinic staffed by sleep consultants. Typically sleep clinics receive referrals from cardiology (electrophysiology), ear, nose, and throat specialists, endocrinology and bariatric surgery clinics. The patient journey typically starts with seeing a physician who feels the need for further evaluation by a sleep consultant. Patients then undergo the complete evaluation in a sleep clinic using patient self-report measures such as the Epworth Sleepiness Scale (ESS) [14] STOP BANG [15]. Diagnosis is established either *via* home sleep apnea testing (HSAT) using portable devices or an in-lab diagnostic polysomnogram (PSG) with a full EEG montage as indicated.

HSAT is typically offered to patients between the ages of 18 and 65 year, who have high pretest probability of moderate-to-severe OSA, along with the absence of comorbid sleep disorders or any other medical conditions that might compromise the test's accuracy. Polysomnogram is ordered in patients with congestive heart failure, neuromuscular disease, and moderate-to-severe pulmonary diseases, specifically those requiring supplemental oxygen. AASM practice guidelines are used to score and read the sleep studies.

The robust approach and screening help increase the identification of sleep-disordered breathing in at-risk individuals in order to advance the treatment of a wide spectrum of general medical conditions. The standardized, cost-effective approach primarily seen in tertiary healthcare centers helps elaborate and deepen the coordination of care among providers.

OSA is approached as a chronic disease requiring long-term, multidisciplinary management. Once the diagnosis is established, the patients are included in deciding an appropriate treatment strategy that may include positive airway pressure devices, oral appliances, behavioral treatments, surgery, and/or adjunctive treatments.

Continuous positive airway pressure (CPAP) and Bilevel positive airway pressures (BiPAP) are readily available and dispensed by sleep clinics. Patients are expected to return to the clinic for follow-up visits to ensure CPAP adherence. Continuous positive airway pressure (CPAP), the gold standard treatment, needs to be used for more than 4 h/night to be effective, but suffers from relatively poor adherence. Worldwide the rate of compliance seems to be about 30-85% [16] with somewhat increase seen with remote monitoring. There is no published data about CPAP compliance in UAE, however, a prospective study of a cohort of 156 patients diagnosed to have OSA based on polysomnography between January 2012 and January 2014 in King Saud University, Riyadh, Kingdom of Saudi Arabia, were followed for 10 months showed a compliance of 80% [12].

Regulation of Driving Licenses in Regard to Sleep-disordered Breathing

Drowsy driving remains one of the greatest risks for fatal motor vehicle accidents. The risk, danger, and often tragic results of drowsy driving are on the rise and are alarming. Drowsy driving is the dangerous combination of driving and sleepiness or fatigue. This usually happens when a driver has not slept enough, but it can also happen because of untreated sleep disorders, medications, drinking alcohol, or shift work. Drowsiness makes an individual lose focus, slow reaction time and affects the ability to decide. According to the National Highway Traffic Safety Administration USA [17], drowsy driving was responsible for 72,000 crashes, 44,000 injuries, and 800 deaths in 2013. However, these numbers are underestimated, and up to 6,000 fatal crashes each year may be caused by drowsy drivers (CDC). The data regarding road safety appears to be published by the national newspapers in UAE namely The National and Gulf News and compiled by an independent website "roadsafetyuae.com". According to this website in 2019, UAE Road Traffic Fatalities decline to 448 as reported by The National, resulting in 4.53 fatalities /100,000 inhabitants. Though documents and guidelines are in place to help motorists, including a thorough cardiometabolic and neurologic health, unfortunately, none of these guidelines strictly regulate drowsy driving.

Dental Services for Sleep Apnea in the UAE

The scope of dental services is typically reserved for mandibular advancement devices (MAD). MADs hold the mandibular jaw forward (known as advancement) in order to keep the tongue from obstructing the airway when the patient falls asleep and loses muscle tone. MADs are indicated for mild to moderate sleep apnea. They can be used for severe cases with the expectation the device may not be as efficacious. Oral appliances are nearly as effective as CPAP in improving OSA and have better adherence [18]. Though the literature has shown that it is not always as effective as the gold standard treatment of CPAP, patients are much more compliant with the MAD because it tends to be less obtrusive and more transportable [18].

Most patients are unaware of MAS as a treatment modality and thus mostly referral based. Patients typically first undergo a polysomnogram (PSG) or home sleep test (HST) ordered by their sleep physician. Once OSA is diagnosed and documented, a dental referral can be made. The dentist then performs a general dental examination to ensure the patient has enough teeth and mandibular range to hold the appliance and tolerate advancement. Typically at least 10mm of advancement is adequate; however, the patient starts at 50% of their maximum range [19]. The first 30 days of treatment are for titrating the appliance slowly to see when the patient starts to feel better or stops snoring. This titration is done either by the patient at home or in the clinic every 1-2 weeks. Once the patient and dentist feel they have reached the point of minimal advancement with maximum results, the patient ideally is sent back to the MD for a follow-up sleep test to assess the effectiveness of the MAD. There are no local guidelines however clinicians adopt those put in place by the American Academy of Dental Sleep Medicine (AADSM). Most insurances including Thiqa will cover this benefit with preauthorization as it is a more affordable treatment than CPAP.

Behavioral Sleep Medicine

Behavioral sleep medicine constitutes a broad array of evidence-based techniques for the treatment of major sleep disorders. Cognitive behavioral therapy for insomnia, (CBTi) is the most well-known behavioral sleep medicine treatment. CBTi is recommended as the first line treatment for chronic insomnia in the Australasian, European and US guidelines (American College of Physicians [20]; European Sleep Society Reiman, 2017; Australasian Sleep Association) [21]. The effectiveness of CBTi is well documented [22, 23] and CBTi has been demonstrated to have superior long-term effectiveness in comparison to pharmacotherapy [24]. CBTi has also been demonstrated to improve mental health symptoms and quality of life in patients presenting with comorbid psychiatric disorders and insomnia [23]. The effectiveness of CBTi has not been specifically examined in the UAE and has not been specifically examined with Muslim participants and more research is needed. However, given the robustness of empirical findings behavioral sleep interventions are likely to be similarly effective in the UAE population. Preliminary data shows that CBTi is likely to be an acceptable intervention amongst Emirati nationals; 68.6% of participants in a sleep intervention for obese Emirati men with type II diabetes completed the study [25].

Culturally Adapting CBTi

In our clinical experience, CBTi interventions sometimes need to be culturally adapted to meet the needs of UAE residents. Many UAE residents maintain a polyphasic sleep schedule. A short daytime nap is culturally congruent with the extreme daytime temperatures in the UAE and Islamic culture. A daytime nap is referred to as Qailulah in Islamic culture and is encouraged in Islamic religious texts [26]. In addition, the sleep schedules of Muslims are influenced by Salat, the obligatory Muslim prayers, which take place five times daily. The first prayer, Fajr, takes place at dawn (appx 1 – 1.5 hours before sunrise) and in the summer months can be as early as 4:30am. Thus, consolidated sleep length varies seasonally depending on the length of the day; many Muslims return to bed after Fajr, and sleep until work time. Prayer timings need to be considered when setting scheduled sleep times and wake times during stimulus control interventions. There is little research examining the impact of split sleep due to the Fajr prayer, although other research suggests that daytime performance and fatigue is dependent upon the total sleep time, regardless of whether sleep is biphasic. One small study in Saudi Arabia including eight participants examined the impact of split sleep due to the Fajr prayer found no difference in daytime sleepiness or sleep architecture as a result of interrupted sleep [27].

BSM practitioners working in the UAE should also have an understanding of cultural and religious beliefs regarding mental health symptoms and sleep disorders. Patients in the UAE are ethnically and culturally diverse, even within Muslims, and vary in their belief systems. Many patients are comfortable with Western biomedical conceptualizations and treatments. Others may believe their symptoms can be attributed to supernatural forces, such as black magic, the evil eye and jinn. The jinn are described in the Qur'an in great detail as beings created by Allah that are capable of possession of humans and interfering in the daily affairs of humans. These beliefs are culturally normative and common. One study of 47 Muslim patients in an outpatient psychiatry clinic in the Netherlands found that 78.7% (n = 37) believed in jinn and 80.9% (n = 38) believed in the evil eye [6]. It is recommended that BSM practitioners explore with patients their attribution for their symptoms of poor sleep and insomnia.

Clinicians practicing in the UAE should also be prepared to work with patients during the Holy Month of Ramadan. During Ramadan, Muslims eat exclusively between sunset and sunrise, and fast during the day; non-Muslims are not expected to fast, however, eating, drinking and smoking in public during fasting hours. The evening meal iftar occurs at sunset and is followed by a morning meal suhoor, which occurs just before sunrise. In the UAE, regular working hours are decreased by two hours per day, many shops and restaurants are closed until after evening prayers, and businesses provide extended post-iftar hours. These changes, accompanied by increased social activities and obligations, can lead to delayed bedtimes, sleep disruption and decreased total sleep time for many. A recent meta-analysis of 24 studies spanning 12 countries, with 646 participants showed a decrease in total sleep time from 7.2 to 6.4 hours per night during Ramadan [28]. Patients may present to clinics seeking strategies to improve sleep during Ramadan. Patients with pre-existing sleep disorders, such as insomnia, may experience a resurgence in symptoms after Ramadan. This may be particularly true for individuals who are evening chronotypes.

Mental Health and Sleep

Mental health diseases and sleep are closely related. Patients presenting to sleep clinics have been reported to have significant rates of mental health disorders [29]. Poor sleep is a risk factor, predictor and a symptom of most mental health disorders with both quantity and quality of sleep being affected. Depressive disorders are characterized by subjective sleep disturbance mainly manifesting as insomnia though hypersomnia may also be experienced. In hypo/manic episodes there is decreased need for sleep with sleep onset latency. Studies have also shown presence of sleep disturbance in the inter-episode period in bipolar disorders [30]. Similar to mood disorders, sleep disturbance is also one of the diagnostic criteria of anxiety disorders including generalized anxiety and post-traumatic stress disorders. Patients with anxiety and panic disorders can have alterations in sleep initiation and maintenance. Conversely mood disorders are found in up to half [31] and anxiety disorders in more than one third of patients with chronic sleep problems [32]. Sleep problems such as sleep latency, decreased sleep efficiency and reduction in total sleep time can occur in psychotic disorders such as schizophrenia. These problems are thought to contribute to both emergence and relapse of delusional and hallucinatory experiences. The relationship between sleep and substance use is bidirectional with sleep problems leading to substance use and substance use affecting sleep latency, duration and quality of sleep. Poor quality sleep is also a common complaint of patients with personality disorders and is often a manifestation of interaction between dysfunctional personality traits and environmental stresses. Both acute and chronic stress can have prominent effects on sleep architecture and circadian rhythm.

Psychotropic medication used for treatment of mental health problems can also affect the experience of sleep and the sleep wake cycle. Antidepressants such as fluoxetine and venlafaxine, which have activating properties can disrupt sleep by increasing REM latency and suppressing REM sleep whilst others with sedative effects such as mirtazapine, amitriptyline and trazodone enhance sleep by improving sleep efficiency but can cause daytime somnolence. Vivid dreams, nightmares, restless legs, bruxism, diaphoresis, increase in BMI are other concerns experienced with some antidepressant medication. The majority of the first and second generation antipsychotics cause at least some degree of sedation and are therefore used clinically, off label, for sleep problems. It is prudent to be aware that antipsychotics can in the long run adversely affect sleep through weight gain with risk of obstructive sleep apnea.

Barriers

In the UAE, as anywhere else in the world, stigma linked to mental health is prevalent. Patients may be unwilling to consult with mental health providers, even if the reason for referral is insomnia [33]. This is compounded in expatriate communities with fear of adverse outcomes at work including fear of losing one's job with disclosure of mental health problems. Another factor which hinders patients seeking clinical help is the lack of parity in insurance coverage for physical and mental health problems with the majority of non-citizens having to pay at least partly out of pocket. Cultural barriers such as viewing mental health and sleep problems as metaphysical in nature, conceptualizing symptoms as being caused by evil eye along with mistrust of mental health services and concerns about dependence on psychotropic medication often lead patients turning to traditional healers (Mutawa). Reassuringly the trend appears to be changing with expansion of services in the region.

Despite the promise of behavioral sleep medicine interventions in the UAE, there are barriers to their implementation. One barrier to obtaining and implementing CBTi in the UAE and broader Gulf Region is the lack of availability of trained providers [33]. This is true even in the United States, where 88% of BSM certified practitioners are located [34]. To our knowledge, there are no psychologists certified in behavioral sleep medicine in the UAE [17]. A second barrier is lack of knowledge regarding the role of behavioral therapies in the management of chronic insomnia on behalf of both physicians and patients. One qualitative study in Saudi Arabia found that physicians were unaware of clinical guidelines for the management of insomnia [33]. In addition, physicians reported that patients expected pharmacotherapy as an outcome of their consultation rather than a referral for behavioral therapy [33].

RECOMMENDATIONS

UAE patients presenting to sleep clinics with primary sleep complaints should receive mental health screening as part of their initial evaluation. Behavioral sleep medicine should be easily accessible as a first line treatment option for patients, with psychiatric referrals readily available. Initial behavioral health evaluations should examine in addition to the patient's presenting sleep concern, their cultural and religious beliefs, as well as psychosocial context. Treatment recommendations should include culturally specific targeted interventions which incorporate these variables. In the long term, it would be beneficial to develop local/regional culturally specific guidelines for the implementation of behavioral sleep medicine therapies.

Mental health stigma may prevent patients from seeking the care that they need, even if the reason for referral is not directly related to mental health. Referring providers are encouraged to educate patients on the behavioral management of sleep concerns. In addition, the method in which services are delivered is especially important. Patients are likely to benefit from integrated behavioral health models in which psychological and psychiatric services are embedded within a sleep medicine clinic, rather than referral to distinct mental health services. Finally, it is important to note that treatment targeting disordered sleep may help to improve general mental health, and for patients with poor sleep and comorbid mental health concerns, a behavioral sleep medicine referral may be a more acceptable treatment alternative

CONCLUSION

In this review, the challenges unique to the diagnosis and management of sleep disorders in the UAE have been highlighted. Developing regional guidelines and enhancing public health educational measures are key. With the growth of medical schools, fellowship training positions, international academic affiliations and medical tourism, advancement in the field of sleep medicine is promising.

CONSENT FOR PUBLICATION

Not applicable.

CONFLICT OF INTEREST

The authors declare no conflict of interest, financial or otherwise.

ACKNOWLEDGEMENT

Declared none.

REFERENCES

[1]   Central Intelligence Agency. (2020). United Arab Emirates. In the world factbook. Retrieved Jan 20th 2021, from. https://www.cia.gov/library/publications/the-world-factbook/geos/br.html

[2]   Arora T, Alhelali E, Grey I. Poor sleep efficiency and daytime napping are risk factors of depersonalization disorder in female university students. Neurobiol Sleep Circadian Rhythms 2020; 9100059
[http://dx.doi.org/10.1016/j.nbscr.2020.100059] [PMID: 33364526]

[3]   Ahmed AE, Al-Jahdali F, AlALwan A, *et al.* Prevalence of sleep duration among Saudi adults. Saudi Med J 2017; 38(3): 276-83.
[http://dx.doi.org/10.15537/smj.2017.3.17101] [PMID: 28251223]

[4]   Fatani A, Al-Rouqi K, Al Towairky J, *et al.* Effect of age and gender in the prevalence of excessive daytime sleepiness among a sample of the Saudi population. J Epidemiol Glob Health 2015; 5(S1) (Suppl. 1): S59-66.
[http://dx.doi.org/10.1016/j.jegh.2015.05.005] [PMID: 26099548]

[5]   Abedalqader F, Alhuarrat MAD, Ibrahim G, *et al.* The correlation between smart device usage & sleep quality among UAE residents. Sleep Med 2019; 63: 18-23.
[http://dx.doi.org/10.1016/j.sleep.2019.04.017] [PMID: 31600657]

[6]   Lim A, Hoek HW, Ghane S, Deen M, Blom JD. The attribution of mental health problems to jinn: an explorative study in a transcultural psychiatric outpatient clinic. Front Psychiatry 2018; 9: 89.
[http://dx.doi.org/10.3389/fpsyt.2018.00089] [PMID: 29643820]

[7]   Netzer NC, Stoohs RA, Netzer CM, Clark K, Strohl KP. Using the Berlin Questionnaire to identify patients at risk for the sleep apnea syndrome. Ann Intern Med 1999; 131(7): 485-91.
[http://dx.doi.org/10.7326/0003-4819-131-7-199910050-00002] [PMID: 10507956]

[8]   Al Shaikh Y, Haytham Shieb M, Koruturk S, Alghefari A, Hassan Z, Mussa B. The symptoms and risk of sleep apnea among adults in the United Arab Emirates. Ann Thorac Med 2018; 13(3): 168-74.
[http://dx.doi.org/10.4103/atm.ATM_245_17] [PMID: 30123336]

[9]   Wali S, Abaalkhail B. Prevalence of restless legs syndrome and associated risk factors among middle-aged Saudi population. Ann Thorac Med 2015; 10(3): 193-8.
[http://dx.doi.org/10.4103/1817-1737.160839] [PMID: 26229562]

[10]   Wali SO, Alsafadi S, Abaalkhail B, *et al*. Risk factors of primary and secondary restless legs syndrome among a middle-aged population in Saudi Arabia: A community-based study. Ann Thorac Med 2018; 13(3): 175-81.
[http://dx.doi.org/10.4103/atm.ATM_344_17] [PMID: 30123337]

[11]   Almeneessier AS, Al-Jebrin S, Labani R, *et al*. Medical specialty visits and diagnoses received by Saudi patients prior to a diagnosis of narcolepsy. Sleep Breath 2019; 23(2): 603-9.
[http://dx.doi.org/10.1007/s11325-019-01807-5] [PMID: 30820852]

[12]   BaHammam AS. Knowledge and attitude of primary health care physicians towards sleep disorders. Saudi Med J 2000; 21(12): 1164-7.
[PMID: 11360092]

[13]   BaHammam A, Al-Jahdali H, AlHarbi A, AlOtaibi G, Asiri S, AlSayegh A. Saudi regulations for the accreditation of sleep medicine physicians and technologists. Ann Thorac Med 2013; 8(1): 3-7.
[http://dx.doi.org/10.4103/1817-1737.105710] [PMID: 23440260]

[14]   Johns MW. A new method for measuring daytime sleepiness: the Epworth sleepiness scale. Sleep 1991; 14(6): 540-5.
[http://dx.doi.org/10.1093/sleep/14.6.540] [PMID: 1798888]

[15]   Chung F, Yegneswaran B, Liao P, *et al*. STOP Questionnaire. Anesthesiology 2008; 108(5): 812-21.
[http://dx.doi.org/10.1097/ALN.0b013e31816d83e4] [PMID: 18431116]

[16]   Barbé F, Durán-Cantolla J, Capote F, *et al*. Long-term effect of continuous positive airway pressure in hypertensive patients with sleep apnea. Am J Respir Crit Care Med 2010; 181(7): 718-26.
[http://dx.doi.org/10.1164/rccm.200901-0050OC] [PMID: 20007932]

[17]   Tefft BC. Prevalence of Motor Vehicle Crashes Involving Drowsy Drivers, United States, 2009-2013 (Technical Report). Washington, D.C.: AAA Foundation for Traffic Safety 2014.

[18]   Ramar K, Dort LC, Katz SG, *et al*. Clinical practice guideline for the treatment of obstructive sleep apnea and snoring with oral appliance therapy: an update for 2015: an American Academy of Sleep Medicine and American Academy of Dental Sleep Medicine clinical practice guideline. J Clin Sleep Med 2015; 11(7): 773-827.
[http://dx.doi.org/10.5664/jcsm.4858] [PMID: 26094920]

[19]   Marklund M, Verbraecken J, Randerath W. Non-CPAP therapies in obstructive sleep apnoea: mandibular advancement device therapy. Eur Respir J 2012; 39(5): 1241-7.
[http://dx.doi.org/10.1183/09031936.00144711] [PMID: 22075487]

[20]   Qaseem A, Kansagara D, Forciea MA, Cooke M, Denberg TD. Management of chronic insomnia disorder in adults: a clinical practice guideline from the American College of Physicians. Ann Intern Med 2016; 165(2): 125-33.
[http://dx.doi.org/10.7326/M15-2175] [PMID: 27136449]

[21]   Ree M, Junge M, Cunnington D. Australasian Sleep Association position statement regarding the use of psychological/behavioral treatments in the management of insomnia in adults. Sleep Med 2017; 36 (Suppl. 1): S43-7.
[http://dx.doi.org/10.1016/j.sleep.2017.03.017] [PMID: 28648226]

[22]   van Straten A, van der Zweerde T, Kleiboer A, Cuijpers P, Morin CM, Lancee J. Cognitive and behavioral therapies in the treatment of insomnia: A meta-analysis. Sleep Med Rev 2018; 38: 3-16.
[http://dx.doi.org/10.1016/j.smrv.2017.02.001] [PMID: 28392168]

[23]   Wu JQ, Appleman ER, Salazar RD, Ong JC. Cognitive behavioral therapy for insomnia comorbid with psychiatric and medical conditions: a meta-analysis. JAMA Intern Med 2015; 175(9): 1461-72.
[http://dx.doi.org/10.1001/jamainternmed.2015.3006] [PMID: 26147487]

[24]   Mitchell MD, Gehrman P, Perlis M, Umscheid CA. Comparative effectiveness of cognitive behavioral therapy for insomnia: a systematic review. BMC Fam Pract 2012; 13(1): 40.
[http://dx.doi.org/10.1186/1471-2296-13-40] [PMID: 22631616]

[25]   Mussa BM, Schauman M, Ramalingam V, Skaria S, Abusnana S. Personalized intervention to improve stress and sleep patterns for glycemic control and weight management in obese Emirati patients with type 2 diabetes: a randomized controlled clinical trial. Diabetes Metab Syndr Obes 2019; 12: 991-9.
[http://dx.doi.org/10.2147/DMSO.S201142] [PMID: 31388307]

[26]   BaHammam A. Sleep from an islamic perspective. Ann Thorac Med 2011; 6(4): 187-92.
[http://dx.doi.org/10.4103/1817-1737.84771] [PMID: 21977062]

[27]   BaHammam A, Spence DW, Sharif MM, Pandi Perumal S. Sleep architecture of consolidated and split sleep due to the dawn (Fajr) prayer among Muslims and its impact on daytime sleepiness. Ann Thorac Med 2012; 7(1): 36-41.
[http://dx.doi.org/10.4103/1817-1737.91560] [PMID: 22347349]

[28]   Mo'ez Al-Islam EF, Jahrami HA, Alhayki FA, *et al.* BaHammam AS. Effect of diurnal fasting on sleep during Ramadan: a systematic review and meta-analysis. Sleep Breath 2019; •••: 1-2.

[29]   DeZee KJ, Hatzigeorgiou C, Kristo D, Jackson JL. Prevalence of and screening for mental disorders in a sleep clinic. J Clin Sleep Med 2005; 1(2): 136-42.
[http://dx.doi.org/10.5664/jcsm.26307] [PMID: 17561627]

[30]   Harvey AG, Talbot LS, Gershon A. Sleep disturbance in bipolar disorder across the lifespan. Clin Psychol Sci Pract 2009; 16(2): 256-77.
[http://dx.doi.org/10.1111/j.1468-2850.2009.01164.x] [PMID: 22493520]

[31]   Benca RM, Okawa M, Uchiyama M, *et al.* Sleep and mood disorders. Sleep Med Rev 1997; 1(1): 45-56.
[http://dx.doi.org/10.1016/S1087-0792(97)90005-8] [PMID: 15310523]

[32]   Staner L. Sleep and anxiety disorders. Dialogues Clin Neurosci 2003; 5(3): 249-58.
[http://dx.doi.org/10.31887/DCNS.2003.5.3/lstaner] [PMID: 22033804]

[33]   Dobia A, Ryan K, Abutaleb M, Edwards A. Perceptions of physicians in Saudi Arabia on the use of international clinical guidelines for managing primary insomnia. PLoS One 2019; 14(8)e0220960
[http://dx.doi.org/10.1371/journal.pone.0220960] [PMID: 31398230]

[34]   Thomas A, Grandner M, Nowakowski S, Nesom G, Corbitt C, Perlis ML. Where are the behavioral sleep medicine providers and where are they needed? A geographic assessment. Behav Sleep Med 2016; 14(6): 687-98.
[http://dx.doi.org/10.1080/15402002.2016.1173551] [PMID: 27159249]

CHAPTER 7

Sleep Medicine in Hong Kong – Development, Knowledge Gaps and Future Challenges

K.L. Choo[1,*], A.M. Li[2], J.W. Chan[3,4], V.K.H. Lam[4] and Y.K. Wing[3,4]

[1] Department of Medicine, North District Hospital, Hong Kong SAR, China; Past President, Hong Kong Society of Sleep Medicine, Hong Kong SAR, China

[2] Department of Pediatrics, Prince of Wales Hospital, The Chinese University of Hong Kong, Hong Kong SAR, China.

[3] Department of Psychiatry, Faculty of Medicine, The Chinese University of Hong Kong, Shatin, N.T., Hong Kong SAR, China

[4] Li Chiu Kong Family Sleep Assessment Unit, Shatin Hospital, Department of Psychiatry, Faculty of Medicine, The Chinese University of Hong Kong, Hong Kong SAR, China

Abstract: The development of sleep medicine in Hong Kong has often been driven by clinical needs. The 1980s saw a surge of interest in sleep apnoea and brought multiple specialties together to study the diagnosis and management of sleep-related breathing disorders. Sleep and mood disorders often go hand in hand. With circadian disruption and sleep deprivation impacting the general population, including our paediatric age groups, the lack of quality sleep is a public health concern. Unfortunately, training in sleep medicine has been fragmented from undergraduate curricula to specialty training requirements. Sleep service standardisation is just beginning, although progress has been slow. Due to the lack of a specialty board, the Hong Kong Society of Sleep Medicine is providing a platform for interdisciplinary collaboration especially in training and education for both healthcare professionals and the general public, while the university-affiliated departments will provide the lead for multi-disciplinary research.

Keywords: Sleep medicine, Service development, Training, Research, Challenges, Hong Kong.

INTRODUCTION

Sleep medicine is a new medical arena with multidisciplinary involvement. We will review the historical development of sleep medicine and services in Hong Kong, followed by the elaboration of challenges in sleep medicine development in

* **Corresponding author K.L. Choo:** Department of Medicine, North District Hospital, Hong Kong SAR, China; E-mail: kahlin.choo@gmail.com

Hrayr P. Attarian, Marie-Louise M. Coussa-Koniski & Alain Michel Sabri (Eds.)

three clinical specialties (respiratory medicine, pediatrics, and psychiatry) as well as technologist training in Hong Kong.

EARLY SLEEP RESEARCH AND SLEEP LABORATORIES IN HONG KONG

Overnight polysomnography (PSG) was first conducted in the sleep laboratories of the two local university-affiliated hospitals (Prince of Wales Hospital, PWH, and Queen Mary Hospital, QMH respectively) in the 1980s. PWH reported early laboratory-diagnosed Chinese narcolepsy patients in a retrospective study [1] that confirmed a high association with HLA DR2 similar to the Western population [2]. The prevalence rate of narcolepsy in Hong Kong Chinese was later found to be 0.034% in a population-wide study [3].

Obstructive Sleep Apnoea Cases with Multidisciplinary Input

With improved understanding and characterisation of sleep apnoea syndrome by Guilleminault [4] and the introduction of Continuous Positive Airway Pressure (CPAP) by Sullivan [5], obstructive sleep apnoea syndrome (OSAS) cases were identified and reported locally [6, 7]. At the beginning, sleep testing required the collaboration of psychiatrists who were running sleep laboratories and pulmonologists who were managing severe OSAS patients with complications, such as cor pulmonale and respiratory failure. Otolaryngologists were also being consulted for snoring and providing surgical treatment such as tonsillectomy and uvulopalatopharyngoplasty (UPPP) [8]. Since the 1990s, drug-induced sleep video nasoendoscopy was performed to enhance the understanding of OSAS patients' upper airway dynamics [9]. Skeletal surgery [10] was also introduced by local Maxillofacial Surgeons to widen the upper airway [11].

RESPIRATORY SLEEP MEDICINE IN HONG KONG

With the availability of computerised PSG systems and CPAP treatment, an increasing number of respiratory services in public hospitals started providing sleep diagnostic and treatment services in the 1990s. Between 1997 and 2000, two community studies that determined the prevalence of OSAS among middle-aged adults in Hong Kong were conducted at QMH. Based on PSG, it was estimated that 9% of middle-aged men had OSA, while 4.1% were symptomatic with daytime sleepiness [12]. Prevalence of OSAS was lower among middle-aged women at 2.1% [13]. With age, however, there was a 12-fold rise among women from the fourth to the sixth decade. The University of Hong Kong (HKU) researchers have gone on to study cardiometabolic complications [14 - 16] and underlying pathogenetic mechanisms of OSA.

Sleep Service Challenges

Attended overnight PSG is labour-intensive. The first full-time sleep technologist was recruited and trained by the Chinese University of Hong Kong (CUHK) before undergoing overseas training in 1986. (Please see the latter paragraphs on the sleep technologist training) However, few public hospitals were funding technical positions for sleep technologists to work full time in the sleep laboratory. Instead, most hospitals operated sleep services in beds or rooms attached to inpatient wards and relied on night-shift nurses to conduct unattended overnight PSG. Without designated staff, it was difficult to perform manual non-invasive positive airway pressure titration for indicated patients or manual scoring of PSG tracings. There was also a lack of protected time for physicians to score or review PSG studies. Support for patients receiving long-term home CPAP treatment was not always available. As a result, the average waiting time for adult PSG testing in public hospitals often exceeds a year.

The situation of supply not meeting demand is complicated by commercial CPAP suppliers' attempts to fill the gap. Self-financed home unattended PSG and auto-adjusting CPAP trials without prior diagnosis or titration report review by physicians are not uncommon. Since there is no statutory body monitoring the quality of sleep testing or reporting in Hong Kong, OSA could be over-or misdiagnosed. Poor initial CPAP experience is known to adversely affect patients' CPAP acceptance and treatment compliance.

Role of Home Sleep Assessment Tests (HSAT)

To meet the ever-increasing demand for early diagnosis and treatment of OSAS patients, a randomised controlled trial (RCT) was conducted by the PWH Medical Department to compare ambulatory approach (HSAT and home auto CPAP titration) with the hospital-based approach. The home-based approach was found to be non-inferior to the hospital-based approach in terms of CPAP usage and clinical outcomes. Patients with suspected OSAS benefited from a shorter waiting time to testing while hospitals could reserve inpatient beds for acutely ill patients rather than ambulatory OSAS patients [17].

Public Medical (Hospital Authority) Sleep Laboratory Service Model for Adult Obstructive Sleep Apnoea

The year 2020 saw the implementation of a 24-hour sleep laboratory service model for adult sleep apnoea at two public (Hospital Authority, HA) hospitals.

The respective roles of sleep technologists in conducting and scoring PSG, nurses in supporting home CPAP treatment, and doctors in analysing PSG reports and formulating a differential diagnosis and management plan were finally recognised. These sleep centres commit to performing home sleep assessment tests and home CPAP titration in addition to overnight PSG and in-laboratory CPAP titration. As more hospitals will receive funding to implement this service model, it is hoped that patients' access to a comprehensive sleep service would improve and public sleep diagnostic and treatment services would become sustainable.

Respiratory Sleep Medicine training

Training would not be complete without adequate clinical exposure and a standard curriculum. A comprehensive sleep medicine fellowship training programme should specify minimum training duration and ideally include an attachment to the diverse specialties involved in the diagnosis and treatment of sleep disorders. Currently, sleep medicine is embedded in the Respiratory Medicine training programme for Hong Kong College of Physicians. However, there is no specification on the duration of sleep medicine training required for a Respiratory trainee.

PAEDIATRIC SLEEP MEDICINE IN HONG KONG

In Hong Kong, most paediatric units have facilities to conduct sleep assessments, but very few utilise an interdisciplinary approach, and even fewer put any emphasis on research. The current demand for sleep diagnostic services greatly outweighs the supply available, waiting time for 9-12 months is the norm. As our knowledge on childhood sleep disorders enhances, there is a need to provide a comprehensive, top-notched multidisciplinary sleep service and research for children in Hong Kong.

The Burden of Pediatric Sleep Problems

Good sleep should entail adequate duration and optimal quality. Over the past decade, concerns have been raised across the globe on the increasing number of children and adolescents whose sleep is inadequate. This problem is a major public health concern. The growing tendency to sleep less is due to a combination of factors, namely social, technological, and academic. The latter is most true for Hong Kongers! A decrease in sleep duration in 6-11 years old has been documented by a local research group where weekday sleep duration significantly decreased from 9.2 to 8.9 hours over 10 years [18]. On the other hand, we have evidence that a condition like obstructive sleep apnoea (OSA) which affects one's sleep quality is also prevalent. Among primary school-aged children, an OSA prevalence of up to 5% has been reported [19]. Sleep problems are also prevalent among infants, toddlers, and preschoolers in Hong Kong. Cross-cultural studies by *J Mindell et al.* documented the shortest sleep duration in our youngsters. Furthermore, mothers in Hong Kong were most likely to think their child has a sleep problem [20, 21].

THE SERIOUSNESS OF PEDIATRIC SLEEP PROBLEMS IS NOT RECOGNIZED

Despite the significant consequences associated with inadequate sleep and sleep disorder like OSA, these problems are under-recognised and undertreated in our locality, and possibly in many other cities in the Asia Pacific. This is a result of a lack of public awareness of the importance of sleep, a fragmented sleep service with each unit having its approach and policy, and inadequate training of health professionals. The sleep-related message needed to support good quality and adequate sleep is not being successfully conveyed to the public. People have often taken sleep for granted and especially so in our locality where academic performance trumps the importance of adequate and optimal sleep! The widely available and affordable electronic devices are not helping the situation. Although delaying school start times would be able to help bring the benefit to students, there was a lot of resistance in Hong Kong at which parents and teachers are more concerned about extra-curricular activities and attendance to after-school tutorials [22]. Although sleep education may increase the sleep knowledge of adolescents, their sleep habits were hardly changed [23]. We need a robust and workable strategy that can effectively channel information about sleep, and positively influence the sleep perceptions and choices made by the public and health care professionals.

THE WAY FORWARD IN PAEDIATRIC SLEEP MEDICINE

There is a need for more effort to include sleep-related education in all paediatric residency programmes [24]. It is only until recently that the Hong Kong College of Paediatricians approved and accredited the sub-specialty respiratory training programme, in which sleep medicine exposure constitutes a compulsory component. A lack of accreditation of sleep centres and quality monitoring remains a hurdle in establishing internationally recognised training units in Hong Kong. Likewise, sleep medicine is rarely covered in the medical school curriculum [25]. Sleep medicine training should start as early as in the medical school years. Under the sub-specialty of respiratory medicine, the College of Paediatricians should develop a public-health-based communication strategy, where professionals can share experiences and knowledge can be effectively disseminated to the public. The involvement of different stakeholders will be important to make sure all needs are considered and false information demystified. Research should be given a high priority within the health authority hierarchy and funding made available to intensify and encourage world-class research which can then be translated to better clinical practice.

SLEEP MEDICINE AND PSYCHIATRY IN HONG KONG

Sleep Problems are Common in Psychiatry

Sleep disturbances are common in psychiatric practice. Sleep disturbances were reported by over 90% of patients with depression [26], 30-80% of patients with schizophrenia [27], and up to 70-90% of patients with anxiety disorders [28]. There is a paradigm shift of recognising that sleep disturbances have a bidirectional relationship with mental illness [29]. In Hong Kong, our study reported that a significant proportion of depressed patients continue to complain about sleep disturbance despite their treatment [30], including nightmare [31] and insomnia [32], which would also predict poorer outcomes of depression. Similarly, the presence of insomnia and nightmare also predicted a higher risk of suicide in schizophrenia [33]. On the other hand, treatment of psychiatric disorders can lead to sleep disturbances, for example, the associations between antidepressants and restless legs syndrome and nightmares, Z-hypnotics, and sleep-walking [34]. Psychotropic drugs (*e.g.* second-generation antipsychotics) may also increase the metabolic risk with a higher risk of obstructive sleep apnea [35].

Circadian Disruptions and Psychiatric Illnesses

Emerging pieces of evidence are suggesting that circadian disruptions may underlie the pathophysiology of mood disorders [36]. There is a likewise bidirectional relationship between circadian rhythm and mental health, such that circadian disruptions of sleep and endocrine functions were often seen in depression, while environmental circadian disruption such as jet lag, shift work, exposure to artificial light at night can precipitate or exacerbate affective symptoms [37]. Eveningness (a circadian preference towards a late bedtime and late rise time) was found in 20% of patients with major depressive disorder and was associated with more severe depressive symptoms, insomnia, suicidality, and a high rate of non-remission of depression [32]. Collectively, the evidence suggests there is a close linkage between sleep disturbances, circadian rhythm, and mental illness, an in-depth understanding of their relationships is imperative in patient care.

Sleep Interventions are Effective but Mostly not Readily Accessible

There is a need to provide independent target treatment for insomnia in the context of comorbid psychiatric conditions [38]. Prescriptions of benzodiazepines and non-benzodiazepines hypnotics were common, which were up to 40% and 28% in local psychiatric out-patients respectively [32, 33]. However, not only residual insomnia remained very frequent and problematic, the polypharmacy and long-term use of Z-hypnotics led to complex sleep behavior including sleepwalking and sleep-related eating disorder [32 - 34]. Similarly, nightmares are associated with a psychiatric disorder, increase risk of mood disorders, and suicide [32]. The lifetime and 1-year prevalence of recurrent nightmares was 22.5% and 21.7% in a local cohort of psychiatric outpatients in Hong Kong [39]. Mounting evidence has shown that cognitive behavioural therapy for insomnia (CBT-I) is suggested as the first-line treatment for chronic insomnia in adults [40] and imagery rehearsal therapy (IRT), which consists of restructuring the theme of the nightmares were useful in combating nightmares. With regard to the circadian rhythm, chronotherapeutics (which refers to the controlled exposure to environmental stimuli that act on biological rhythms in order to achieve therapeutic effects in the treatment of psychiatric conditions) have been applied in psychiatric patients [41]. The most investigated circadian treatment is bright light therapy, as light is the strongest stimulus for the entrainment to the external environment [42]. The efficacy of bright light therapy has been demonstrated in both seasonal [43] and non-seasonal depression [44]. The treatment should be considered especially in the population where pharmacological treatment is less desirable, such as adolescents, pregnant women, elders, and patients with complex medical comorbidities. However, there is a lack of accessibility for most psychotherapeutic and chronotherapeutic interventions that will purposely be targeting the sleep and circadian disturbances in the psychiatric practice in Hong Kong.

Current evidence suggests effective treatments are available for the common sleep complaints and circadian misalignments, and these treatments likely also benefit the co-existing psychiatric disorders. The clinical significance lies in the accurate and comprehensive assessment of sleep and circadian symptoms in patients with psychiatric illness and the personalization of treatment plans to tailor the individual needs. In this regard, there is also a need to have a comprehensive diagnostic polysomnographic investigation of sleep and circadian disturbances in psychiatric patients. The development of digital sleep intervention may help to improve the accessibility and scalability of the psychotherapeutic intervention in the future.

In-attended Sleep Study and Psychiatry

The development of sleep medicine in psychiatry was closely related to the early vision and building of a dedicated sleep unit for attended polysomnography in the department of Psychiatry, PWH, CUHK, by Emeritus Professor Char- Nie Chen in the late 1980s. The subsequent relocation and expansion of the sleep laboratory from PWH to the current site at Shatin Hospital allowed the development of a comprehensive sleep service to investigate the spectrum of sleep problems across ages. Thus, the department of psychiatry, CUHK has a longstanding close collaboration with other disciplines especially Paediatrics on a number of joint research projects and service development [18, 19, 22, 23]. The sleep laboratory has also served as a referral centre for a number of sleep disorders including narcolepsy and REM sleep behaviour disorder (RBD), a distinct parasomnia characterized by recurrent dream-enactment behaviors and REM sleep without atonia (RSWA) [45]. More than 90% of patients with iRBD were found to develop α-synucleinopathies, including Parkinson's disease (PD), dementia of Lewy bodies (DLB), and multiple system atrophy (MSA) within 15 years [45]. In collaboration with neurologists, the study of RBD patients has extended to investigate the familial aggregation and the close association with psychiatric disorders in the context of neurodegeneration [46, 47].

The Way Forward - Need to Develop Sleep Medicine in Psychiatry

There is a need to develop a sleep medicine sub-specialty in psychiatry. In contrary to both Hong Kong College of Physicians (Respiratory Medicine) and Hong Kong College of Pediatricians, the Hong Kong College of Psychiatrists has no formal recognition of sleep and circadian medicine training in the curriculum. Currently, there is only piecemeal training for local psychiatrists concerning the importance of sleep-wake and circadian influences in psychiatric disorders as well as the close association of sleep disorders such as RBD, psychiatric disorders, and future neurodegeneration. There is a timely need to integrate sleep medicine training as an integrated assessment, therapeutic strategy, and future prognostic marker in psychiatry.

SLEEP TECHNOLOGISTS TRAINING IN HONG KONG

A sleep technologist is recognized as a separate and distinct allied health profession with a vital role in assisting the evaluation and follow-up care of patients with sleep disorders [48]. Sleep technologist has a diverse role in performing the sleep studies, providing patient care service or managing a sleep laboratory. Standardization of practice, quality assurance, continuing education, promotion of sleep medicine to the public, and professionalism of sleep technologists are also important for the development of sleep medicine in Hong Kong. The current training opportunity for sleep technologists is inadequate to meet our service needs. For example, sleep technology is not yet recognized as a nursing specialty under the major public health provider, Hospital Authority, and there is also no structured formal educational programme offered by a tertiary institution in Hong Kong. Nevertheless, there are several training routes to acquire the knowledge and skills of sleep technology. It includes in-house training and mentorship from experienced staff, self-initiating learning, seeking a local clinical attachment from a standard sleep laboratory, and attending the sleep training courses/ conference that are organized by local or overseas institutions such as the Hong Kong Society of Sleep Medicine or American Association of Sleep Technologists. Nonetheless, this brings concern about the variable standard of practice in sleep laboratories.

Credentialing and Continuing Education

The first Registered Polysomnographic Technologist (RPSGT) was granted in Hong Kong in 1993 [49]. By 2015, there were 76 RPSGT in Hong Kong, and currently, there are 44 active RPSGT credential holders. They come from different health care professionals and work in various specialties, such as the department of Medicine (28.9%), Psychiatry (17.8%), Electro-Diagnostic Unit (15.6%), Otolaryngology (13.3%) and Paediatrics (11.1%), *etc.* Most of them are part-time workers (64.6%) in providing both sleep service and other clinical duty in their service unit and over half of the sleep technologists were nursing staff (54.2%) [50].

With the growth of local sleep services, there is increasing demand for more formal sleep technologists training, a Registered Polysomnographic Sleep Technologists Committee was first established in 2009 under the Hong Kong Society of Sleep Medicine. The committee has about 10 voluntary committee members and aims to promote sleep technology, enhance communication and standardize sleep laboratory practice in the field. As there is no accredited organization for sleep technologists in Hong Kong, the future development of accrediting sleep medicine physicians and technologists may be a major step toward the development of sleep medicine practices in all Asian countries [51].

SLEEP SPECIALIST TRAINING AND INTERNATIONAL SLEEP MEDICINE EXAMINATION

In the absence of a sleep specialty board in Hong Kong, the Hong Kong Society of Sleep Medicine (HKSSM) was founded in 1993 by Psychiatrist Professor Chen Char-Nie (CUHK) and Respiratory Physician Professor Mary Ip (HKU). HKSSM, served by a multidisciplinary council of specialists (including Paediatricians, Pulmonologists, Otolaryngologists, and Psychiatrists) organises regular clinical and scientific meetings. The society also conducts regular public education seminars and supports an RPSGT group that organizes workshops and RPSGT continuing education activities [52]. As a founding member of the Asian Society of Sleep Medicine, HKSSM is also a member of the World Sleep Society (WSS).

Since 2013, HKSSM has worked with World Sleep Federation and later, WSS, to organize two International Sleep Medicine Examinations for doctors [52]. HKSSM Examination Committee not only organized certificate courses to help candidates prepare for the examination but also conducted a series of tutorials led by different specialists during the year leading to the examinations. So far, 22 doctors (including Otolaryngologists, Paediatricians, Pulmonologists, and Psychiatrists) have passed the examination and received the International Sleep Specialist designation awarded by WSS. Thirteen applicants have shown interest in the third examination in 2020. However, due to the COVID-19 pandemic, preparations for the examination had been put on hold.

FUTURE DEVELOPMENT OF SLEEP MEDICINE IN HONG KONG

The future development of sleep medicine in Hong Kong will face a lot of challenges including the need to integrate sleep medicine curriculum into the undergraduate medical and healthcare professional curriculum as well as the development of sleep-focused training among various specialties. Although the current medical colleges in Hong Kong are much clinical specialty-based, sleep medicine serves as a strong reminder that medicine and human suffering/disease will cut across "historically created" disciplines and "require" multi-disciplinary involvement. Indeed, the nature of sleep problems often comes with comorbid sleep, medical, psychiatric, and social/lifestyle problems that will affect all ages. For example, insomnia is highly comorbid with OSA, RBD with future neurodegeneration, childhood OSA and adult cardiovascular problems, sleep deprivation with lifestyle issues are just a few common examples. Thus, there is a need to enhance inter-disciplinary collaboration, and the establishment of an integrated Sleep Assessment Unit in each hospital would facilitate cross-disciplinary collaboration for the specialty-based doctors. While an independent sleep specialty board like that of the American Academy of Sleep Medicine may be an ideal distant goal, the need for continuing collaboration of various specialties through integrated sleep services within and across disciplines underscores the vital role of HKSSM as an important platform for liaison and exchange and, further enhancement of research-services integration and public health education in promoting sleep health literacy, the future development of sleep medicine in Hong Kong will continue to grow amidst the many challenges ahead.

CONCLUSION

It has been more than three decades since the first sleep laboratories were established in Hong Kong. Despite early interests and research in various sleep-related disorders by psychiatrists and respiratory physicians, sleep medicine remained a niche in many specialties, with inconsistent coverage in respective training curricula. Recent plans to implement the public sleep laboratory service model for adult OSA patients' diagnosis and treatment have been making slow progress. There is no current accreditation for sleep laboratories and examination for doctors is still voluntary. To keep RPSGT abreast of latest sleep medicine developments, HKSSM has been taking on the role of providing ongoing education. We must recognise that quality sleep underlies good physical and mental health, particularly for the paediatric population when early detection and treatment could prevent disease in adulthood. Finally, understanding our intrinsic circadian rhythm, promoting healthy lifestyle habits and pursuing nonpharmacological approaches to maintain quality sleep should be universal goals. With evolving knowledge and the advent of wearable technology, the mysteries of sleep will continue to be unravelled and this would undoubtedly require inter-specialty collaboration in research, education and future service development.

CONSENT FOR PUBLICATION

Not applicable.

CONFLICT OF INTEREST

The authors declare no conflict of interest, financial or otherwise.

ACKNOWLEDGEMENT

Declared none.

REFERENCES

[1]   Wing YK, Chiu HFK, Ho CKW, Chen CN. Narcolepsy in Hong Kong Chinese - a preliminary experience. Aust N Z J Med 1994; 24(3): 304-6.
      [http://dx.doi.org/10.1111/j.1445-5994.1994.tb02177.x] [PMID: 7980215]

[2]   Choo KL, Guilleminault C. Narcolepsy and idiopathic hypersomnolence. Clin Chest Med 1998; 19(1): 169-81.

[http://dx.doi.org/10.1016/S0272-5231(05)70440-8] [PMID: 9554226]

[3]   Wing YK, Li RHY, Lam CW, Ho CKW, Fong SYY, Leung T. The prevalence of narcolepsy among Chinese in Hong Kong. Ann Neurol 2002; 51(5): 578-84.
[http://dx.doi.org/10.1002/ana.10162] [PMID: 12112103]

[4]   Guilleminault C, Tilkian A, Dement WC. The sleep apnea syndromes. Annu Rev Med 1976; 27(1): 465-84.
[http://dx.doi.org/10.1146/annurev.me.27.020176.002341] [PMID: 180875]

[5]   Sullivan C, Berthon-Jones M, Issa FG, Eves L. Reversal of obstructive sleep apnoea by continuous positive airway pressure applied through the nares. Lancet 1981; 317(8225): 862-5.
[http://dx.doi.org/10.1016/S0140-6736(81)92140-1] [PMID: 6112294]

[6]   Ip M. SSY, Lam WK, Obstructive Sleep Apnoea Syndrome - A Rare Entity in Hong Kong Chinese? Journal of Hong Kong Medical Association 1989; 41(2): 191-4.

[7]   Chiu HF, Lee S, Ho KW, Leung CC, Chen CN. Sleep apnoea syndrome--a study of 5 cases. Singapore Med J 1990; 31(5): 466-8.
[PMID: 2259945]

[8]   Fujita S, Conway W, Zorick F, Roth T. Surgical correction of anatomic azbnormalities in obstructive sleep apnea syndrome: uvulopalatopharyngoplasty. Otolaryngol Head Neck Surg 1981; 89(6): 923-34.
[http://dx.doi.org/10.1177/019459988108900609] [PMID: 6801592]

[9]   Abdullah VJ, Wing YK, van Hasselt CA. Video sleep nasendoscopy: the Hong Kong experience. Otolaryngol Clin North Am 2003; 36(3): 461-471, vi.
[http://dx.doi.org/10.1016/S0030-6665(02)00176-7] [PMID: 12956094]

[10]   Riley RW, Powell NB, Guilleminault C. Obstructive sleep apnea syndrome: A surgical protocol for dynamic upper airway reconstruction. J Oral Maxillofac Surg 1993; 51(7): 742-7.
[http://dx.doi.org/10.1016/S0278-2391(10)80412-4] [PMID: 8509912]

[11]   Tsui WK, Yang Y, Mcgrath C, Leung YY. Mandibular distraction osteogenesis versus sagittal split ramus osteotomy in managing obstructive sleep apnea: A randomized clinical trial. J Craniomaxillofac Surg 2019; 47(5): 750-7.
[http://dx.doi.org/10.1016/j.jcms.2019.01.046] [PMID: 30777736]

[12]   Ip MSM, Lam B, Lauder IJ, *et al.* A community study of sleep-disordered breathing in middle-aged Chinese men in Hong Kong. Chest 2001; 119(1): 62-9.
[http://dx.doi.org/10.1378/chest.119.1.62] [PMID: 11157585]

[13]   Ip MSM, Lam B, Tang LCH, Lauder IJ, Ip TY, Lam WK. A community study of sleep-disordered breathing in middle-aged Chinese women in Hong Kong: prevalence and gender differences. Chest 2004; 125(1): 127-34.
[http://dx.doi.org/10.1378/chest.125.1.127] [PMID: 14718431]

[14]   Ip MSM, Lam B, Ng MMT, Lam WK, Tsang KWT, Lam KSL. Obstructive sleep apnea is independently associated with insulin resistance. Am J Respir Crit Care Med 2002; 165(5): 670-6.
[http://dx.doi.org/10.1164/ajrccm.165.5.2103001] [PMID: 11874812]

[15]   Ip MSM, Tse HF, Lam B, Tsang KWT, Lam WK. Endothelial function in obstructive sleep apnea and response to treatment. Am J Respir Crit Care Med 2004; 169(3): 348-53.
[http://dx.doi.org/10.1164/rccm.200306-767OC] [PMID: 14551167]

[16]   Lam JCM. A randomized controlled trial of nCPAP on insulin sensitivity in obstructive sleep apnea. Eur Respir J 2010; 35(1): 138-45.
[http://dx.doi.org/10.1183/09031936.00047709] [PMID: 19608589]

[17]   Hui DS, Ng SS, To KW, *et al.* A randomized controlled trial of an ambulatory approach versus the hospital-based approach in managing suspected obstructive sleep apnea syndrome. Sci Rep 2017; 7(1): 45901.
[http://dx.doi.org/10.1038/srep45901] [PMID: 28374832]

[18] Wang G, Zhang J, Lam SP, *et al.* Ten-Year Secular Trends in Sleep/Wake Patterns in Shanghai and Hong Kong School-Aged Children: A Tale of Two Cities. J Clin Sleep Med 2019; 15(10): 1495-502.
[http://dx.doi.org/10.5664/jcsm.7984] [PMID: 31596215]

[19] Li AM, So HK, Au CT, *et al.* Epidemiology of obstructive sleep apnoea syndrome in Chinese children: a two-phase community study. Thorax 2010; 65(11): 991-7.
[http://dx.doi.org/10.1136/thx.2010.134858] [PMID: 20965935]

[20] Mindell JA, Sadeh A, Wiegand B, How TH, Goh DYT. Cross-cultural differences in infant and toddler sleep. Sleep Med 2010; 11(3): 274-80.
[http://dx.doi.org/10.1016/j.sleep.2009.04.012] [PMID: 20138578]

[21] Mindell JA, Sadeh A, Kwon R, Goh DYT. Cross-cultural differences in the sleep of preschool children. Sleep Med 2013; 14(12): 1283-9.
[http://dx.doi.org/10.1016/j.sleep.2013.09.002] [PMID: 24269649]

[22] Chan NY, Zhang J, Yu MWM, *et al.* Impact of a modest delay in school start time in Hong Kong school adolescents. Sleep Med 2017; 30: 164-70.
[http://dx.doi.org/10.1016/j.sleep.2016.09.018] [PMID: 28215242]

[23] Wing YK. CN, Yu MWM, Lam SP, Zhang JH, Li SX, Kong APS, Li AM., A multi-level and multi-modal school-based sleep education programme on adolescent sleep and health- A cluster randomized controlled trial. Pediatrics 2015; 135: e635-43.
[http://dx.doi.org/10.1542/peds.2014-2419] [PMID: 25687152]

[24] Mindell JA, Bartle A, Ahn Y, *et al.* Sleep education in pediatric residency programs: a cross-cultural look. BMC Res Notes 2013; 6(1): 130.
[http://dx.doi.org/10.1186/1756-0500-6-130] [PMID: 23552445]

[25] Mindell JA, Bartle A, Wahab NA, *et al.* Sleep education in medical school curriculum: A glimpse across countries. Sleep Med 2011; 12(9): 928-31.
[http://dx.doi.org/10.1016/j.sleep.2011.07.001] [PMID: 21924951]

[26] Thase ME. Antidepressant treatment of the depressed patient with insomnia. J Clin Psychiatry 1999; 60 (Suppl. 17): 28-31.
[PMID: 10446739]

[27] Cohrs S. Sleep disturbances in patients with schizophrenia : impact and effect of antipsychotics. CNS Drugs 2008; 22(11): 939-62.
[http://dx.doi.org/10.2165/00023210-200822110-00004] [PMID: 18840034]

[28] Richards A, Kanady JC, Neylan TC. Sleep disturbance in PTSD and other anxiety-related disorders: an updated review of clinical features, physiological characteristics, and psychological and neurobiological mechanisms. Neuropsychopharmacology 2020; 45(1): 55-73.
[http://dx.doi.org/10.1038/s41386-019-0486-5] [PMID: 31443103]

[29] Freeman D, Sheaves B, Waite F, Harvey AG, Harrison PJ. Sleep disturbance and psychiatric disorders. Lancet Psychiatry 2020; 7(7): 628-37.
[http://dx.doi.org/10.1016/S2215-0366(20)30136-X] [PMID: 32563308]

[30] Li SX, Lam SP, Chan JWY, Yu MWM, Wing YK. Residual sleep disturbances in patients remitted from major depressive disorder: a 4-year naturalistic follow-up study. Sleep 2012; 35(8): 1153-61.
[http://dx.doi.org/10.5665/sleep.2008] [PMID: 22851811]

[31] Li SX, Lam SP, Yu MWM, Zhang J, Wing YK. Nocturnal sleep disturbances as a predictor of suicide attempts among psychiatric outpatients: a clinical, epidemiologic, prospective study. J Clin Psychiatry 2010; 71(11): 1440-6.
[http://dx.doi.org/10.4088/JCP.09m05661gry] [PMID: 21114949]

[32] Chan JWY, Lam SP, Li SX, *et al.* Eveningness and insomnia: independent risk factors of nonremission in major depressive disorder. Sleep 2014; 37(5): 911-7.
[http://dx.doi.org/10.5665/sleep.3658] [PMID: 24790269]

[33]   Li SX, Lam SP, Zhang J, *et al.* Sleep Disturbances and Suicide Risk in an 8-Year Longitudinal Study of Schizophrenia-Spectrum Disorders. Sleep 2016; 39(6): 1275-82.
[http://dx.doi.org/10.5665/sleep.5852] [PMID: 27091530]

[34]   Lam SP, Fong SYY, Ho CKW, Yu MWM, Wing YK. Parasomnia among psychiatric outpatients: a clinical, epidemiologic, cross-sectional study. J Clin Psychiatry 2008; 69(9): 1374-82.
[http://dx.doi.org/10.4088/JCP.v69n0904] [PMID: 19193338]

[35]   Sharafkhaneh A, Giray N, Richardson P, Young T, Hirshkowitz M. Association of psychiatric disorders and sleep apnea in a large cohort. Sleep 2005; 28(11): 1405-11.
[http://dx.doi.org/10.1093/sleep/28.11.1405] [PMID: 16335330]

[36]   McClung CA. How might circadian rhythms control mood? Let me count the ways..... Biol Psychiatry 2013; 74(4): 242-9.
[http://dx.doi.org/10.1016/j.biopsych.2013.02.019] [PMID: 23558300]

[37]   Walker WH II, Walton JC, DeVries AC, Nelson RJ. Circadian rhythm disruption and mental health. Transl Psychiatry 2020; 10(1): 28.
[http://dx.doi.org/10.1038/s41398-020-0694-0] [PMID: 32066704]

[38]   Harvey AG, Murray G, Chandler RA, Soehner A. Sleep disturbance as transdiagnostic: Consideration of neurobiological mechanisms. Clin Psychol Rev 2011; 31(2): 225-35.
[http://dx.doi.org/10.1016/j.cpr.2010.04.003] [PMID: 20471738]

[39]   Li SX, Zhang B, Li AM, Wing YK. Prevalence and correlates of frequent nightmares: a community-based 2-phase study. Sleep 2010; 33(6): 774-80.
[http://dx.doi.org/10.1093/sleep/33.6.774] [PMID: 20550018]

[40]   Chan NY, Chan JWY, Li SX, Wing YK. Non-pharmacological Approaches for Management of Insomnia. Neurotherapeutics 2021; 18(1): 32-43.
[http://dx.doi.org/10.1007/s13311-021-01029-2] [PMID: 33821446]

[41]   Benedetti F, Barbini B, Colombo C, Smeraldi E. Chronotherapeutics in a psychiatric ward. Sleep Med Rev 2007; 11(6): 509-22.
[http://dx.doi.org/10.1016/j.smrv.2007.06.004] [PMID: 17689120]

[42]   Czeisler CA, Allan JS, Strogatz SH, *et al.* Bright light resets the human circadian pacemaker independent of the timing of the sleep-wake cycle. Science 1986; 233(4764): 667-71.
[http://dx.doi.org/10.1126/science.3726555] [PMID: 3726555]

[43]   Pjrek E, Friedrich ME, Cambioli L, *et al.* The Efficacy of Light Therapy in the Treatment of Seasonal Affective Disorder: A Meta-Analysis of Randomized Controlled Trials. Psychother Psychosom 2020; 89(1): 17-24.
[http://dx.doi.org/10.1159/000502891] [PMID: 31574513]

[44]   Chan JWY. LS, Li SX, Chau SWH, Chan SY, Chan NY, Zhang JH, Wing YK. Adjunctive bright light treatment with gradual advance in unipolar major depressive disorder with evening chronotype – a randomized controlled trial. Psychol Med 2022; 52(8): 1448-57.
[http://dx.doi.org/10.1017/S0033291720003232] [PMID: 32924897]

[45]   Galbiati A, Verga L, Giora E, Zucconi M, Ferini-Strambi L. The risk of neurodegeneration in REM sleep behavior disorder: A systematic review and meta-analysis of longitudinal studies. Sleep Med Rev 2019; 43: 37-46.
[http://dx.doi.org/10.1016/j.smrv.2018.09.008] [PMID: 30503716]

[46]   Liu Y, Zhang J, Lam SP, *et al.* A case–control–family study of idiopathic rapid eye movement sleep behavior disorder. Ann Neurol 2019; 85(4): 582-92.
[http://dx.doi.org/10.1002/ana.25435] [PMID: 30761606]

[47]   Wing YK, LS Zhang J, Leung E, *et al.* Reduced Striatal Dopamine transmission in REM Sleep Behaviour Disorder co-morbid with depression. Neurology 2015; 84: 516-22.
[http://dx.doi.org/10.1212/WNL.0000000000001215] [PMID: 25568298]

[48] (AAST), AAoST. Retrieved on August 15, 2021 Website. https://www.aastweb.org/what-is-a-sleep-technologist

[49] Technologists BoRP. Retrieved on August 15, 2021 Website:. https://www.brpt.org/recertify/

[50] Committee RPST. Sleep Laboratory Manpower Survey (Technical Personnel) 2017, the Hong Kong Society of Sleep Medicine.

[51] BaHammam AS, Han F, Gupta R, *et al.* Asian accreditation of sleep medicine physicians and technologists: practice guidelines by the Asian Society of Sleep Medicine. Sleep Med 2021; 81: 246-52.
[http://dx.doi.org/10.1016/j.sleep.2021.02.041] [PMID: 33735652]

[52] Choo KL. Development of Sleep Medicine in Hong Kong. Hong Kong Medical Diary 2021; 26(4): 23-5.

Sleep Medicine in China

Liyue Xu[1], Chenyang Li[1] and Fang Han[1,*]

[1] Division of Sleep Medicine, Peking University People's Hospital, Beijing, China

Abstract: As the world's most populous country, China has a high prevalence of sleep disorders, posing a huge public health burden. After 30 years of development, more and more professionals, patients, and public health policymakers are recognizing the importance of sleep. Although sleep problem is recognized in the Traditional Chinese Medicine area, modern sleep medicine starts from the diagnosis and treatment of obstructive sleep apnea. By 2017, about 2,000 sleep centers had been established nationwide which can diagnose and treat OSA, narcolepsy, restless legs syndrome, REM sleep disorder, and other sleep diseases. Research in different sleep fields has emerged in the recent 20 years. However, there are gaps between the sleep service capacity and the demand from patients due to the lack of sleep professionals as well as the medical insurance coverage. Education and training of both physicians and technicians still have a long way to go. Understanding the development and challenges will help us maintain the development of sleep medicine in China.

Keywords: Sleep disorders, Sleep medicine, China, Practice.

China is a developing country with 1.4 billion people. With the rapid development of the economy during the past decades, sleep health is getting more and more attention in China, and it has been included in the Healthy China Initiatives 2019-2030. One of its aims is to increase the average sleep time from 6.5 hours to longer than 7 hours. In addition, China's Brain Plan launched in the year 2021 includes both basic sleep and human sleep disorders research projects, which will promote the research level in China.

EPIDEMIOLOGICAL DATA

In recent years, with the rapid changes in lifestyle and the aging of the population, the incidence of sleep disorders is increasing rapidly in China. It was estimated that about 15% of the population suffers from chronic insomnia [1], which is the most common sleep disorder. The number of patients with obstructive sleep apnea

* **Corresponding author Fang Han:** Division of Sleep Medicine, Peking University People's Hospital, Beijing 100044, China; Telephone: +86-10-88324206; Fax: 86-10-88324207; E-mail: hanfang1@hotmail.com

Hrayr P. Attarian, Marie-Louise M. Coussa-Koniski & Alain Michel Sabri (Eds.)

(OSA) in China exceeds 170 million, which ranks the first in the world [2]. Using a questionnaire survey followed by portable screen testing, the population study indicated that the prevalence of sleep apnea with an apnea-hypopnea index (AHI) >5 and daytime sleepiness is 3.5%-4.8% in the Chinese population over 30 years old [3]. Later, another study showed that Han people have a higher prevalence than some minorities such as Zhuang people [4]. Higher prevalence was seen in obese people, males, post-menopause women, and subjects from urban [4]. The special facial structure may contribute to the high sleep apnea incidence [5, 6].

Narcolepsy has long been considered a rare disease in China. A population-based epidemiology study reported a prevalence of 0.034% (95% confidence interval: 0.01-0.12%) in Hongkong Chinese, which belongs to the south of China [7]. However, if this could represent the Northern part of China remains unclear, as the HLA gene distribution and environmental factors that may trigger narcolepsy differ between the two regions. In September 1998, collaborations were developed between Peking University People's Hospital's sleep lab and the neurology service of Beijing Children's Hospital [8], a gradually increased incidence of presentation of narcolepsy cataplexy in the pediatric neurology clinic, with a range of 0.04%-0.063% [8]. This increasing incidence may be attributed to the increasing awareness of this disease. In 2011, we reported that the incidence of childhood narcolepsy increased several folds in China following the H1N1winter flu pandemic (pH1N1) [9].

The prevalence of RLS was reported to be 0.69% to 7.2% in Chinese adults [10 - 12], depending on the survey methodology and population. It is widely recognized that like other eastern Asians, RLS prevalence is low in Chinese. With the development of sleep medicine, data from more epidemiological and clinical practice imply that this might not be right. REM behavior disorder (RBD) was reported in 0.38% of elder Chinese (≥70 years old) in Hong Kong [13]. Other sleep disorders, such as central hypersomnia, dyssomnia, and sleep-related movement disorders, are relatively less recognized and may be considered as rare, but still cannot be ignored in such a rapidly changing society with a large population, the medical care, and economic burden of sleep disorders are heavy.

DEVELOPMENT OF SLEEP MEDICINE IN CHINA

Many philosophical and theoretical questions about sleep and dream have been written in traditional Chinese medicine literature [14]. Varied approaches, including traditional herbs, auto-hypnosis, exercises, and acupuncture, have been used to treat insomnia since ancient times. They are now still used as the first-line treatment for insomnia by many physicians in China. However, the practice of modem sleep medicine in China starts with the recognition of sleep apnea [15].

The first diagnosis of OSA in China was in 1981 by Dr. HUANG Xi-zhen through observation at Peking Union Hospital. Unfortunately, the patient did not receive any treatment and died during sleep several years later. The first polysomnography (PSG) system was modified from an electroencephalograph (EEG) machine by Dr. Huang's group in 1983. Five cases of sleep apnea syndrome were published in the Chinese Journal of Internal Medicine in 1985, which implied that OSA was recognized by the Chinese medical community [16]. In 1986, Dr. Huang set up the first sleep lab in China after six-month training at the sleep center of Stanford University. However, the development of sleep medicine was very slow. There were only 4-5 sleep labs in China by the year 1997.

During the past ten to fifteen years, with the rapid development of the economy, the demand for sleep services in China grows fast. According to a sampling survey conducted in the year 2017 by the Chinese Sleep Research Society, it was estimated that there were around 2000 sleep labs or centers inside hospitals providing sleep diagnostic and therapeutic services across the countries, and most of these labs were set up during the past ten years. In addition, there are emerging private sleep services too. After the year 2018, there is a 20% increase in sleep services nationwide due to the adjustment of the government policy. Physicians with a pulmonary medicine background account for two-thirds (67%) of the sleep practitioners, others include ENT (25%), dentists, traditional Chinese Medicine, neurology, and psychiatry. In-lab PSG was the main diagnostic tool for sleep disorders, 66% of hospitals are equipped with home sleep test (HST) devices, however, only 14% of them were applied at home, and the majority were used in other wards inside the hospital. The usage of HST has been increasing in recent years [17, 18].

There is a dynamic change in treatment procedures for sleep apnea. The first CPAP machine was used in 1987 in China. Since then, this number increased gradually. A rapid increase was seen in 1995 due to the availability of a CPAP machine made in China. In the early days of the 1990s, the majority of the OSAS patients were treated using ENT surgical procedures, especially UPPP. In recent years, the PAP machine becomes the first choice for most adult OSA patients. However, compared with a big population and the high prevalence, the absolute number of PAP users is relatively low. Dentists got involved in sleep apnea management at the beginning of sleep practice, as people realized that Chinese has a special facial structure as a risk of sleep apnea [5, 6]. Custom-made or commercialized oral appliances are available in the market.

Sleep medicine has not been recognized as an independent specialty yet in China, most of the sleep labs start from dealing with sleep-disordered breathing only, as the labs are mainly under the department of respiratory medicine and ENT. Patients with insomnia disorder generally go to neurological or psychiatric clinics. In recent years, with more involvement of sleep medicine by neurologists and psychiatrists, more non-respiratory sleep disorders are recognized and managed. More sleep labs develop to multiple disciplinary sleep centers managing varieties of sleep disorders. There are around 20 independent divisions of sleep medicine across China, leading clinical practice, education, and research in the sleep area.

In addition to training, one step to standardize sleep medicine practice is to use clinical guidelines or expert consensus (Table **1**) to educate and regulate the clinical practice. The Sleep Breathing Disorder Assembly of the Chinese Thoracic Society published the first guideline for sleep breathing disorders in 2002 [19] and updated it in 2012 [20]. To deal with the influence of the COVID-19 pandemic, telemedicine in sleep medicine is getting more popular, and an expert consensus on remote management of sleep apnea using telemedicine was published in the National Medical Journal China [21]. There is also a new trend using the emerging technology in sleep disorders management. An early sleep apnea screening system based on internet and oximetry was developed by Celki Co around 2005. Now more wearable devices and APPs targeting the population develop, but few were validated by sleep labs. The commercialized 5G technology develops quickly and helps the transmission of sleep signals including video and sound spontaneously in time, this will bring revolutionary changes to sleep practice in the future.

SLEEP EDUCATION AND SLEEP RESEARCH

The build-up of the sleep education system in medical schools started from the inclusion of the sleep apnea chapter into the medical textbook at Peking University in 2002, then in the medical school across the whole country. A sleep medicine textbook for the postgraduate student was published in 2016. Milestones in establishing a formal infrastructure for sleep education and training include: (1) a sleep medicine textbook for residency was recognized by the Ministry of Health China in 2019; (2) a 3-6 months of a sleep training project for physicians and technologists was established inside the Chinese Thoracic Society as a part of PCCMs fellowship training program; (3) In 2019, sleep fellowship training and specialist certification system were recognized by Chinese Government as an independent program in the newly established medical accreditation system. Peking University will start the recruitment of sleep fellows in 2022, as the first in China.

Sleep research work started from basic research areas, and CSRS was initiated by basic scientists. The Natural Science Foundation China (NSFC) is the major research agency supporting sleep research. There were few sleep projects get supported before 2001. In 2009, the Department of Health Science was set up inside the NSFC, and sleep research was classified as an independent supported area in both Respiratory Medicine Branch and Neurological Department, later in Psychiatry Department, together with the more financial support to medical research, more sleep research programs get supported (Fig. **1**). Other research agencies like The Ministry of Science and Technology listed sleep disorders in the chronic disease research programs and the Brain Plan; local research agency at provincial levels also support sleep programs.

Sleep research work in China covers different areas. Publications about sleep research are increasing. Fig. (**2**) shows the number of publications on sleep from 1990 to 2020 in China. Basic researchers found out different neurological circuits and circadian rhyme controlling sleep-wake cycles [22, 23]. Intermitted hypoxia mimicking sleep apnea comorbidities is the most studied in clinical research projects. China has abundant sleep patient resources, SAVE study recruited more than two-thirds of the sleep apnea patients from China [17]. A large narcolepsy cohort helped reveal the link between H1N1 virus infection and narcolepsy onset) [9]. The RBD studies based on the cohort in Hongkong are well-recognized internationally [24]. Traditional Chinese Medicine would be a unique resource for exploring.

INTERNATIONAL COOPERATION

International exchange and cooperation are important to promote sleep research and practice. The first generation of basic sleep researchers was trained in Europe including France and the former Soviet. Almost all of the new generations of sleep researchers have an overseas training background. Many of their mentors received distinguished contribution rewards by CSRS. The mini-fellow training program by AASM helped train more than 10 sleep doctors from China, and the ISTRP by WSS has 13/23 from China enrolled from 2020-2022. CSRS established cooperation with the Australian Sleep Association for academic meeting exchange. The Sino-German sleep cooperation started in 2008, and had 5 times bilateral meetings supported by NSFC&DFG, also organized one symposium for a young student, and established one joint sleep center. Dr. Guilleminault from Stanford University helped the Chinese sleep community in many aspects. The first national sleep apnea conference was organized by the Chinese Medical Association in 1998, and Dr. Kingman Strohl from Case Western Reserve University gave the keynote speech and published the review paper in the Chinese Journal of Respiration and Tuberculosis, the official journal of Chinese Thoracic Society, which largely promoted the recognition of sleep apnea. The successful cooperation between Peking University and Stanford

University on narcolepsy and KLS research does not only increase awareness but also promotes the clinical care of hypersomnia. The restless legs syndrome questionnaire was introduced by Dr. Wayne. Henning, and reminded the sleep society that RLS in China was not as rare as we thought, an ongoing joint genetic study with a German group on Chinese RLS may add new findings to the RLS research area. Joint studies on the telemedicine system between China with Dr. Penzel in Germany and Dr. Kuna, Dr. Pack at the University of Pennsylvania help the patients during the COVID-19 pandemic very much. The support by Dr. Phyllis Zee from Northwestern University benefits the establishment of the circadian rhythm sleep disorder diagnostic and therapeutic system in China.

As a member of SAGIC group [25], China contributes sleep apnea patients with ethnic background different from the white and black population in other centers, which is an advantage for cross-ethnic comparison, as the successful comparisons between Chinese and white narcolepsy patients [26].

ACADEMIC AND PATIENT ORGANIZATIONS

There are two major sleep medicine organizations in China. The Chinese Sleep Research Society (CSRS) is a multidisciplinary society with members from basic research to clinical medicine including pulmonary medicine, ENT, dental medicine, psychology, neurology, psychiatry, TCM, and other fields. Since 1994 when the society was founded, members of CSRS have increased from 100 to over 4000. CSRS is a founding member of the Asian Sleep Research Society (1994), and a member of the World Sleep Society. CSRS holds its academic meeting annually, with around 2000 attendees for the 2020 meeting. The Sleep Medicine Committee in the Chinese Medical Doctor Association was established in 2012 and focused mainly on sleep professionals' training.

Chinese Medical Association is the major professional medical society consisting of Societies of different medical specialties in China. Sleep assembly was set up inside the Chinese Thoracic Society and the Chinese Neurology Society, respectively. The former (established 2000) focuses on sleep disordered breathing, and the latter on non-respiratory sleep disorders. Sleep sections inside ENT Society and Pediatric Society are also active. Accordingly, there are sleep academic societies at the provincial levels. As sleep medicine is a multi-disciplinary area, there are overlaps in regard to their academic activities among these Assemblies and Sections.

In addition, some Chinese sleep researchers working in other countries formed the Overseas Chinese Sleep Research Society in 2002, and it cooperates with CSRS, and meet informally during APSS and other international sleep meetings.

The patient organizations are under development. There are routine educational programs for sleep apnea patients, however, only narcolepsy patient organization is established with the involvement of several hundreds of patients and their families, focusing on the effort for the introduction of new medications. Chinese Sleep Research Society has supported patients with Kleine-Levin syndrome (KLS) and narcolepsy to observe the activities of patient organizations in the USA, and offered support to attend the European Narcolepsy Network conference in 2019 and 2020. Sleep experts are also helping to promote the construction of the patient network in China.

CHALLENGES

Sleep medicine in China is facing significant challenges. It is estimated that there are at least 60 million with symptomatic sleep apnea in China. However, less than one percent of these patients have been diagnosed and treated using PAP machine. Enlarging the diagnostic and therapeutic capacity to meet the gap between limited service and increasing demand is a challenge to the sleep community in China. The recognition and management of non-respiratory sleep disorders need to improve.

There is a shortage of sleep practitioners including both physicians and technicians. Currently, RPSGT has not been recognized as a profession. Only a few sleep centers have nurses. Most of the physicians in China have to take care of patients other than sleep disorders in their original specialty. As a result, physicians' focus on the practice of sleep medicine is limited. To overcome this obstacle, continued medical educational programs designed under the umbrella of sleep medicine for sleep knowledge, skill and competency training are needed.

Insurance coverage for the diagnosis and treatment of sleep disorders will be the key for a wide public benefit. Through the effort by the Sleep Section of the Chinese Thoracic Society, the Beijing city government health care insurance system finally approved that PSG was a reimbursable diagnostic test. This policy was soon followed by other provinces. However, the PAP machines are still paid from patients' pocket (about 1000USD/APAP machine).

In addition, the lack of drugs limited the treatment of sleep disorders in China. No China FDA approved medications for narcolepsy in the Chinese market are available at present. All available including methylphenidate and antidepressants are used off-label. Emerging techniques such as hypoglossal nerve stimulation are not yet available in China.

Table 1. Guidelines and Expert Consensuses for Sleep Disorders in China.

Year	Title	Working Group
2002, 2012	Guidelines for the diagnosis and treatment of obstructive sleep apnea hypopnea syndrome (draft) in 2002, updated in 2011	Sleep Respiratory Diseases Group, Respiratory Diseases Branch of Chinese Medical Association
2013	Expert consensus on clinical diagnosis and treatment of obstructive sleep apnea-related hypertension	Chinese Medical Doctor Association Hypertension Professional Committee, Chinese Medical Association Respiratory Disease Branch Sleep Disorders Group
2015	Guidelines for the diagnosis and treatment of narcolepsy in China	Chinese Medical Association Neurology Branch; Chinese Medical Association Neurology Branch Sleep Disorders Group; Chinese Medical Science and Technology Committee Neurology Professional Committee Sleep Disorders Group
2017	Expert consensus on the clinical application of non-invasive positive pressure ventilation for sleep breathing disorders (draft)	Sleep Related Breathing Disorders Group of Chinese Thoracic Society
2017	China rapid eye movement sleep behavior disorder diagnosis and treatment guidelines	Sleep Disorders Society, Chinese Society of Neurology
2017	Expert consensus on clinical application of non-invasive positive pressure ventilation at home	Sleep Related Breathing Disorders Group of Chinese Thoracic Society
2018	Guideline for the evaluation and treatment of insomnia in Chinese adults (2017)	Chinese Society of Neurology, Sleep Disorder Society, Chinese Society of Neurology
2018	Expert consensus on Chinese adult polysomnography technology operation specification and clinical application	Sleep Disorders Professional Committee of Neurologist Branch of Chinese Medical Doctor Association, Sleep Disorders Professional Committee of Chinese Sleep Research Association, Sleep Disorders Group of Neurology Branch of Chinese Medical Association
2020	Chinese guideline for the diagnosis and treatment of childhood obstructive sleep apnea (2020)	Working Group of Chinese Guideline for the Diagnosis and Treatment of Childhood OSA, Subspecialty Group of Pediatrics, Society of Otorhinolaryngology Head and Neck Surgery, Chinese Medical Association, Subspecialty Group of Respiratory Diseases, Society of Pediatrics, Chinese Medical Association, Society of Pediatric Surgery, Chinese Medical Association, Editorial Board of Chinese Journal of Otorhinolaryngology Head and Neck Surgery

(Table 1) cont.....

Year	Title	Working Group
2021	Guidelines for the diagnosis and treatment of restless legs syndrome in China (2021)	Sleep Science Group of Chinese Medical Doctor Association Neurologist Branch, Sleep Disorders Society, Chinese Society of Neurology, Sleep Disorder Professional Committee of Chinese Sleep Research Association
2021	Expert consensus on the clinical practice of telemedicine in adults with obstructive sleep apnea hypopnea syndrome	Sleep Respiratory Disorder Working Committee of the Respiratory Physician Branch of the Chinese Medical Doctor Association, "Hua Tuo Project" Sleep Health Project Expert Committee

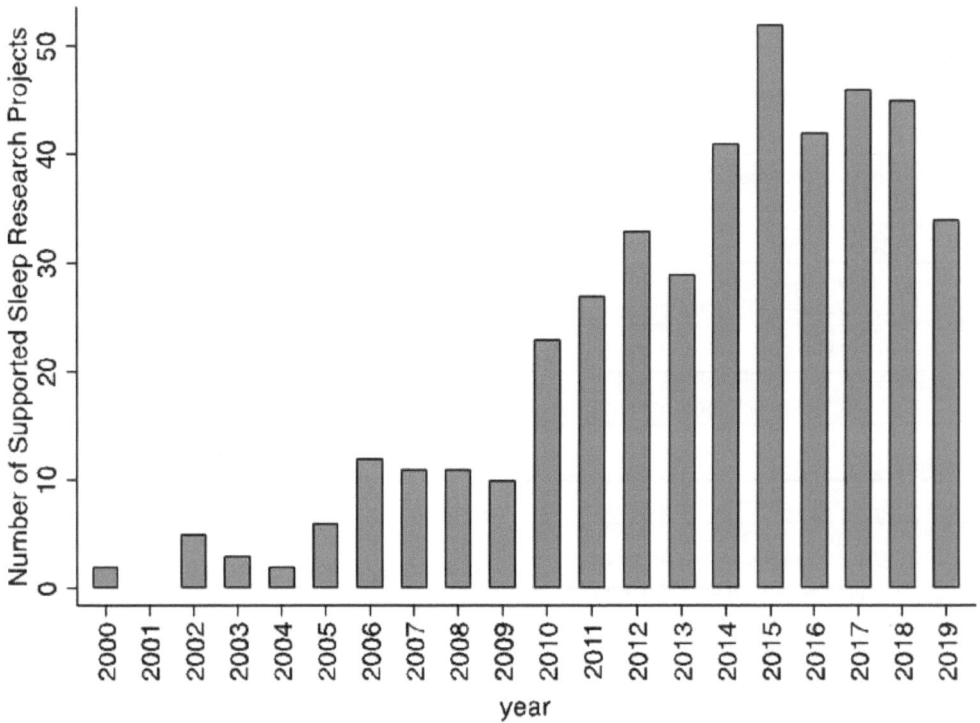

Fig. (1). Number of Supported Sleep Research Projects from 2000 to 2019 in China. Data was obtained from the website of National Natural Science Foundation of China by searching for word of "sleep".

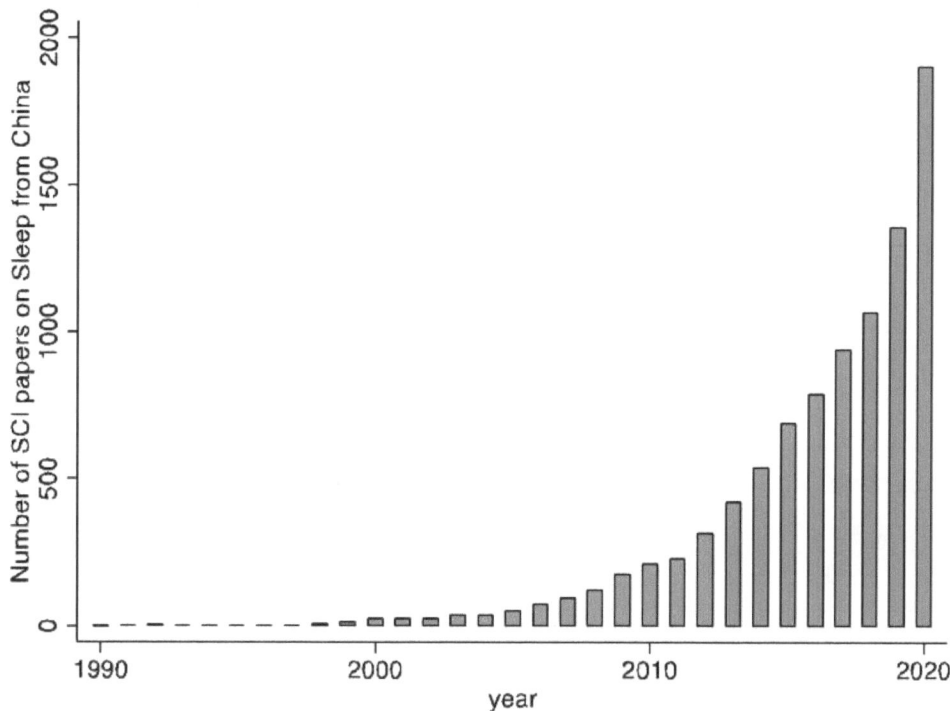

Fig. (2). The number of published papers about sleep from 1990 to 2020. Data was obtained from Web of Science by searching for key word of "sleep" in China.

CONCLUSION

As the world's most populous developing country, China has a large number of people with sleep disorders. Sleep medicine in China has developed rapidly over the past two decades, with more than 2,000 sleep laboratories across the country. However, we are facing a great challenge. There are gaps between the sleep service capacity and the demand from patients due to the lack of sleep professionals as well as the medical insurance coverage. Education and training of both physicians and technicians still have a long way to go. The development of affordable positive airway pressure (PAP) machine and the coverage of PAP machine by health care insurance are the two key issues to make this treatment available to more patients.

CONSENT FOR PUBLICATION

Not applicable.

CONFLICT OF INTEREST

The authors declare no conflict of interest, financial or otherwise.

ACKNOWLEDGEMENT

Declared none.

REFERENCES

[1]   Cao XL, Wang SB, Zhong BL, *et al.* The prevalence of insomnia in the general population in China: A meta-analysis. PLoS One 2017; 12(2): e0170772.
        [http://dx.doi.org/10.1371/journal.pone.0170772] [PMID: 28234940]

[2]   Benjafield AV, Ayas NT, Eastwood PR, *et al.* Estimation of the global prevalence and burden of obstructive sleep apnoea: a literature-based analysis. Lancet Respir Med 2019; 7(8): 687-98.
        [http://dx.doi.org/10.1016/S2213-2600(19)30198-5] [PMID: 31300334]

[3]   Ip MSM, Lam B, Lauder IJ, *et al.* A community study of sleep-disordered breathing in middle-aged Chinese men in Hong Kong. Chest 2001; 119(1): 62-9.
        [http://dx.doi.org/10.1378/chest.119.1.62] [PMID: 11157585]

[4]   Liu J, Wei C, Huang L, *et al.* Prevalence of signs and symptoms suggestive of obstructive sleep apnea syndrome in Guangxi, China. Sleep Breath 2014; 18(2): 375-82.
        [http://dx.doi.org/10.1007/s11325-013-0896-2] [PMID: 24072550]

[5]   Richard W W. Lee M, PhD; Sivabalan Vasudavan, BDSc, MDSc, MPH; David S. Hui, MB, BS, MD3; Tania Prvan, PhD; Peter Petocz, PhD; M. Ali Darendeliler, PhD; Peter A. Cistulli, MD, PhD. Differences in Craniofacial Structures and Obesity in Caucasian and Chinese Patients with Obstructive Sleep Apnea. sleep 2010; 33(8): 1075-80.

[6]   Xu L, Keenan BT, Wiemken AS, *et al.* Differences in three-dimensional upper airway anatomy between Asian and European patients with obstructive sleep apnea. Sleep 2020; 43(5): zsz273.
        [http://dx.doi.org/10.1093/sleep/zsz273] [PMID: 31735957]

[7]   Wing YK, Li RHY, Lam CW, Ho CKW, Fong SYY, Leung T. The prevalence of narcolepsy among Chinese in Hong Kong. Ann Neurol 2002; 51(5): 578-84.
        [http://dx.doi.org/10.1002/ana.10162] [PMID: 12112103]

[8]   Han F, Chen E, Wei H, *et al.* Childhood narcolepsy in North China. Sleep 2001; 24(3): 321-4.
        [http://dx.doi.org/10.1093/sleep/24.3.321] [PMID: 11322715]

[9]   Han F, Lin L, Warby SC, *et al.* Narcolepsy onset is seasonal and increased following the 2009 H1N1 pandemic in china. Ann Neurol 2011; 70(3): 410-7.
        [http://dx.doi.org/10.1002/ana.22587] [PMID: 21866560]

[10]   Shi Y, Yu H, Ding D, Yu P, Wu D, Hong Z. Prevalence and risk factors of restless legs syndrome among Chinese adults in a rural community of Shanghai in China. PLoS One 2015; 10(3): e0121215.
        [http://dx.doi.org/10.1371/journal.pone.0121215] [PMID: 25803876]

[11]   Li LH, Chen HB, Zhang LP, Wang ZW, Wang CP. A community-based investigation on restless legs syndrome in a town in China. Sleep Med 2012; 13(4): 342-5.
        [http://dx.doi.org/10.1016/j.sleep.2011.09.008] [PMID: 22172960]

[12]   Ma JF, Xin XY, Liang L, *et al.* Restless legs syndrome in Chinese elderly people of an urban suburb in Shanghai: A community-based survey. Parkinsonism Relat Disord 2012; 18(3): 294-8.
        [http://dx.doi.org/10.1016/j.parkreldis.2011.11.014] [PMID: 22154296]

[13]   Chiu HFK, Wing YK, Lam LCW, *et al.* Sleep-related injury in the elderly--an epidemiological study in Hong Kong. Sleep 2000; 23(4): 1-5.

[http://dx.doi.org/10.1093/sleep/23.4.1e] [PMID: 10875558]

[14]   Y LS. Chinese philosophical and medical views on chronobiology and sleep. 1995.

[15]   Han F. Development of sleep medicine in China. Chin Med J (Engl) 2009; 122(12): 1462-3.
[PMID: 19567172]

[16]   Huang XZ, Liu XL, Chen SC. [Sleep apnea: a report of 5 cases]. Zhonghua Nei Ke Za Zhi 1985;
24(2): 83-86, 125.
[PMID: 3987449]

[17]   McEvoy RD, Antic NA, Heeley E, *et al.* CPAP for Prevention of Cardiovascular Events in Obstructive
Sleep Apnea. N Engl J Med 2016; 375(10): 919-31.
[http://dx.doi.org/10.1056/NEJMoa1606599] [PMID: 27571048]

[18]   Xu L, Han F, Keenan BT, *et al.* Validation of the Nox-T3 Portable Monitor for Diagnosis of
Obstructive Sleep Apnea in Chinese Adults. J Clin Sleep Med 2017; 13(5): 675-83.
[http://dx.doi.org/10.5664/jcsm.6582] [PMID: 28356181]

[19]   The Sleep Assembly of the Chinese Respiratory Society Clinical practice guideline: diagnosis and
management of obstructive sleep apnea syndrome (draft). Zhonghua Jie He He Hu Xi Za Zhi 2002;
25(4): 195-8. [in Chinese].

[20]   The Sleep Assembly of the Chinese Respiratory Society Clinical practice guideline: diagnosis and
management of obstructive sleep apnea syndrome. Zhonghua Jie He He Hu Xi Za Zhi 2012; 35(1): 9-
12. [in Chinese].

[21]   Expert consensus on clinical practice of telemedicine in adult obstructive sleep apnea hypopnea
syndrome. Zhonghua Yi Xue Za Zhi 2021; 101(22): 1657-64. [in Chinese].

[22]   Ren S, Wang Y, Yue F, *et al.* The paraventricular thalamus is a critical thalamic area for wakefulness.
Science 2018; 362(6413): 429-34.
[http://dx.doi.org/10.1126/science.aat2512] [PMID: 30361367]

[23]   Qu WM, Xu XH, Yan MM, Wang YQ, Urade Y, Huang ZL. Essential role of dopamine D2 receptor in
the maintenance of wakefulness, but not in homeostatic regulation of sleep, in mice. J Neurosci 2010;
30(12): 4382-9.
[http://dx.doi.org/10.1523/JNEUROSCI.4936-09.2010] [PMID: 20335474]

[24]   Liu Y, Zhang J, Lam SP, *et al.* A case–control–family study of idiopathic rapid eye movement sleep
behavior disorder. Ann Neurol 2019; 85(4): 582-92.
[http://dx.doi.org/10.1002/ana.25435] [PMID: 30761606]

[25]   Rizzatti FG, Mazzotti DR, Mindel J, *et al.* Defining extreme phenotypes of OSA across international
sleep centers. Chest 2020; 158(3): 1187-97.
[http://dx.doi.org/10.1016/j.chest.2020.03.055] [PMID: 32304773]

[26]   Maski K. Understanding Racial Differences in Narcolepsy Symptoms May Improve Diagnosis. Sleep
2015; 38(11): 1663-4.
[http://dx.doi.org/10.5665/sleep.5130] [PMID: 26446120]

CHAPTER 9

Current Practice of Sleep Medicine in Lebanon

Marie-Louise M. Coussa-Koniski[1,*], **Christy Costanian**[1] and **Alain Michel Sabri**[2]

[1] *School of Medicine, Lebanese American University, Beirut, Lebanon*

[2] *Department of Otolaryngology-Head & Neck Surgery, SSMC-Mayo Clinic, Abu Dhabi, UAE*

Abstract: There are several major universities and medical schools in Lebanon, including the American University of Beirut School of Medicine & Medical Center, Lebanese American University/Medical Center, Lebanese University, Universite Saint Joseph/Hotel Dieu de France, Beirut Arab University, University of Balamand, Saint Georges University/Medical Center, Holy Spirit University of Kaslik and others. Many of these medical centers and schools of medicine offer a solid medical education as well as post-graduate training in various fields of medicine that are related to sleep medicine. These include Pulmonary and Critical Care Medicine, General/Bariatric Surgery, Neurology, Otolaryngology, Head and Neck Surgery, Dentistry, Oral & Maxillofacial Surgery, Orthodontics, Psychiatry, Nutrition/dietetics and other related specialties.

As will be further elaborated in this chapter, there are multiple particularities related to the diagnosis and management of patients who have sleep disorders in Lebanon. Even though the field is developing, there are certainly opportunities for further advancement and development.

Keywords: Awareness campaigns, CPAP, Insurance reimbursement, Insomnia, Ministry of Health, Multidisciplinary sleep disorders team, Obstructive sleep apnea, Patient education, Polysomnograms, Sleep centers, Uvulo-palatopharyngoplasty (UPPP).

INTRODUCTION

Lebanon has a long history of education in general and particularly medical education. The Phoenician alphabet, a precursor to most modern languages, was launched to the world from Phoenecia, modern day Lebanon, around 2000 BCE by Cadmus of Tyre, whose sister Europa was kidnapped and taken to Europe (Greece more specifically). Europe, the continent was subsequently named after

* **Corresponding author Marie-Louise M. Coussa-Koniski:** School of Medicine, Lebanese American University, Beirut, Lebanon; Tel: + 961 1 200800; E-mail: marielouise.coussa@laumcrh.com

Hrayr P. Attarian, Marie-Louise M. Coussa-Koniski & Alain Michel Sabri (Eds.)

her. Beirut hosted the first law school in history (Law School of Berytus: Roman 3rd century AD). Lebanon has witnessed the establishment multiple educational institutions of higher learning, many founded in the 18th century and early 19th, that have spread knowledge and graduated leaders in all fields of science and humanities.

<u>Healthcare Services in Lebanon</u>: are provided by different categories of third party payers.

• A large percentage of the working population are covered by the National Health Social Security (NHSS) and "Mutuelle des fonctionnaires de l'état" corresponding to 23.4% of in and outpatients health expenditure as of 2017, this coverage is valid as long as the person is working and paradoxically it stops at retirement leaving these advanced age persons without medical coverage.

Moreover, because there are always delays in covering new tests or treatments and because sleep Medicine is new in Lebanon, costs of sleep diseases-related tests and treatments are not covered by the local NHSS.

• Ministry of public health and military schemes (Army, Internal Security Forces, General Security, State Security, and Customs) covers 21.4% of in and outpatients' health expenditure as of 2017 and follow NHSS criteria hence they do not cover costs of sleep diseases-related tests and treatments.

• The private sector provides 21.4% of healthcare services through Private insurance or patients self paying particularly in cities and large towns, they cover the costs of tests and treatments related to sleep diseases.

WHAT TYPE OF FACILITIES PROVIDE CARE AND WHAT TYPE OF PRACTITIONERS ARE INVOLVED IN SLEEP MEDICINE?

• Until the year 2000, there were barely no sleep specialists and consequently no dedicated sleep laboratories services. Sleep problems such as insomnia, parasomnias….were generally handled by psychiatrists.

Awareness of the medical community about sleep apnea, which needs a multidisciplinary involvement, was very low.

• With the recent improved understanding and awareness of sleep medicine due to a significant increase of research and publications worldwide; and with the return of trained sleep specialists, several sleep disorders centers and clinics were implemented progressively. Their size is small with a 2-3 beds capacity and sometimes they are co-managed by Pulmonologists and neurologists or Psychiatrists or ENT specialists with an interest in sleep medicine.

The majority of these specialized sleep labs are located in Universities Medical Centers mainly private and in Beirut (11-12 Sleep Centers) and major cities 7-8 (Byblos, Tripoli, Saida, Zahlé, Tyr 1-2 in each town).

The majority of these sleep centers provide clinical diagnosis and suggestions for treatment but frequently no regular follow up and treatment supervision is done. This gap is often filled by the company which sells the machine. This procedure impacts on compliance and long-term results of the treatment.

• Beside these centers several companies located even in remote areas are performing home sleep tests or offering their services to hospitals by non-trained people at much lower prices than the Universities' sleep centers, they are usually commercial companies more interested in selling costly CPAP machines and financial benefits. These practices escape to any quality control and accreditation by scientific societies or regulatory bodies.

• Another aspect of sleep medicine in Lebanon is that despite the limited number of beds in sleep laboratories, the overall occupancy rate is far from being high most probably due to the fact that these centers are private and patients have to pay themselves for the costs.

• Surgical management: The majority of sleep and snoring surgeries are performed by Otolaryngologist/Head and Neck surgeons in the form of Septoplasty, Turbinate Reduction surgery including Radiofrequency and Submucosa Resection, and the traditional Uvulopalato/pharyngoplasty (UPPP). Some Otolaryngologists perform office Radiofrequency treatment to the soft palate and the tongue base (many of these tongue are performed in the operating room). Tongue surgery (reduction), sliding genioplasty, LAUP, and hyoid suspension are not popular at all and hardly performed. Most of these have mostly been abandoned worldwide as well for obstructive sleep apnea. There are few Oral/Maxillofacial surgeons who perform Craniofacial Skeleton surgeries such as Maxillomandibular Advancement procedure, however, rare. There are many dental/orthodondics groups that provide the oral dental mandibular advancement appliance which can be an adjunct to other surgical procedures or is often used on its own in carefully selected cases. The hypoglossal nerve stimulator is not performed yet in Lebanon. There are very few, if any, true organized multidisciplinary sleep disordered teams.

• Bariatric surgery is very popular in Lebanon due to the increasing rate of obesity: the prevalence of obesity in Lebanon in 2019 was 44%, however, awareness about pre and post op evaluation and follow up regarding sleep disorders is low. Multiple centers produce excellent results in bariatric surgery which presumably would have a positive impact on sleep apnea from anecdotal reports.

Sleep Medicine Training

• There is no comprehensive sleep Medicine fellowship training program with accreditation of sleep Medicine as an independent medical specialty.

• The number of sleep specialists presently working in Lebanon is 20-25, they were trained in the US with an American board in sleep Medicine or in Europe with a specialist diploma. The majority of them are Pulmonologists but also a few are Otolaryngology-Head & Neck Surgery specialists, Neurologists, Psychiatrists and Dentists with a subspecialty in sleep medicine and are practicing in university centers.

Recently few Family Physicians started taking care of these patients.

• Sleep Medicine is taught in the universities as part of the Pulmonary, Neurology, ENT, or Psychiatry modules.

• In an attempt to create an individualized sleep medicine entity, the Lebanese Pulmonary Society is working to create a sleep disorders group who will be involved in creating practice guidelines, a regulatory body and delivering continuing education.

Sleep Technologists

There is no individualized, structured and formal sleep technologist training nor a recognized diploma.

Most of the sleep studies are done by either respiratory therapists or in-house trained and mentored experienced staff or biomedical technicians working for the commercial companies, leading to variable standards of practice in sleep laboratories.

Pediatric Sleep Medicine

Although it is estimated that 30% of children may have a sleep disorder at some point during childhood, the research in pediatric population in Lebanon is still in a neonatal stage with a lack of sleep Pediatricians and lack of diagnostic labs.

M. El Habbas *et al.* 2014 [1] showed a significant relationship between unhealthy diet and sleep disorders and its association with poor academic performance, behavioral problems, poor mental and physical health.

Clinical and Research knowledge Gap

Lebanon is a small low-income country in the MENA region. In 2019, the MOPH reported current health expenditure was at 936 USD per capita while 15-65 years had a literacy rate of 99.8% in 2018, and the population aged 14 years and younger was 26% of the total in 2019

Despite the above challenges, there has been significant growth in sleep research and publications in Lebanon since 2000. The worsening of the economic, and political impact of the COVID-19 pandemic has increased the understanding of the numerous adverse health outcomes and the importance of sleep for overall well-being.

The development of the Lebanese Insomnia scale (LIS-18) ((S.Hallit *et al*; 2019) [2] and its evaluation in epidemiologic studies (M.Chahoud; March 2017) [3], (Riachi M. *et al* 2012) [4] validation of the Arabic Version of the Epworth Sleepiness Scale.

Data on the prevalence of sleep disorders in the general Lebanese adult population are scarce and limited to certain geographical areas in the country (Urban areas, special selected samples of the population, cross sectional, epidemiological, bias…). Research in several areas such as: the prevalence of sleep disorders, Insomnia, sleep in psychiatry, in diabetic patients is increasing.

Chami HA .*et al.* [5], in a pilot study on 501 participants from the Greater Beirut area, aged between 35-65 years, reported a prevalence of 44.5% of insomnia symptoms more than 15 nights/month and 34.5% with insomnia disorder classified by ICSD-3 and DSM-5 criteria, significantly higher in prevalence than that reported in developed countries and associated with high prevalence of anxiety (16.7%) and mood disorders (12.6%). This high prevalence has been associated with war and exposure to war trauma. To add, females, those with lower education level and comorbidities, were significantly positively associated with insomnia symptoms in this sample. On the other hand, older age, low family income and unemployment were related to insomnia disorder and have been also associated with the tumultuous geopolitical conditions of the country. In addition, high noise pollution previously reported in greater Beirut which is" 65-79 dBA", higher than levels recommended by the World Health Organization"45-55 dBA" could be also contributing [5]. The findings of this study conducted before the worsening of the political, social and economic situation are already alarming.

As an extension of their aforementioned study, Chami and colleagues [6] studied sleep duration and its associated factors among adults in Beirut and Mount Lebanon. Taken together, the findings of Chami *et al.* [5, 6] emphasize the importance of tackling social determinants of health that in turn, may be related to sleep duration and insomnia, especially since the onset of the financial crisis in October 2019.

Given the unique stressors that this subgroup faces, studies examining sleep disorders in university students in Lebanon were also conducted. Kabrita *et al* [7], Kabrita and Hajjar-Muca [8] and Assaad *et al.* [9], showed that sleep problems in this population are common and they impact on the daily performance, risky behaviors and psychological wellbeing.

Another cross sectional study "Assessing sleep quality of Lebanese high school students in relation to lifestyle: pilot study" (R. Chahine, 2018) [10], concluded that 76.5% of teen agers have poor sleep patterns in Beirut)

These results have important implications for programs to improve academic performance by targeting sleep habits of students.

Isolation and stress brought on by the COVID 19 pandemic recently may negatively impact psychological well-being and impair sleep quality. In a cross-sectional study among healthcare workers who were at the frontlines of the COVID 19 response at a private university hospital in Lebanon, Zarzour *et al.* [11], found that participants reported poor sleep quality. But no studies were done on the sleep abnormalities related to the COVID-19 infection itself.

Large Population-based Studies about Obstructive Sleep Apnea (OSA) in Lebanon are Lacking

H.A Chami *et al.* [5] in their above mentioned cross sectional pilot survey using the Berlin Questionnaire reported that the prevalence of Sleep Apnea was 33.3% higher than that reported in other studies, with same methods, around the world but only 5% were diagnosed by a physician.

A. Choucair *et al.*, 2019 [12] in a cross sectional study showed that physician-diagnosed sleep apnea was 11% compared to the risk of sleep apnea assessed by the Epworth Sleepiness Scale and the STOP-BANG questionnaires were 30.10% and 39.20% respectively.

Another study assessed the epidemiological characteristics of OSA in a retrospective hospital-based historical cohort of adults patients referred for sleep evaluation by polysomnography at a referral center in Beirut (Marie-Louise

Coussa – Koniski *et al* 2019) [13] and showed that despite high prevalence of severe OSA (43%) and symptoms (97%) in these patients, the referral rates were low underlying again low awareness of the medical community, moreover, women presented more atypical symptoms which could explain low representation of women in this cohort and contribute to the under evaluation of OSA in women and lower referral rates.

F.R.Talih *et al.*, 2017 [14] showed in a prospective study using the Berlin Questionnaire and the Epworth Sleepiness Score that the risk of OSA is increased in hospitalized psychiatric patients which has detrimental effects on these patients. Again only a minimal percentage of them received a previous diagnosis of Sleep Apnea underlying the under diagnosis of sleep disorders among psychiatric patients.

Al Sadik *et al.* 2012. BAU [15] aimed to evaluate the dentofacial characteristics in a sample of Lebanese OSA patients and correlate them according to severity and sites of obstruction, A cephalometric study.

D.Khawla *et al.*, 2017 [16] showed that sleep duration impacts on the development of diabetes and overweight in a sample of North Lebanese population.

M.Riachi *et al.*, 2017 [17] evaluated the factors predicting CPAP adherence in Obstructive Sleep apnea Syndrome.

M-L. Coussa-Koniski, A.Sabri *et al.*, are preparing a publication about the association of OSA and Ehler-Danlos Syndrome.

Finally a "Handbook of healthcare in the Arab world" published in 2021 shows very few data on Sleep Medicine in Lebanon, hoping that this book will shed light on the work done in this country in the field of sleep medicine despite all the challenges.

What is Needed?

Lebanon has undergone the epidemiological transition with risk factors shifted from poor sanitation to unhealthy diets and a sedentary lifestyle. Therefore, rates of non-communicable disease have soared in the past 20 years. The prevalence of hypertension in 2019 was at 53%, followed by obesity at 44% and followed by CVD at 29.7% [1]. The age-standardized incidence rates for major cancers were reported to be 200 per 100,000 all being risk factors for Sleep apnea with significant economic impact [18].

In this regard sleep Medicine services are certainly underdeveloped hence the large number of undiagnosed patients, suffering from Sleep Related Breathing Disorders (SRBD) and other sleep diseases. Despite the limited number of beds available to conduct polysomnograms, the overall occupancy rate is low. In addition complications of sleep diseases and their suggestive symptoms are poorly known. For example, studies show that up to 20% of road traffic accidents in the world are sleep-related. Every year more than 1000 people die due road traffic crashes in Lebanon, but no studies were done to evaluate the role of somnolence. (https://wwwq.grsproadsafety.org/programes/countries/Lebanon/).

CONCLUSION

Sleep Medicine in Lebanon as well as the medical corps face several challenges despite the availability of advanced medical institutions and well trained physicians and staff:

• No certified sleep technicians or training programs.

• Lack of coverage of the diagnostic tests and treatments of sleep disease, compounded by the current political, economic and financial crisis which impacts on the quality of care as patients are frequently lost to follow up.

• Consequently technical support, after-sales services and end users education are limited to very few suppliers which also impact negatively on the compliance to the treatment.

• Competition by commercial CPAP suppliers without expertise but with financial objectives, doing home sleep tests at much lower prices and delivering treatments without medical opinion.

• Discrepancy in the availability and delivery of care between cities and rural areas.

• Absence of regulatory bodies and quality control.

• Lack of awareness of the medical community of the necessity of an interdisciplinary approach, with low referral rates to sleep specialists.

• Lack of awareness amongst the population about sleep disorders and the serious consequences on the health of patients. Scarcity of national awareness and educational campaigns.

• In many instances, lack of an organized structures and research/clinical funding to assist clinicians in conducting their research.

• Women access to care.

• Need for more prospective large scale studies and a national more detailed and comprehensive database.

• Regulation of driving licenses.

• Absence of Obstructive Sleep Apnea Multidisciplinary teams where the sleep experts including pulmonary physician, neurologists, otolaryngologists, psychologists/psychiatrists, bariatric surgeons, dentists/orthodontists, dieticians and sleep technologists work together to discuss individualized therapy for our patients.

• Offer other alternative therapies for sleep apnea such as hypoglossal nerve stimulators and the Oral Mandibular advancement appliance [19, 20].

A collaborative organized work with the various aforementioned sleep specialists, hospitals, health authorities-governmental agencies/ministry of health and insurance companies is urgently needed to further advance the important public health challenge that is sleep apnea and improve the delivery of healthcare in this field to a wider segment of the population by providing education, awareness campaigns, equipment and funding. Additionally University training programs are encouraged to include sleep Medicine in the curriculum and to train specialists, sleep technicians and offer continuous medical education and research in this important subspecialty [21].

CONSENT FOR PUBLICATION

Not applicable.

CONFLICT OF INTEREST

The authors declare no conflict of interest, financial or otherwise.

ACKNOWLEDGEMENT

Declared none.

REFERENCES

[1]   El Habbas Maya, Rajab Mariam, Ziad Fouad, Abou Merhi Bassem. Sleep Disorders in Lebanese Children: prevalence, relation with dietary habits and impact on children behaviors Int J of current res in life sciences; 2014; 3(12): 076-82.

[2]   Hallit S, Sacre H, Haddad C, *et al.* Development of the Lebanese insomnia scale (LIS-18): a new scale to assess insomnia in adult patients. BMC Psychiatry 2019; 19(1): 421.
        [http://dx.doi.org/10.1186/s12888-019-2406-y] [PMID: 31881985]

[3]   Chahoud M, Chahine R, Salameh P, Sauleau EA. Reliability, factor analysis and internal consistency calculation of the Insomnia Severity Index (ISI) in French and English among Lebanese adolescents. 2017. eNeurologicalsci 2017; 7: 9-14.

[4]   Riachi M, Juvelekian G, Sleilaty G, Bazerbachi T, Khayat G, Mouradides C. Validation of the Arabic Version of the Epworth Sleepiness Scale: multicenter study. Rev Mal Resp 2012; 29(5): 697-704.
[http://dx.doi.org/10.1016/j.rmr.2011.12.017] [PMID: 22682596]

[5]   Chami HA, Bechnak A, Isma'eel H, *et al*. Sleepless in Beirut: Sleep Difficulties in an Urban Environment With Chronic Psychosocial Stress. J Clin Sleep Med 2019; 15(4): 603-14.
[http://dx.doi.org/10.5664/jcsm.7724] [PMID: 30952222]

[6]   Chami HA, Ghandour B, Isma'eel H, Nasreddine L, Nasrallah M, Tamim H. Sleepless in Beirut: sleep duration and associated subjective sleep insufficiency, daytime fatigue, and sleep debt in an urban environment. Sleep Breath 2020; 24(1): 357-67.
[http://dx.doi.org/10.1007/s11325-019-01833-3] [PMID: 31028521]

[7]   Kabrita C, Hajjar-Muça T, Duffy J. Predictors of poor sleep quality among Lebanese university students: association between evening typology, lifestyle behaviors, and sleep habits. Nat Sci Sleep 2014; 6(Jan): 11-8.
[http://dx.doi.org/10.2147/NSS.S55538] [PMID: 24470782]

[8]   Kabrita C, Hajjar-Muça T. Sex-specific sleep patterns among university students in Lebanon: impact on depression and academic performance. Nat Sci Sleep 2016; 8(Jun): 189-96.
[http://dx.doi.org/10.2147/NSS.S104383] [PMID: 27382345]

[9]   Assaad S, Costanian C, Haddad G, Tannous F. Sleep patterns and disorders among university students in Lebanon. J Res Health Sci 2014; 14(3): 198-204.
[PMID: 25209906]

[10]   Chahine R, Farah R, Chahoud M, Harb A, Rami Tarabay E. Sauleau,R.Godbout. Assessing sleep quality of Lebanese high school students in relation to lifestyle: pilot study. Easter. Mediterr. Health J. 2018 2018; 28(8): 722-8.

[11]   Zarzour M, Hachem C, Kerbage H, Richa S, Choueifaty DE, Saliba G. Anxiety and sleep quality in a sample of Lebanese healthcare workers during the COVID -19 outbreak. Encephale 2021; (Sept): S0013700621001895.
[PMID: 34728067]

[12]   Choucair Aurelie. Diana Malaeb, Souheil Hallit, Elissar Dagher. University St Esprit Kaslik. 2021.

[13]   Coussa-Koniski ML, Saliba E, Welty FK, Deeb M. Epidemiological characteristics of obstructive sleep apnea in a hospital-based historical cohort in Lebanon. PLoS One 2020; 15(5): e0231528.
[http://dx.doi.org/10.1371/journal.pone.0231528] [PMID: 32413035]

[14]   Talih F, Ajaltouni JJ, Tamim HM, Kobeissi FH. Risk of obstructive sleep apnea and excessive daytime sleepiness in hospitalized psychiatric patients. 2017. Neuropsyvchiatric disease and treatment. 13:1193-1200.

[15]   Al Sadik Oussama Abu Baker. Dentofacial characteristics of Obstructive Sleep Apnea patients in relation to severity and obstruction sites 2012 BAUedulb

[16]   Khawla D, Rima H, Sleiman F, Al-Isakandarani M, Koubar M, Hoteit M. Insufficient Sleep is a contributor to overweight and type 2 diabetes in adults. 2017. Intern. J.of Diab Res;. 6(4): 83-90.

[17]   Riachi M, Najm S, Iskandar M, Choucair J, Ibrahim I, Juvelekian G. Sleep Breath 2017; 21: 295-302.
[http://dx.doi.org/10.1007/s11325-016-1408-y] [PMID: 27638725]

[18]   https://wwwq.grsproadsafety.org/programes/countries/Lebanon/

[19]   Olson MD, Junna MR. Hypoglossal Nerve Stimulation Therapy for the Treatment of Obstructive Sleep Apnea. Neurotherapeutics 2021; 18(1): 91-9.
[http://dx.doi.org/10.1007/s13311-021-01012-x] [PMID: 33559036]

[20]   Metz JE, Attarian HP, Harrison MC, *et al.* High-Resolution Pulse Oximetry and Titration of a Mandibular Advancement Device for Obstructive Sleep Apnea. Front Neurol 2019; 10: 757.
[http://dx.doi.org/10.3389/fneur.2019.00757] [PMID: 31379712]

[21]   Attarian HP, Sabri AN. When to suspect obstructive sleep apnea syndrome. Postgrad Med 2002; 111(3): 70-6.
[http://dx.doi.org/10.3810/pgm.2002.03.1137] [PMID: 11912998]

CHAPTER 10

Sleep Medicine in Armenia

Haykuhi Hovakimyan[1,2] and **Samson G. Khachatryan**[1,2,*]

¹ Department of Neurology and Neurosurgery, National Institute of Health, Yerevan, Armenia

² Sleep Disorders Center, Somnus Neurology Clinic, Yerevan, Armenia

Abstract: Sleep medicine is a young branch of Armenian medicine. In this chapter, we presented the history of sleep medicine development in Armenia. After brief initial information about Armenia as a country, references to sleep and sleep disorders in medieval Armenian folklore and medicine are given. An overview of the current situation with sleep medicine in Armenia is presented. A special attention is given to the spectrum of sleep-related specialists who work(ed) in Armenia, and to the domains of sleep medicine available. Acknowledgement of world sleep experts who helped and contributed to the development of sleep medicine and sleep research in Armenia follows. Also, we discuss different organizations operating in the field of sleep in Armenia, their activities and pursued goals. Importantly, the main results of a sleep disorders prevalence study in Armenia are presented. At the end, we summarize the problems and issues accumulated in the field of sleep medicine in Armenia.

Keywords: Armenia, Folklore, History, Sleep, Sleep medicine, Somnology.

INTRODUCTION

The Republic of Armenia is a developing parliamentary state with the capital Yerevan and ten regions - administrative divisions called marzes. Armenia is an ancient country geographically located on Armenian Highlands in South Caucasus and served as a connecting state between Europe and Asia for centuries. Prunus armeniaca (Armenian plum), the Latin scientific name for apricot, is one of the symbols of the country and is even represented as one of three colors of the national flag. The population of Armenia is 2.9 mln according to the World Bank's 2019 report [1]. The official language is Armenian which is a separate branch of the Indo-European language group. The Armenian language is widely used also in the Armenian diaspora which refers to the Armenians leaving outside of Armenia. Approximately 7 mln Armenians are living out of motherland in around 100 countries of the world.

* **Corresponding author Samson G. Khachatryan:** Chairman, Department of Neurology and Neurosurgery, National Institute of Health, President, Armenian Sleep Disorders Association, Titogradyan 14, Yerevan 0087, Armenia, Tel: +37491519641; E-mail: drsamkhach@gmail.com

Hrayr P. Attarian, Marie-Louise M. Coussa-Koniski & Alain Michel Sabri (Eds.)

According to the Armenian health system evaluation, the life expectancy in Armenia at birth is higher than the average of the Commonwealth of Independent States (CIS), similar to neighboring Georgia, but it is inferior to the average of the developed European countries.

Armenia's population can receive medical care on two main levels - primary and secondary. The primary level of healthcare is represented by the outpatient clinics. Despite many gaps, the Armenian healthcare system is trying to improve the quality and the effectiveness of patient treatment in this area. This is done through a system of qualification and accreditation programs. The secondary level of medical care includes hospitals and specialized clinics. Usually, the diagnostic methods used on this level are more difficult to access due to relatively low availability and affordability. Currently, the functioning of the Armenian healthcare system improves. The COVID-19 pandemic, despite causing serious load and strain to Armenia's health system, also played a positive role in making it more flexible and diversified.

The study of sleep and its disorders is an important feature for the medical field in any country. Stressing the importance of sleep disorders in the general medical field and relevant medical disciplines brings a lot more success than ignoring its role. Countries with well-established sleep medicine benefit from better public health indicators and improved productivity of employees and students.

Implementing the sleep hygiene rules and conducting sleep importance propaganda inevitably influences the population's general health. Knowing these benefits, a developing country with a low level of physicians' sleep-related qualification and lack of sleep medicine's technical capabilities should seek to develop sleep medicine. Although sleep medicine globally is a rather young specialist field and started to separate as medicine's branch from the late 1970s to early 1980s with standard recommendations of sleep scoring, while by 1990s there already existed a unified internationally accepted classification of sleep disorders [2 - 4]. Armenia had no traditions of sleep medicine before the Soviet Union had collapsed. The country had to develop its own health system thereafter being expectedly focused on more urgent medical fields like cardiovascular, oncology, infectious and surgical fields. Understandably, only after those directions are changed to a better condition the country could have thought about sleep medicine. In this chapter, we are focusing on Armenia's historical and cultural contributions, the development and current situation with sleep medicine in the country, the management of sleep disorders, and the future of sleep medicine in Armenia.

SLEEP AND CULTURE

Sleep has been the focus of humanity's attention since ancient times. To this day, it continues to be one of the most mysterious phenomena in nature and in human physiology. Sleep and various manifestations associated with sleep have been studied for many centuries by a variety of scholars in the field of philosophy, theology, and medicine. It could not help but find its deserved place in the field of art, such as literature, art, and music, *etc.* In different times, sleep and sleep-related manifestations appeared in the work of a variety of authors [5].

Armenian culture is also no exception. Research into Armenian literature revealed one interesting fact related to sleep. In Armenian national epic poem called "The Daredevils of Sassoun" or "Davit of Sassoun", a characteristic depiction of Klein-Levin syndrome was found and described, which is probably the first-ever description of this syndrome, as the poem dates back to the eighth century C.E [6].

In the 15th century C.E., the Armenian medieval physician and naturalist Amirdovlat Amasiatsi emphasized the role of sleep and the importance of the sleep-wake period for a human being. Amirdovlat was a famous doctor and pharmacist during that period. Having studied his works, one can see that in the Middle Ages medicine in Armenia and the region was quite progressive. In his works, he described human anatomy, hygiene, pathology, and pharmacology. He also has works dedicated to causes of the pathologies and different diseases, symptoms that characterize the clinical picture, treatment, and care of the patient, explored medical features of various plants, their prevalence, location, and application for treatment of diseases. He dedicated a whole chapter to sleep in his "Ogut Bzhshkutyan" ("The Benefits of Medicine") book and frequently referred to its importance in many other chapters. He wrote his works in Middle Armenian, also in Greek, Arabic, Persian, French, Turkish, and used to refer to the works of other medical scholars (Fig. **1**). Gurunluoglu et al. carried out an important summary of Amirdovlat's scientific and medical works, presenting his valuable heritage to the international medical community [7].

Such works allow us to conclude that with a deeper and more detailed cultural research of ancient medicine and other fields, we can find a lot of hidden and interesting information about the understanding of sleep function and its disorders in older times.

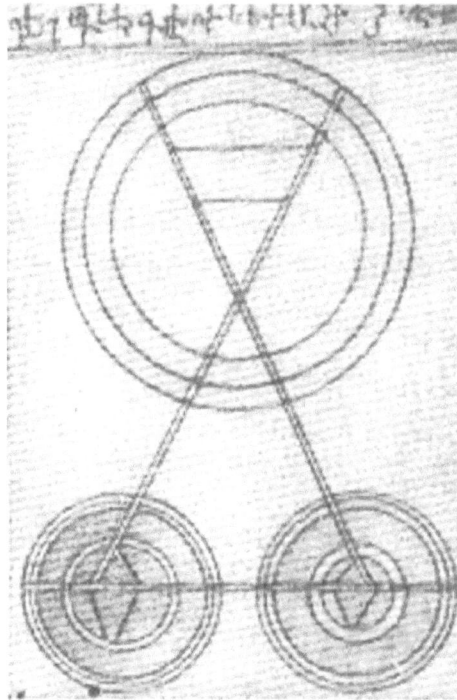

Fig. (1). Visual pathways described by Amirdovlat Amasiatsi in his "The Benefits of Medicine" book. 15th century C.E.

Sleep Medicine Development in Armenia

Although sleep medicine as a separate field was not present in Armenia, the development of neurology and especially epileptology in the 1990s stimulated some more knowledge of sleep disorders and their diagnostic approaches. The development of epileptology in Armenia, promoted by late Prof. Vahagn Darbinyan, was essential for younger Armenian neurologists to get introduced also with sleep and its effects on epilepsy, its patterns on EEG recording, the role of sleep deprivation as a provoking mechanism of abnormal EEG activity. The improvement of epilepsy practice brought also a necessity to differentiate between epileptic and non-epileptic phenomena connected to sleep. Witnessing the interesting interactions between sleep and epilepsy, and facing sleep apnea management issues during stroke patient management the author (S.K.) was inspired for later involvement in this field. The first edition of Kryger's "Principles and Practice of Sleep Medicine" book [8] found on the shelves in their Neurology department opened additional insights to understand the structure and importance of sleep medicine as an independent medical specialty field with big potential to develop. These intentions were further shaped by the initiatives coming from the Armenian Medical Association's president Dr. Parounak

Zelveian, who as a cardiologist, interested in the connection of sleep apnea and hypertension, was putting efforts to involve other specialists and to support the development of the sleep medicine in Armenia.

Training in Sleep Medicine and Sleep Research

Only a few specialists to date had appropriate training in sleep medicine and/or sleep research abroad. The author - Dr. Samson Khachatryan (S.K.) - had several trainings in sleep at various centers and institutions. Most notably he was granted the American Academy of Sleep Medicine Mini-Fellowship Program for International Scholars (2006) spent at the Cleveland Clinic Foundation's Sleep Disorders Center (mentored by Dr. Nancy Foldvary-Schaefer) [9]. His training was kindly supported also by the Armenian Medical Association (ArMA).

Other very important trainings by Armenian sleep specialists included Dr. Marina Petrosyan's research fellowship visit to Athens Univesity's Sleep Center. Dr. Samson Khachatryan visited New-York Cornell Medical Center's Comprehensive Sleep and Epilepsy Centers (with Dr. Charles Pollack, Prof. Arthur Spielman - sleep, and Dr. Cynthia Harden - epilepsy), Sleep and EEG laboratory at InselSpital, University of Bern (with Prof. Johannes Mathis), Sleep Center of Innsbruck University Clinic (mentored by Prof. Birgit Hogl) and European Sleep Research Society's (ESRS) research training grant spent at Lugano Regional Medical Center's Epilepsy and Sleep Center (led by Prof. Mauro Manconi). Supported by the latter program Ms. Lilit Ghahramanyan – a clinical psychologist from Armenia – visited the Freiburg Sleep Center (Prof. Dieter Riemann) to improve her knowledge and skills in sleep disorders, especially insomnia research and cognitive-behavioral therapy for insomnia (CBT-I). She later spent a year in Bern at InselSpital's sleep center (Profs. Claudio Bassetti, Johannes Mathis, Wolfgang Schmitt) with her sleep research program on "Anhedonia and insomnia" supported by a Swiss government research grant. Ms. Haykuhi Hovakimyan – a clinical psychologist - was also awarded a training grant from ESRS, which was postponed due to the COVID-19 situation. She will be trained in the Freiburg Sleep Center, as well.

From 2007-2010 ESRS was conducting a 4-year Marie-Curie project entitled "Training in Sleep Research and Sleep Medicine", and considering its unique format it was a great opportunity for the author (S.K.) to participate in its last edition and establish close connections with a large group of prominent tutors – leaders of sleep research in Europe, also visiting the Centre of Neuroscience of Lyon and spending some time with the "Physiopathologie des réseaux neuronaux du cycle veille-sommeil" team, led by Prof. Pierre-Herve Luppi. It gave him a valuable chance to get introduced to experimental sleep research, the organization of many important projects to have ideas for the possible future implementation of basic sleep research in Armenia. One of this Project's greatest achievements was creating perfect networking environment for young sleep researchers from across Europe. Many of them have become well-known specialists in their countries and professional fields and keep close connections with each other stimulating ongoing international collaborations.

Despite the difficult phase of formation, sleep medicine in Armenia had and continues to have persons who at different times and to a different extent were involved in sleep disorders management or sleep-related research (Table 1).

Table 1. Specialists from Armenia with different involvement and interests in sleep disorders and/or sleep medicine practice.

Name Surname	Specialty	Sleep Medicine/Research Field
Vahagn Darbinyan	Neurology, epileptology	Parasomnias
Ada Tadevosyan	Psychiatry	Sleep and stress
Arthur Shukuryan	Otolaryngology	Sleep apnea
Nubar Aslanyan	Biochemistry	Chronobiology
Samson Khachatryan	Neurology, sleep medicine, epileptology (ESRS certified somnologist)	Comprehensive sleep medicine practice
Marina Petrosyan	Pulmonology	Sleep-related breathing disorders
Parounak Zelveian	Cardiology, hypertension	Sleep apnea and hypertension
Hrant Ter-Poghosyan	Orthodontics	Sleep apnea, sleep bruxism
Zaruhi Tavadyan	Neurology, movement disorders	Sleep in movement disorders
Lilit Ghahramanyan	Clinical psychology	Insomnia, CBT-I, Behavioral sleep medicine
Gegham Khandanyan	Otolaryngology	Sleep apnea
Zhirayr Arabyan	Pediatric otolaryngology	Pediatric sleep apnea
Astghik Baghdasaryan	Pediatric pulmonology, allergology	Pediatric sleep apnea

Sleep Specialists Visiting Armenia

Prof. Karl Doghramji was among the first sleep specialists to visit Armenia and deliver a great overview lecture in 2006. With the efforts of ArMA and its neurology division led by Dr. Samson Khachatryan, a two-day symposium on sleep disorders was held in Yerevan (2007) with the involvement of leading sleep researchers and academics (Profs. Claudio Bassetti, Diego Garcia-Borreguero, Markku Partinen, Thomas Pollmacher, Jean Krieger). It raised bigger attention to the sleep medicine field and gave to the listeners a perfect overview of the most important topics in sleep disorders. Later, other prominent sleep researchers, clinicians, and academics visited Armenia, through years helping to promote and keep sleep awareness high in the country (Hrayr P. Attarian, Sudhansu Chokroverty, Jan Ulfberg, Peter Halasz, Lori Panosian, Helen Baghdoian, Ralph Lydic, Wolfgang Oertel, Sonia Nevsimalova, Rodolfo Soca, Mikhail Poluektov, Roman Buzunov, Sahak Mahseredjian, Lia Maisuradze) supported by sleep technologists of Armenian origin (Vardan Shahmuradyan, Armen Sargsyan).

Prof. Hrayr P. Attarian (Northwestern University) had a great involvement in helping Armenian colleagues with article writing and participated in some important sleep-related publications which were key to present some of the Armenian sleep research efforts on the international level [6, 10]. Prof. Jan Ulfberg helped with the first epidemiological study of sleep and its disorders in the Armenian population [11].

Professors Helen Baghdoian and Ralph Lydic are helping Dr. Khachatryan's efforts with the establishment of basic sleep research in Armenia.

Through visits to various foreign sleep centers, the introduction and practical involvement into different "schools" were important to feel the quintessence of the American and European sleep medicine traditions, practice, and research. These were incorporated into the initial steps of sleep medicine practice implementation in Armenia. The sleep technicians in Armenia were trained by the sleep specialist (S.K.) as there was no specific local training program. Experienced Armenian diaspora sleep technology specialists - Dr. Vardan Shahmuradian and Dr. Armen Sargsyan - used their invaluable efforts in improving the technological side of sleep practice in Armenia.

Unfortunately, the introduction of sleep disorders medicine was initially met by ignorance and low demand from the local medical field. The available few sleep specialists were conducting many seminars and round-table meetings with different medical specialists trying to raise interest in the problem of sleep and its disorders. The establishment of equipped sleep center furthered this process and helped in making clinical somnology more familiar to physicians and more applicable in their clinical practice. Polysomnography started to find its place among neurological diagnostic studies while home-based sleep apnea testing boosted the diagnosis and treatment of obstructive sleep apnea (OSA) and made it more popular among cardiologists, pulmonologists, ENTs, and other physicians. In 2008 a manual of practical recommendations for ENT specialists was published for the diagnosis and treatment options of obstructive sleep apnea. In 2019 a guideline on the management of insomnia was developed by the Armenian

Ministry of Health (moderated by Dr. Samson Khachatryan), based on internationally available evidence and local peculiarities. However, it still needs to be implemented, which is a common issue for the guidelines in the Armenian medical field.

More recently, there were important changes to the procedural side of expert medical assessment related to sleep disorders. Narcolepsy and sleepwalking were officially recognized in the military service expertise and involved polysomnography as a diagnostic tool to support the diagnosis. Some other expertise systems (disability assessment, justice practice, police recruitment and retirement) were similarly revised. There is also constant interest in the field from the dental community, mainly in orthodontics. A few specialists are involved in the dental management of sleep apnea and sleep-related bruxism.

Sleep Facilities and Services in Armenia

Currently, there are three laboratories/centers providing sleep diagnostics and sleep disorders management to patients in need. They are all located in the capital of Armenia - Yerevan. Two of these are mostly focused on sleep apnea diagnosis and management using home sleep apnea testing, and only rarely attended studies. The third one - Sleep and Movement Disorders Center of Somnus Neurology Clinic is the only facility in Armenia providing multi-component sleep management. Our center is located at a large multidisciplinary hospital and is in good professional interaction with relevant departments (neurology, cardiology, pulmonology, ENT, *etc.*). Its staff is composed of neurologists, a clinical psychologist, a psychiatrist, and sleep technicians. This one-bed sleep center provides sleep diagnostic studies in the form of polysomnography, EEG-monitoring (combined studies), MSLT, MWT, and actigraphy. Several home sleep apnea testing devices are available, and help to facilitate OSA diagnosis in a priori clear and uncomplicated adult cases and are also used for pediatric OSA diagnosis. CPAP-titration is used mostly in the form of out-of-center auto-titration. Manual titration and split-night studies are rarely used. The diagnostic studies are done mostly for adults, but children are also frequently investigated at the center in collaboration with pediatric hospital specialists.

Several sleep-assessment scales (Epworth Sleepiness Scale, Pittsburgh Sleep Quality Index, and Berlin Questionnaire) are translated into Armenian, validated, and used in clinical practice and research projects [12 - 14]. Some other scales are also under validation (Karolinska Sleepiness Scale, Parkinson Disease Sleep Scale - 2, RBD-I, *etc.*). Sleep diaries and sleep logs are routinely utilized alongside quality of life instruments. Cognitive-behavioral therapy for insomnia (CBT-I) is available since the beginning of the Center's work and its demand increases with time so is the practice. Sleep treatments include various PAP modalities (CPAP, BPAP, Auto-PAP) with devices usually rented by the patients, and blue light therapy. No sleep telemedicine is available at the moment, although it is being considered for implementation in the future.

Being also an academic site for the Department of Neurology and Neurosurgery of the Armenian National Institute of Health (ANIH) makes the Somnus Sleep Center a site for sleep education for residents and fellows of neurology and other relevant departments of ANIH, and also for neurologists passing their 5-year CME accreditation program. Thus, sleep disorders as a focused topic are involved in these curricula, prompting more dissemination of general knowledge for sleep and its disorders among Armenian clinicians.

Armenian Sleep Disorders Association (ARSDA)

Armenian Sleep Disorders Association (ARSDA) [15] was founded in 2011 by Dr. Samson Khachatryan and is the only organization in Armenia aimed at dissemination and development of sleep medicine and sleep research. With the establishment of ARSDA, the Armenian sleep field gained another milestone to voice sleep problems to the public, to authorities, and to proceed with some important projects. ARSDA's main goal is to raise awareness about sleep, its disorders, and pathological manifestations in society and among professional groups (medical professionals, psychologists, and other related specialists).

From the beginning of its activities, ARSDA tried to maintain its goals through various activities and special programs, cooperations with students, residents, specialists from different medical areas, local and international medical, educational, healthcare organizations.

Among the main activities stands out the door-to-door survey that was held in 2015-2017 with the participation of active members of ARSDA, including practicing doctors, medical students, neurology and cardiology residents, psychologists, *etc.* The survey aimed at assessing the prevalence of various sleep habits, complaints, and disorders in the Armenian population.

On October 10, 2019, in collaboration with ANIH, ARSDA hosted a round table discussion entitled "The role of sleep medicine in healthcare system". It was organized jointly by ARSDA, ANIH, and the Assembly of National Sleep Societies (ANSS) of ESRS. Representatives from Romania and Russia presented their experience and model of development of sleep medicine in their countries. The above-mentioned epidemiological data and trends of sleep disorders in Armenia were also discussed at the meeting. It ended with a general round-table discussion and suggestions towards the development and acknowledgment of sleep medicine by the Armenian healthcare system. Different government and insurance organizations were invited to participate not attended by some of them. Based on this meeting's materials a joint position statement was prepared for publication in the newly established Armenian Journal of Health and Medical Sciences – the official journal of ANIH.

This was a pilot event of the "Beyond Boundaries" project which was proposed by the ANSS Executive Committee and aimed at helping European countries with underdeveloped sleep medicine to find solutions, fill some important gaps, educate specialists, *etc.*, and could be tailored to particular needs. In this case, the meeting was dedicated to raising awareness of many problems accumulated in Armenia's sleep medicine and served as a good model to evaluate the Project's positive potential and limitations, helping to shape it further. It included also the next day's educational seminar titled "Sleep Research and Sleep Medicine" attended by a variety of specialists related to sleep.

The ANSS Executive Committee group, visiting Armenia, included a pleiad of prominent European sleep specialists, including Barbara Gnidovec Strazisar (ANSS President, Slovenia), Ysbrand van der Werf (The Netherlands), Lyudmila Korostovtseva (ANSS secretary, Russia), Johan Verbraecken (Belgium), Oana Deleanu (Romania) who were joined by Dr. Samson Khachatryan – also an ANSS board member - as a host from ARSDA/ANIH. For the first time, the events were supported on the level of Director of ANIH, Dr. Alexander Bazarchyan and Vice-Minister of Health, Ms. Lena Nanushyan.

Every year with participation in the World Sleep Day activities since 2008 the issue of sleep and its disorders was raised in Armenia by Dr. Samson Khachatryan numerous times and in different formats. From seminars and other educational events to press conferences and TV appearances, the World Sleep Day activities in Armenia gained important media coverage and medical field attention. In 2020, right before the pandemic-related restrictions were applied, Dr. Samson Khachatryan and his team continued to hold various meetings. This activity was marked by receiving a Distinguished Activity Award from the World Sleep Society for his efforts to disseminate knowledge about sleep and its disorders in Armenia.

The end of 2020 was quite difficult for Armenia, because a war erupted, after which Armenian soldiers, alongside various psychological traumas, acquired also problems with sleep. Thus, as a World Sleep Day 2021 activity, special seminars were organized for military medical personnel and separately for soldiers. It was dedicated to the improvement of sleep disorders knowledge among specialists and the dissemination of sleep hygiene rules among soldiers, carefully conducted by

Haykuhi Hovakimyan. At the moment, ARSDA continues its active work, accentuating the importance of sleep in maintaining and improving health and quality of life.

EPIDEMIOLOGY OF SLEEP DISORDERS IN ARMENIAN POPULATION

Sleep disorders are common worldwide, with insomnia and sleep apnea being the most frequently encountered entities [16 - 18]. As it was already mentioned above, ARSDA conducted several epidemiological studies to assess the prevalence of different sleep complaints, sleep disorders, and their comorbidities in the Armenian population.

One of the most important epidemiological studies was the multi-site, rural, and urban population-based door-to-door survey conducted by ARSDA in 2015-2017 [11].

We studied sleep-wake time, average sleep duration, sleep-related habits, and complaints, including insomnia, excessive daytime sleepiness, sleep-related breathing disorders (snoring, sleep apnea), restless legs syndrome, and other sleep problems.

One thousand and one participants aged 18 years and above were included in this study. The survey was conducted at four different sites in the country taking into account geographic specificity and altitude: Bagratashen (rural/North/lowest), Yerevan (urban/West/low-to-average), Akner (rural/South/high), Ayrk/Verin Shorzha (rural/East/highest).

The survey form contained twenty-seven questions assessing sleep time, important co-morbidities, insomnia, restless legs syndrome, snoring and apnea, excessive daytime sleepiness, and sleep-related behaviors. The results show that the mean sleep duration was 6.7 hours. Insomnia and daytime sleepiness were the most prevalent sleep disorders in the Armenian population (Fig. **2**).

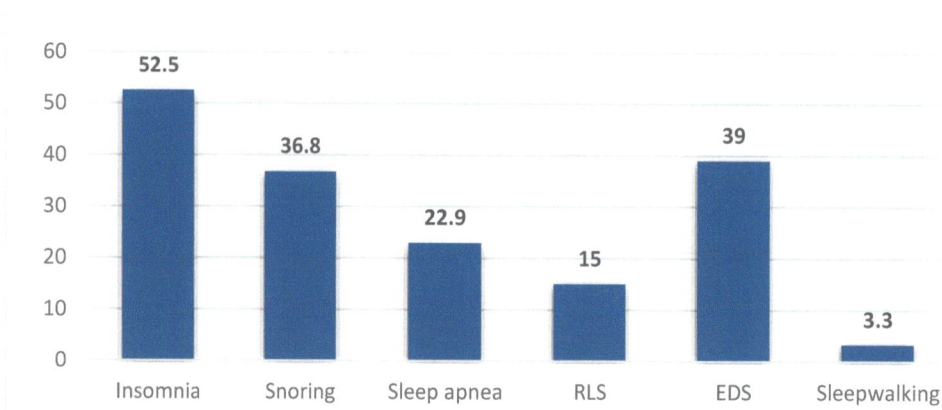

Fig. (2). Prevalence of sleep disorders in Armenia (%). RLS – restless legs syndrome, EDS – excessive daytime sleepiness.

In 2013-2014 ARSDA conducted a survey to assess sleep-related habits and prevalence of sleep disturbances among medical students [19]. This anonymous assessment was carried out by a questionnaire, which contained questions related to main sleep habits. Sleep latency, daytime sleepiness, sleep-related behavioral and movement complaints, sleep hygiene, and participation in medical duties were assessed. Overall 295 medical students with a mean age of 19.8 years completed the questionnaire. As the results show, Armenian medical students prefer to study mostly in the evenings and late at night (43.4%). Mean sleep duration was 6.7 hours and daytime sleepiness was the most common complaint. Those with shorter sleep duration (6 hours or less, 36.1%) mentioned more problems with memory and concentration (p= 0.016). Interestingly, the academic performance among more senior medical students (years 6 and 7, n=49) correlated with sleep duration, but such a result was not seen in the general sample.

An earlier telephone survey was conducted among 1269 adults in Yerevan, who were evaluated for the prevalence of restless legs syndrome (7.9%) [20].

During all these years, within its frame of activities ARSDA regularly conducts other sleep-related prevalence studies in collaboration with clinical and educational institutions, such as specialized sleep disorders clinic and medical universities: 1) study of sleep problems and sleep disorders during COVID-19 lockdown, 2) sleep-related symptoms among Armenian military servicemen after the recent war in Artsakh, 3) traffic accidents related to sleep at the wheel and its connections to sleep apnea and excessive daytime sleepiness [21 - 23].

Clinical and Basic Sleep Research

Overall, sleep research in Armenia is represented by clinical research. Basic or experimental research is not done and was lacking since Soviet Armenian times. It is surprising considering that several well-established research institutes of biochemistry, physiology, and molecular biology were active in fundamental research and continue producing quality output, but none of them ever focused on sleep. However, there is a Memorandum of Understanding signed recently by the Institute of Molecular Biology and Department of Neurology and Neurosurgery of Armenian National Institute of Health, to plan and explore possible collaboration and projects in neuroscience, including sleep research.

The situation is somewhat better with clinical sleep research, with some researchers doing active research in respective fields. It is mostly focused on sleep in epilepsy, sleep in Parkinson's disease, obstructive sleep apnea in cardiology, pulmonology, and ENT. Studies on OSA profiling among the Armenian population, included in Dr. Marina Petrosyan's Doctor of Medical Sciences research program, were an important achievement for Armenian sleep medicine [24 - 27].

A large direction of research is being conducted around sleep and epilepsy interaction. Led by S.K. this is a multidirectional research study, which involves in the process also young investigators, medical students, and clinical psychologists, helping them to participate in a research project and also to present some pieces of this work at various congresses [28]. Some important data for the general sleep research field were obtained from this study, *e.g.* confirmation of RLS and the first description of sleep bruxism both having higher prevalence among epilepsy patients compared to the general population [10].

Another important research direction related to sleep is the work of Dr. Zaruhi Tavadyan, who is focused on non-motor symptoms of Parkinson's disease. Sleep disorders form an important part of this study.

Other research activities of our group included sleep during COVID-19 lockdown (mentioned above), and "RLS and altitude". The latter was incorporated into the prevalence study of sleep disorders in the general population of Armenia. The RLS and altitude study is planned and performed in collaboration with Prof. Jan Ulfberg (Sweden) [29].

CHALLENGES AND GAPS OF SLEEP MEDICINE IN ARMENIA

Currently, sleep medicine as a field is still far from being established. This is mostly coming from the lack of coverage for sleep disorders, their diagnostics, and treatment from government-supported and private medical insurance programs.

In general, the following are obvious obstacles to the development of sleep medicine in Armenia:

- Lack of knowledge about sleep medicine as a field and ignoring many sleep disorders among doctors and related professionals.

- Low referral rate from relevant medical specialties.

- Pediatric sleep medicine is underdeveloped, but slowly moving forward, an agreement with a big children's hospital in Yerevan was reached to build a pediatric sleep laboratory.

- Many sleep medicines are not available in Armenia (*e.g.* modafinil, methylphenidate, suvorexant, zolpidem, sodium oxybate, bupropion, pitolisant, *etc.*) or are strictly controlled making them unattractive to industry to register.

- Overall, patients with narcolepsy have serious problems with finding their drugs abroad.

- PAP-therapy device import is hampered by customs rules applying taxes to respiratory therapy devices.

- No major sleep industry manufacturer is represented in Armenia.

- "Sleep at the wheel" as an important health issue is not appropriately addressed by authorities.

- The local tech support usually is unfamiliar with the devices used in sleep medicine (diagnostic and PAP-therapy), while sending the devices abroad for repair is costly.

- Some cultural difficulties exist in the way of implementing cognitive-behavioral therapy for insomnia, PAP-therapy adaptation, scale-based assessments, and sleep diary-keeping.

- A big problem exists with the reimbursement of sleep diagnostics and treatments, as many companies consider sleep disorders as chronic and do not reimburse, while government reimburses only severe cases and sometimes expertise. This issue will be addressed in various ways in the coming years.

- From an educational point of view, there is a big need to improve curricula for many specialty fields, including appropriate and updated information about sleep medicine, which will inevitably improve the patients' diagnosis and communication between specialists.

As seen above, there are still important issues in the sleep medicine field in Armenia. These include educational gaps, lack of governmental support, and issues related to availability and cultural acceptance.

FUTURE PERSPECTIVES

With increased attention from the government to sleep medicine as an important health issue influencing social life, there will be possibilities to remove some obstacles mentioned in the chapter and increase the importance of sleep health for the Armenian society. Finally, with the increased involvement of young specialists and researchers, sleep medicine will develop and establish itself as an important medical field in Armenia.

CONSENT FOR PUBLICATION

Not applicable.

CONFLICT OF INTEREST

The authors declare no conflict of interest, financial or otherwise.

ACKNOWLEDGEMENT

Declared none.

REFERENCES

[1]   The World Bank. https://data.worldbank.org/indicator/SP.POP.TOTLaccessed on July 18, 2021

[2]   Rechtschaffen A, Kales A. (1968) A Manual of Standardized Terminology, Techniques and Scoring System for Sleep Stages of Human Subjects. Public Health Service, Washington DC, US Government Printing Office.

[3]   Pelayo R, Dement WC. History of Sleep Physiology and Medicine. In: Kryger M.H., Roth T., Dement W.C., editors (2016) Principles and Practice of Sleep Medicine, Sixth edition, Elsevier, 3-15.

[4]   American Academy of Sleep Medicine. International classification of sleep disorders, revised: Diagnostic and coding manual. Chicago, Illinois: American Academy of Sleep Medicine 2001.

[5]   Shapiro CM, Boquiren F, Boquiren V, Sherman D. Sleep in art and literature. In: Kryger, M.H., Avidan, A.Y., Berry, R.B., (2010) Atlas of Clinical Sleep Medicine. 1st Edition. Elsevier, 1-7.

[6]   Khachatryan SG, Attarian HP. Possible description of Kleine-Levin syndrome in "The Daredevils of Sassoun" Armenian medieval epic poem. Sleep Med 2020; 73: 246-9.
        [http://dx.doi.org/10.1016/j.sleep.2020.07.006] [PMID: 32861982]

[7]   Gurunluoglu A, Gurunluoglu R, Hakobyan T. A medieval physician: Amirdovlat Amasiatsi (1420–1495). J Med Biogr 2019; 27(2): 76-85.
        [http://dx.doi.org/10.1177/0967772016682726] [PMID: 28092465]

[8]   Kryger MH, Roth T, Dement WC, Eds. editors (1989) Principles and Practice of Sleep Medicine, Saunders Company, W. B.

[9]   Sleep medicine news and updates. J Clin Sleep Med 2006; 02(03): 366-70..
       [http://dx.doi.org/10.5664/jcsm.26604]

[10]   Khachatryan SG, Ghahramanyan L, Tavadyan Z, Yeghiazaryan N, Attarian HP. Sleep-related movement disorders in a population of patients with epilepsy: prevalence and impact of restless legs syndrome and sleep bruxism. J Clin Sleep Med 2020; 16(3): 409-14.
       [http://dx.doi.org/10.5664/jcsm.8218] [PMID: 31992428]

[11]   Khachatryan S, Ghahramanyan L, Stepanyan A, Darabyan A, Isayan M, Hovakimyan H, *et al.* 2020.Prevalence of sleep disorders in the adult population of Armenia: an epidemiological study.

[12]   Isayan, M., Hovakimyan, H., & Khachatryan, S. (2020, September). Validation of the Armenian version of the Epworth sleepiness scale. In Journal of Sleep Research (Vol. 29, pp. 279-279). 111 River ST, Hoboken 07030-5774, NJ USA: Wiley.

[13]   Hovakimyan, H., Isayan, M., & Khachatryan, S. (2020, September). Validation of the Armenian version of the Pittsburgh sleep quality index. In Journal of Sleep Research (Vol. 29, pp. 241-241). 111 River ST, Hoboken 07030-5774, NJ USA: Wiley.

[14]   Hovakimyan, H., Isayan, M., & Khachatryan, S. (2020, September). Validation of the Armenian version of the Berlin questionnaire. In Journal of Sleep Research (Vol. 29, pp. 241-242). 111 River ST, Hoboken 07030-5774, NJ USA: Wiley.

[15]   Armenian Sleep Disorders Association, Official website, https://armsleep.org/ accessed on July 18, 2021.

[16]   Grandner MA. Sleep, health, and society. Sleep Med Clin 2017; 12(1): 1-22.
       [http://dx.doi.org/10.1016/j.jsmc.2016.10.012] [PMID: 28159089]

[17]   Kansagra S. Sleep disorders in adolescents. Pediatrics 2020; 145 (Suppl. 2): S204-9.
       [http://dx.doi.org/10.1542/peds.2019-2056I] [PMID: 32358212]

[18]   Benjafield AV, Ayas NT, Eastwood PR, *et al.* Estimation of the global prevalence and burden of obstructive sleep apnoea: a literature-based analysis. Lancet Respir Med 2019; 7(8): 687-98.
       [http://dx.doi.org/10.1016/S2213-2600(19)30198-5] [PMID: 31300334]

[19]   Ghahramanyan L, Karamyan A, Budumyan A, Khachatryan S. (2016, September). Sleep complaints, sleep habits and their association with academic performance among medical students in Armenia. In Journal of Sleep Research (Vol. 25, pp. 375-376). 111 River ST, Hoboken 07030-5774, NJ USA: Wiley-blackwell.

[20]   Khachatryan SG, Tavadyan ZD, Margaryan HS, Mouradyan HS, Zelveian PA. O0040 Prevalence of restless legs syndrome in the general adult population of Yerevan, Armenia. Sleep Med 2007; 8(8): S57-8.
       [http://dx.doi.org/10.1016/S1389-9457(07)70222-8]

[21]   Khachatryan S, Isayan M, Hovakimyan H, Vardanyan L. (2020). Effects of novel coronavirus pandemic and self-isolation on sleep disorders. Journal of Sleep Research. Vol. 29, p. 188. 111 River ST, Hoboken 07030-5774, NJ USA: Wiley.

[22]   Isayan M, Hovakimyan H, Khachatryan S. (2020, September). The prevalence of sleep-related car accidents in Armenia. In JOURNAL OF SLEEP RESEARCH (Vol. 29, pp. 189-190). 111 River ST, Hoboken 07030-5774, NJ USA: Wiley.

[23]   Hovakimyan H, Khurshudyan E, Grigoryan K, Ghunyan G, Tunyan T, Khachatryan S. Prevalence of sleep disturbances and the role of flashbacks among military servicemen after acute stress related to war. 7th Congress of the European Academy of Neurology, Virtual, Volume. Eur J Neurol 2021; 28 (Suppl. 1): 653.

[24]   Petrosyan M, Perraki E, Simoes D, *et al.* Exhaled breath markers in patients with obstructive sleep

apnoea. Sleep Breath 2008; 12(3): 207-15.
[http://dx.doi.org/10.1007/s11325-007-0160-8] [PMID: 18074162]

[25] Khandanyan G, Shukuryan A, Khachatryan S, Zelveian P. P0093 Estimation of prevalence of patients at risk for sleep disordered breathing in ENT outpatient clinic attendants (a pilot study). Sleep Med 2007; 8(8): S93.
[http://dx.doi.org/10.1016/S1389-9457(07)70349-0]

[26] Zelveian PH, Buniatian MS, Khachatryan SG, Oschepkova EV, Rogoza AN. Features of night pulse oximetry in patients with arterial hypertension and obstructive sleep pnoea/hypopnea syndrome. New Armenian Medical Journal 2008; 2(3): 49-61.

[27] Zelveian PA, Dgerian LG. [Microalbuminurea as an early indicator of renal lesion in arterial hypertension]. Klin Med (Mosk) 2014; 92(5): 11-7.
[PMID: 25782301]

[28] Isayan M, Vardanyan L, Hovakimyan H, Tavadyan Z, Khachatryan SG. The impact of restless legs syndrome on health-related quality of life in epilepsy. Eur J Neurol 2020; 28 (Suppl. 1): 653.

[29] Khachatryan S, Tavadyan Z, Ulfberg J. (2020, September). Correlation of restless legs syndrome with oxygen saturation: implications for altitude. In JOURNAL of Sleep Research (Vol. 29, pp. 326-326). 111 River ST, Hoboken 07030-5774, NJ USA: Wiley.

CHAPTER 11

Current Practice of Sleep Medicine in Turkey

Caner Sahin[1,*] and **Gozde Orhan Kubat**[1]

[1] Department of ENT, School of Medicine, Alanya Aladdin Keykubat University, Alanya/Antalya, Turkey

Abstract: Sleep Medicine is considered a relatively new specialty in medicine. The practice of sleep medicine in Turkey began in the late 20th century. Sleep medicine in Turkey has developed with the opening of several sleep medicine facilities. The Turkish Medical Association and the Ministry of Health oversee the accreditation of sleep centers as well as certify sleep specialists. The diagnosis and proper treatment of obstructive sleep apnea are important when obtaining driver's licenses and serving in the military. The major hurdles that the sleep medicine community faces in Turkey are financial especially in the current, post COVID-19, and Russian-Ukranian war economic crisis. In addition to these barriers, there are also gaps in knowledge and awareness particularly as it pertains to interethnic differences in sleep disorders' susceptibility.

Keywords: Accreditation, Certification, Financial barriers, Sleep Medicine, Turkey.

INTRODUCTION AND HISTORY

Sleep Medicine is considered a relatively new specialty that is still open to significant transformative changes. More advancements in the field are taking place in the developed world and high income countries than in the developing, middle and low income ones.

The practice of sleep medicine in Turkey began in late 20th century. The earliest studies were performed by physicians of various specialties who had specific interest in sleep medicine. In 1992, the Sleep Research Association was first established at Istanbul Univiersity's Cerrahpasa Faculty of Medicine. Five years later, the Council of Ministers renamed it as Turkish Sleep Research Association. Since then, the Association has become one of the largest and most influential scientific organizations dealing with sleep medicine in the country as well as the one with the largest membership. In the charter convention held in 2007, the name

---

* **Corresponding author Caner Sahin:** Department of ENT, School of Medicine, Alanya Aladdin Keykubat University, Alanya/Antalya, Turkey; Tel: +90 2425106060; Fax: +90 242 510 61 39; E-mail: drcaner2001@gmail.com

Hrayr P. Attarian, Marie-Louise M. Coussa-Koniski & Alain Michel Sabri (Eds.)

of the association was again changed to the "Turkish Sleep Medicine Association". Another organization, "The Sleep Association", was also established in the previous year.

ACCREDITATION AND PRACTICE

Sleep medicine in Turkey has developed with the opening of several accredited sleep medicine facilities in different parts of the country.

Currently, there are 38 facilities providing sleep medicine services accredited by "The Association of Sleep" and another 56 that are accredited by "Turkish Sleep Medical Association". These clinics or facilities are divided into two categories, academic centers and clinical centers. The first group includes sleep medicine laboratories that reside in universities and teaching/research hospitals. The second group encompases sleep laboratories at state hospitals and private clinics and medical centers.

The physician in charge at the sleep disorders center can be from any primary specialty as long as they demonstrate competency and be certified in sleep medicine. The Training Certificate is awarded according to the criteria set by the body accrediting the sleep center (Table **1**). The sleep associations provide both the didactic and clinical education that constitutes the sub-specialty sleep training (Table **2**). The physician in charge must also be a member of the accrediting association. The Ministry of Health then follows up on subsequent accreditation maintenance processes.

Table 1. Requirement for Accreditation of An Academic Sleep Laboratory.

The Sleep Laboratory Must Be located Within a Medical School or an Academic and Research Hospital.	The laboratory Should Perform a Monthly Minimum of 20 Diagnostic and 10 PAP Titrations Studies.
The physician in charge must be certified by and a member of the Sleep Association.	The trainee must submit 100 individual patient studies that they have scored.
The technologist in charge must be likewise certified.	All physicians working at the laboratory should have a minimum of 2 hours a day of training.
The sleep laboratory must have a minimum of 2 beds.	The sleep laboratory should be able to accommodate a variety of sleep complaints and disorders.
The sleep laboratory should be open to run studies and analyze and score records during working hours.	The sleep laboratory should be able to provide samples of daytime studies (MSLT/MWT) that have been conducted and scored on site.

In Turkey, sleep education was not part of the medical school curriculum until 10 years ago. Today, sleep disorders education has been added to the core curriculum of all medical schools, some even provide up to a total of 24 hours of sleep education spread out over the medical school years.

Table 2. Criteria for Sleep Medicine Certification for Physicians.

Clinical Training Must be Completed Within 2 Years of the Didactic Course.	
The Trainee Must Meet the Following Requirements Within 1 Month	Observe the Scoring of 20 PSGs
	Score 30 PSGs
	Observe the PSG hookup of 5 patients
	Perform 5 PSG hookups
	Perform 5 extended EEG studies to monitör for seizure disorders
	Perform 5 PAP titrations
	Perform 3 MSLT studies.
At the conclusion of the month of clinical training. the physician in charge of the center should assess whether the trainee has gained sufficient experience to be certified and provide a written report to the Sleep Association in that regard.	

Furthermore, because sleep medicine is an interdisciplinary speciality. Further sleep education is also provided during certain specialty training *e.g.* Pulmonology, Otolaryngology, Neurology and Psychiatry.

"The Sleep Association" and "The Turkish Sleep Medicine Association" both offer courses for postgraduate sleep training. There are also 2 year certification programs that offer clinical sleep training . Both associations have close to a thousand members. Apart from these two associations, there are 8-10 smaller ones with 50-100 members each. These Ministry of Health accredited associations provide training for sleep technologist.

The Ministry of Health Certified Training Regulation was ratified and published in the Official Constitution No. 28903 on February 04, 2014. The law regulates the certification and registration of training programs by the Ministry of Health. In order to be covered under the above regulation, the specialty must first be determined as a certified training field. The "Regulation on the Improvement and Evaluation of Quality in Health" was published in the Official Gazette No. 29399 and ratified on June 27th 2015 . The coverage of sleep laboratory standards has 8 distinct sections:

1- Physician in charge

2- Technical Staff

3- Administrative Staff

4- Polysomnography Rooms

5- Monitoring room

6- Polysomnography

7- Patient Reporting

8- Archive

Healthcare Coverage

About 98% of people in Turkey are covered by the Social Insurance Institutions(SII). Another 2% depend on private insurance. Over 5 million immigrants receive healthcare coverage under special status insurance through the Ministry of Foreign Affairs.

Guidelines published by the American Academy of Sleep Medicine (AASM) and The European Sleep Research Society (ESRS) are also commonly used in setting laboratory standards. In addition, SSI has its own guidelines on the type of devices that they allow and payment plans for various sleep disorder therapies. . The type of device selected for treatment of sleep related breathing disorder (SBD) is based on "The Social Insurance Institution" guidelines. To make the diagnosis of SBD, a single physician's attestation is sufficient as long as the physician is either an otolaryngologist, neurologist, specialist of chest diseases or psychiatrist. Signatures from 3 specialist physicians are required on the PAP device recommendations. The relevant documents are sent to SSI and examined, and as a result, a fixed amount of payment in Turkish Liras (TL) is provided to the patient to purchase the specific device [1].

Diagnostic Sleep Testing

Diagnostic sleep tests can be performed for any sleep disorder listed in the International Classification of Sleep Disorders (ICSD3). These include all sleep breathing disorders, insomnia, parasomnias, hypersomnias, circadian rhythm sleep-wake disorders and sleep-related movement disorders.

There are 4 types of overnight sleep tests performed in Turkey. Type 4 is the simplest (single air flow monitor and pulse oximetry). Type 3 is cardiorespiratory monitoring with pulse oximetry, airflow monitors, respiratory effort from both thoracic and abdominal belts and sometimes ECG and limb movement monitoring. Type 1 and type 2 are polysomnographies with EEG as well as respiratory and movement monitoring. Type 2 is done at home while type 1 is done in the sleep laboratory or hospital. In Turkey, type 1 testing is most commonly done. This is because SII will only reimburse for studies reporting sleep staging through EEG channels.

SII provides financial support for diagnostic tests and treatments for sleep disorders. In cases where PAP devices are used, SII will pay for a few state approved device types. SII will pay for 20% of the device cost and the patients pay for the difference themselves. Not all the devices are well validated thus creating a major problem. SII also provides some support for surgical treatments, however, cranial nerve stimulators are not covered.

Driving Regulations

Obstructive sleep apnea (OSA) has been identified as an important risk factor in motor vehicle accidents. This risk can be mitigated by treating the OSA with appropriate positive airway pressure (PAP). Based on this, the European Union has changed its driving license directives. Turkey also has changed its requirements to coincide with the EUROPEAN UNION DIRECTIVE 2014/85 [2, 3]. Accordingly, drivers suspected of having moderate or severe OSA should be evaluated by a certified physician before obtaining or renewing their license. They may also be advised to not drive until the diagnosis is confirmed or ruled out. Driver or driver candidates with a confirmed diagnosis of moderate or severe OSA can only obtain a driver's license after an authorized medical specialist confirms that they are receiving adequate treatment, are compliant with it and benefit from it. Drivers diagnosed with moderate or severe OSA and being treated should periodically undergo medical evaluations for the OSA. For Group 1 drivers (those with personal driving licenses), the reevaluation should be at least once every 3 years, for Group 2 (commercial vehicle drivers) the reevaluation should be at least once a year.

In Turkey, individuals with severe OSA (AHI> 30 / hour) or those with moderate OSA (AHI between 15 and 30/hour) and daytime drowsiness cannot obtain a driver's license without receiving treatment first. Turkey's mandatory health report to obtain a driving license consists of 4 parts:

● Part I: Demographics and the individual's photograph.

● Part II: This part is to be filled out by the primary care provider working in health facilities, family health centers, or private health institutions.

● Part III: This part is to be filled out by the relevant specialist physicians working in health facilities or private health institutions.

● Part IV: This part is to be filled by the commission established within the provincial / district health directorate in case a motor vehicle with special equipment is required.

Driver / Driver Candidates will fill in the declaration form and declare to the physician whether they have a "sleep disorder (OSA) and excessive daytime sleepiness". The primary care physician will review the declaration form and examine the driving license candidate who does not report conditions specified in the declaration form, fill in the second part of the medical report according to the examination findings, and prepare the health report. In case the candidate declares suffering from one or more of the conditions listed on the declaration form, the primary care provider will prepare their part of the report and then forward it to the specialist to fill out the third portion.

Obstructive Sleep Apnea and Military Service

The Republic of Turkey has compulsory military service for men over a certain age. Periodic health evaluations, including for sleep disorders are performed on these recruits because excessive daytime sleepiness can lead to attention definition. Screening for OSA is specially important for naval and air force commissioned officers. According to the Turkish Air Force Regulations; pilots with OSA can only qualify for category 4 flights if they have a blood oxygen saturation nadir of 80% or higher and an AHI of less than 15/hour.

People with chronic obstructive pulmonary diseases with severe dysfunction and clinical symptoms or with severe OSA with an AHI of 30/hour or even higher CPAP treatment are exempted from military service.

Patients with obstructive pulmonary diseases such as chronic bronchitis, emphysema, bronchial asthma, and OSA with AHI of 15 to 30 after CPAP treatment receive 1 year deferral from military service.

OSA is increasingly becoming a source of disability and disability-based retirement. Severe OSA disability rate in Turkey is estimated to be 35%. Disability, social security and early retirement applications due to severe OSA are also on the rise.

Challenges to the Practice of Sleep Medicine

Government Social Security covers 98% of Turkish citizens. Enrollees in the Social Security program (SII) contribute to the fund on a monthly basis and on a sliding scale depending on their income and financial circumstances. Sleep Medicine is primarily covered by SII and it determines both diagnostic and therapeutic guidelines for sleep disorders. With increased applications for driving licenses, disability and retirement, there has been a higher demand recently for sleep medicine services. Moreover, 5 million non-citizen immigrants receive medical care free of charge. Approximately 85 million people in Turkey need sleep medicine evaluation and treatment and this has strained the existing sleep medicine resources. The result is a longer wait for appointments at sleep centers. In addition, there has been a decline in the number of sleep study beds which create more problems for healthcare professionals.

In primary care clinics, obesity and daytime sleepiness as well as applications for military service and driver's licenses are triggers for sleep center referrals. Primary care physicians are trained to recognize signs of sleep disorders and legally obligated to refer these patients to sleep centers.

SII policies also affect the economics of sleep centers. SII reimburses only $20 for an overnight sleep test. Starting a sleep laboratory on the other hand costs $ 20,000 and up. Since this is a financially untenable situation, most hospital administrators are not supportive of establishing sleep centers within their institutions. This is primarily because those managing state hospitals are held accountable for their institution's financial wellbeing and sleep centers certainly are not lucrative enterprises. This results into lower number of functioning sleep centers and prolonged wait times and delays in treatment. Home sleep tests are not accepted by SII as evidence for PAP need, therefore, these types of tests currently are used only as screening devices.

Another compounding variable has been the worsening financial difficulties due to the COVID-19 pandemic. Equipment for sleep laboratories are purchased in USD while SII reimburses in TL. The exchange rate between the two currencies has been affecting sleep center's negatively. In addition, SII only replaced equipment once every 10 years. The price of PAP devices ranges from about $ 500- $ 3000, with an estimated average price around $ 850 for CPAP and $1300 for BiPAP. The cost difference is covered by the patient.

Because both hospitals and physicians are reimbursed on a fee for service basis and sleep medicine does not adequately reimburse, most private institutions are moving away from diagnosing and treating sleep disorders. In academic centers, sleep medicine is practiced because it helps specialists build their career.

Sleep laboratories are increasingly being concentrated at academic and research hospitals. Even though most of these were originally established for research purposes, they have become the primary providers for sleep disorder diagnoses-treatments.

The Republic of Turkey is composed of 7 different ethno-geographic regions each with different socioeconomic strata. However, the health-related SII offers only a single, standard approach. It provides free diagnostic testing in every region, regardless of it being an urban or rural environment. It provides payment in TL for treatment as outlined above. Currently, due to the COVID-19 pandemic and the volatile curreny exchange market, there is a financial crisis yet SII continues to only issue the lowest standard payment for PAP devices. Especially during the pandemic and the related currency devaluation, the cost of PAP devices in (TL not USD) has increased but SSI's payment structure has not changed. This has placed a financial burden on patients as they have to pay for the difference themselves.

One of the biggest barriers to getting adequate sleep care is the level of sociocultural development within a specific community. Patients who come from more developed and educated backgrounds, it is more likely they are to comply with treatment. Overall public awareness of sleep disorders is gradually increasing primarily because of driver licensing and other similar regulations dealing with sleep discussed above. In addition, the ability to show patients their oximeter tracings as well as those of respiratory patterns in OSA has increased treatment compliance. In some patients who cannot tolerate CPAP, the more expensive BiPAP has become cost prohibitive due to the devaluation of the TL in comparison to the USD.

Clinical and Research Knowledge Gaps

Kokturk *et al.*, in their epidemiological study, determined the OSA prevalence in Turkey to be 1.9% in men and 0.9% in women [4]. The prevalence of sleep apnea varies, however, among the various ethnic groups. In recent years, more than 5 million immigrants have been living in the country and different ethnicities coexist. In Turkey, unlike countries with more homogeneous populations, accurate epidemiological analysis is hard. Also, different lifestyles and different diets pose different disease risks to people living on the Aegean coast vs. the Mediterranean [5, 6]. In addition, there are physiognomonic differences among different groups. For example; inhabitants of the Black Sea region tend to have unique nasal anatomy that predisposes them to rhinological pathologies while Central Anatolia people tend to have shorter and wider necks predisposing them to OSA. There are ongoing studies on this subject. The extensive influx of refugees in recent years has been a further hindrance to accurate epidemiological studies.

Nevertheless, regional studies on sleep disorders, including insomnia and other non-breathing related sleep disorders have been published in recent years [7 - 9].

Financial constraints have hindered sleep research as well. Most studies need grants either from the EU or the Scientific and Technological Research Council of Turkey (TUBITAK). In order to conduct research, SII requires obtaining written permission for the use of the relevant information. In addition, in order to give this permission, the SSI requires proof that the study is medically necessary. If the study is conducted without obtaining this permission, SII may choose to bill the researcher for the costs associated with the study. Obtaining the said permission can be time-consuming due to bureaucratic hurdles.

The COVID-19 pandemic has reduced the number and frequency of sleep medicine congresses. At the same time, since some of the sleep centers are allocated to pandemic patients, the number of centers that can provide practical training has declined. During the sleep certification process, there is an obligation to work actively in a clinic for 1-6 months. During the pandemic, this aspect of sleep education is interrupted. Therefore there is an increased need for online training opportunities especially in recent years. This is both cost-effective and addresses the decline in physical spaces where training and education take place.

CONCLUSION

In this chapter, we explained differences, economic burden, organization schemes, government rules and restrictions of Sleep Apnea Disease in Turkey.

CONSENT FOR PUBLICATION

Not applicable.

CONFLICT OF INTEREST

The author declares no conflict of interest, financial or otherwise.

ACKNOWLEDGEMENT

We would like to thank Prof. Dr. Bülent Çiftçi and Prof. Dr. Hüseyin Lakadamyalı for their contribution to the article.

REFERENCES

[1]   SII Health Payment Notification. 2020.

[2]   *Oğuz KÖKTÜRK* Classification of Sleep Related Breathing Disorders, Definitions and Obstructive Sleep Apnea Syndrome (Epidemiology and Clinical Features). Turkiye Klinikleri J Pulm Med-Special Topics 2008; 1(1): 40-5.

[3]   McNicholas WT, Ed. New Standards and Guidelines for Drivers with Obstructive Sleep Apnoea Syndrome: Report of the Obstructive Sleep Apnoea Working Group. Brussels: European Commission 2013.

[4]   *Oğuz KÖKTÜRK* Classification of Sleep Related Breathing Disorders, Definitions and Obstructive Sleep Apnea Syndrome (Epidemiology and Clinical Features). Turkiye Klinikleri J Pulm Med-Special Topics 2008; 1(1): 40-5.

[5]   Ozdemir L, Akkurt I, Sümer H, *et al.* The prevalence of sleep related disorders in Sivas, Turkey. Tuberk Toraks 2005; 53(1): 20-7.
[PMID: 15765283]

[6]   Benbir G, Demir AU, Aksu M, *et al.* Prevalence of insomnia and its clinical correlates in a general population in Turkey. Psychiatry Clin Neurosci 2015; 69(9): n/a.
[http://dx.doi.org/10.1111/pcn.12252] [PMID: 25384688]

[7]   Yavuz F, Kabaağıl B, İsmailoğulları S, Zararsız G, Per H. Investigation of the Frequency of Sleep Disorders and its Change According to Classes, Gender and Body Mass Index. J Turk Sleep Med 2019; 6: 88-92.
[http://dx.doi.org/10.4274/jtsm.galenos.2019.46036]

[8]   Tümer A, İlhan B. Incidence of insomnia in young people. OPUS - International Journal of Society Research 2017; 7(13): 426-39.

[9]   National Sleep Epidemiology Survey in the Adult Community (TAPES). http://78.189.53.61/-/uyku/11uykusunu/8_a_demir.pdf [Acces date: August 2014]

CHAPTER 12

Past, Present, and Future Directions of Sleep Medicine in Thailand

Naricha Chirakalwasan[1,2,3,*], **Tayard Desudchit**[2,3,4], **Aroonwan Preutthipan**[3,5,6], **Khunying Nanta Maranetra**[3], **Prapan Yongchaiyudh**[3], **Chairat Neruntarat**[7,8], **Yotin Chinvarun**[3,9] and **Naiphinich Kotchabhakdi**[3,10]

[1] *Division of Pulmonary and Critical Care Medicine, Department of Medicine, Faculty of Medicine, Chulalongkorn University, Bangkok, Thailand*

[2] *Excellence Center for Sleep Disorders, King Chulalongkorn Memorial Hospital, Thai Red Cross Society, Bangkok, Thailand*

[3] *Sleep Society of Thailand, Bangkok, Thailand*

[4] *Division of Pediatric Neurology, Department of Pediatrics, Faculty of Medicine, Chulalongkorn University, Bangkok, Thailand*

[5] *Ramathibodi Hospital Sleep Disorder Center, Ramathibodi, Bangkok, Thailand*

[6] *Division of Pediatric Pulmonology, Department of Pediatrics, Ramathibodi Hospital, Mahidol University, Bangkok, Thailand*

[7] *Department of Otolaryngology, Faculty of Medicine, Srinakharinwirot University, Bangkok, Thailand*

[8] *Sleep Apnea Association, Bangkok, Thailand*

[9] *Neurology division, Department of Medicine, Phramongkutklao Royal Army Hospital and Medical College, Bangkok, Thailand*

[10] *Research Center for Neuroscience and Salaya Sleep Research Laboratory, Institute of Molecular Biosciences, Mahidol University Salaya, Nakornpathom, Thailand*

Abstract: Sleep Medicine is a growing discipline in Thailand. The formal 2-year-sleep medicine fellowship was approved by medical council of Thailand and established under four specialties including internal medicine, psychiatry, pediatrics, and otolaryngology in 2018. Thailand has also established formal sleep technologist courses and certification examinations since 2010. Sleep Society of Thailand was established in 2009 and subsequently other sleep societies were also established. All societies contributed to the development and advancement of sleep medicine in Thailand including the development of national clinical practice guidelines. There are limited numbers of sleep laboratories in the country particularly in government settings. Fortunately, polysomnography conducted at a sleep laboratory in a government hospital

* **Corresponding author Naricha Chirakalwasan:** Division of Pulmonary and Critical Care Medicine, Department of Medicine, Faculty of Medicine, Chulalongkorn University, 1873 Rama IV Road, Pathum Wan, Bangkok 10330, Thailand; Tel: +66-2-256-4000 ext 80741, +66-84-9629502; Email: narichac@hotmail.com

Hrayr P. Attarian, Marie-Louise M. Coussa-Koniski & Alain Michel Sabri (Eds.)

is covered by most of the health care coverage programs. However, CPAP cost is only covered by the civil service welfare system, limited private health insurance, certain state enterprise or government employees. There has been an increasing number of research in the field of sleep medicine in recent years. However, multicenter, multidisciplinary, longitudinal studies in the field of sleep medicine are still lacking. Internationalization in terms of hosting international conferences and awards by the international sleep society has increased the visibility of Thailand regionally and globally. Collaboration among various disciplines is the key to advancing the field forward.

Keywords: Continuous positive airway pressure (CPAP), Polysomnography, Sleep laboratory, Sleep medicine, Sleep medicine research, Sleep Society of Thailand, Thailand.

INTRODUCTION

Sleep medicine is a relatively new discipline in Thailand. It has recently gained more interest and was recognized as a unique entity by the medical council of Thailand in 2018. Concurrently, a formal 2-year-sleep medicine fellowship was approved under four specialties including Medicine, Psychiatry, Pediatrics, and Otolaryngology. However, there is no formal regulation in terms of board requirements for physicians to practice sleep medicine or interpretation of polysomnography. The same lack of regulation is relevant to practice for sleep technologists in Thailand. The nation established guidelines for pediatric and adult obstructive sleep apnea to standardize medical practice for this common sleep disorder. Fortunately, in Thailand, polysomnography conducted at a government hospital is generally reimbursable for most of the health care coverage. However, continuous positive airway pressure (CPAP) is only reimbursable for the civil service welfare system and some limited private health insurance policy. There is more interest in sleep medicine research in recent years with many publications in an international peer-reviewed journal. Thailand is honored to have hosted many international sleep conferences and received world sleep day activity awards for many consecutive years. This chapter will cover the past, present, and future directions of sleep medicine in Thailand.

THE CURRENT PRACTICE OF SLEEP MEDICINE IN THAILAND

Previously till now, sleep medicine practitioners in Thailand are generally intercalated medical specialty including pulmonologist, neurologist or otolaryngologist for adult obstructive sleep apnea and pediatrician for pediatric obstructive sleep apnea, respectively. Psychiatrists, internists, or general practitioners commonly treat insomnia patients. Other sleep disorders could be treated by one of the aforementioned medical specialties [1].

In 2009, a group of medical practitioners who were internationally trained or certified in sleep medicine or with extended experience in managing sleep disorders established the Sleep Society of Thailand (SST) in 2009 [2]. In order to certify the first group of sleep medicine specialist in Thailand, the American Academy of Sleep Medicine (AASM) provided examination material for the first sleep medicine certification. A total of 10 physicians passed the examination and was the first badge to be certified as sleep medicine specialist in Thailand. Subsequently, SST hosted its own certification examination for physicians who met the prerequisite criteria for a number of polysomnography interpretations, sleep disorder consultations, or demonstrable completion of training from an accredited sleep medicine fellowship program abroad. A total of 41 physicians was certified as sleep medicine specialists by SST (26 internists, 8 otolaryngologists, 6 pediatricians, and 1 psychiatrist). A few institutions have started their sleep medicine fellowship program. Chulalongkorn University established the first of the nation's international sleep medicine fellowship program in 2011. To date, there were 16 physicians completed this international sleep medicine fellowship training program (10 international sleep medicine physicians and 6 Thai sleep medicine physicians). Furthermore, 1-year sleep medicine fellowship similarly has been offered at Siriraj hospital. In addition, a Master of Science (MSc) in sleep medicine has also been available at Ramathibodi hospital and Siriraj hospital [3].

Aiming to advance the field of sleep medicine to international standard, in 2018, SST approached the medical council of Thailand and proposed sleep medicine as one of the recognized sleep specialties in Thailand along with a formal sleep medicine fellowship establishment. Eventually, a 2-year-sleep medicine fellowship was approved under four specialties including internal medicine, psychiatry, pediatrics, and otolaryngology. To date, there are a total of 40, 8, 12, and 45 physicians certified as sleep medicine specialists for medicine, psychiatry, pediatrics, and otolaryngology under the medical council of Thailand, respectively. The formally trained 2-year-sleep medicine fellow from medicine was first enrolled in 2019 and graduated in 2021. The one-year sleep in neurology certification program jointly developed by the Sleep Neurology Association and the Thai Neurological Society was first started in 2020. This transition will continuously increase a greater number of formally trained sleep medicine specialists and likely would advance the care of sleep disorders in Thailand.

The ancillary professions are as important for the practice of sleep medicine. Sleep technologist is one of the major drives of sleep medicine field. An inadequate number of sleep technologists is the major drawback of advancing sleep medicine in Thailand and globally. Since 2010, SST has conducted a 5-day basic level sleep technology course annually. In addition, a 4-day advanced level sleep technology course has also been conducted every other year. In order to maintain the standard of sleep technologists in Thailand, SST has been conducting examinations for sleep technologist certification for basic level and advanced level since 2010. To date, a total of 202 and 91 were certified as basic level sleep technologists and advance level sleep technologists, respectively. Like sleep medicine specialists, this certification is not required to practice as a sleep technologist as there is no national regulation to practice sleep medicine in Thailand at the moment.

Sleep Society of Thailand (SST), even though is the largest, is not the only sleep medicine professional society in Thailand. Subsequently, several sleep medicine professional societies were established. Sleep Apnea Association under The Royal College of Otolaryngologists-Head and Neck Surgeons of Thailand was established in 2012. Assembly of Sleep Medicine under Thoracic Society of Thailand under Royal Patronage was established in 2017. Thai Association of Sleep Medicine under The Royal College of Physicians of Thailand was established in 2018. Sleep Neurology Association under The Neurological Society of Thailand was established in 2019. The establishment of these professional societies resulted in the establishment of clinical practice guidelines including "Thai Guideline for Childhood Obstructive Sleep apnea" [4] published in 2013 in cooperation with Sleep Society of Thailand, Pediatric Respiratory and Critical Care Medicine Association, and the Royal College Pediatricians of Thailand and "Clinical Recommendations for Diagnosis and Management of Obstructive Sleep Apnea in Thailand for Adults 2018" [5] in cooperation with Sleep Society of Thailand, Thai Association of Sleep Medicine, Thoracic Society of Thailand, The Neurological Society of Thailand, and The Royal College of Physicians of Thailand. These Clinical Practice Guidelines were developed using rigorous evidence-based methodology with the strength of evidence for each recommendation explicitly stated. The summary of Thai Guidelines for Childhood Obstructive Sleep apnea 2013 and Clinical Recommendations for Diagnosis and Management of Obstructive Sleep Apnea in Thailand for Adults 2018 are shown in Figs. (**1** and **2**) respectively. The Assembly of Sleep Medicine under the Thoracic Society of Thailand under Royal Patronage is in the process of developing clinical practice guidelines for obesity hypoventilation syndrome with a tentative publication date in 2023.

Sleep laboratory is generally the key diagnostic tool for sleep disorders particularly, sleep-disordered breathing such as obstructive sleep apnea. Obstructive sleep apnea is among the most common sleep disorders encountered in Thailand with the prevalence of approximately 15.4% in males and 6.3% in females using AHI $\geq$ 5 events per hour and 4.8% in males and 1.9% in females using AHI $\geq$ 5 events per hour plus symptoms of excessive daytime sleepiness, respectively [6]. For the severity of obstructive sleep apnea, a recent publication from Thailand demonstrated that 71.4% and 14.3% of the obstructive sleep apnea were in severe and moderate severity, respectively [7].

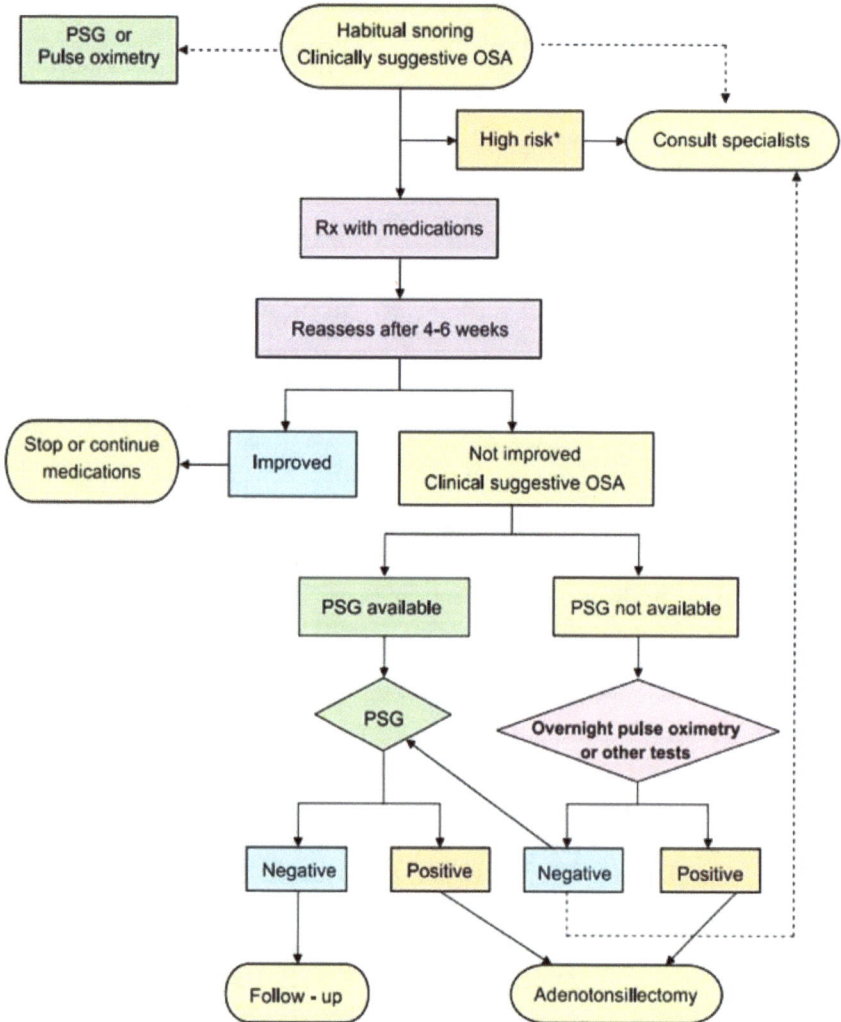

*OSA related complications, age < 3 years, obesity, craniofacial disorders, Down syndrome, cerebral palsy, neuromuscular disorders, chronic lungs, sickle cell, genetic /metabolic /storage diseases.

Fig. (1). Algorithm for management of childhood obstructive sleep apnea.

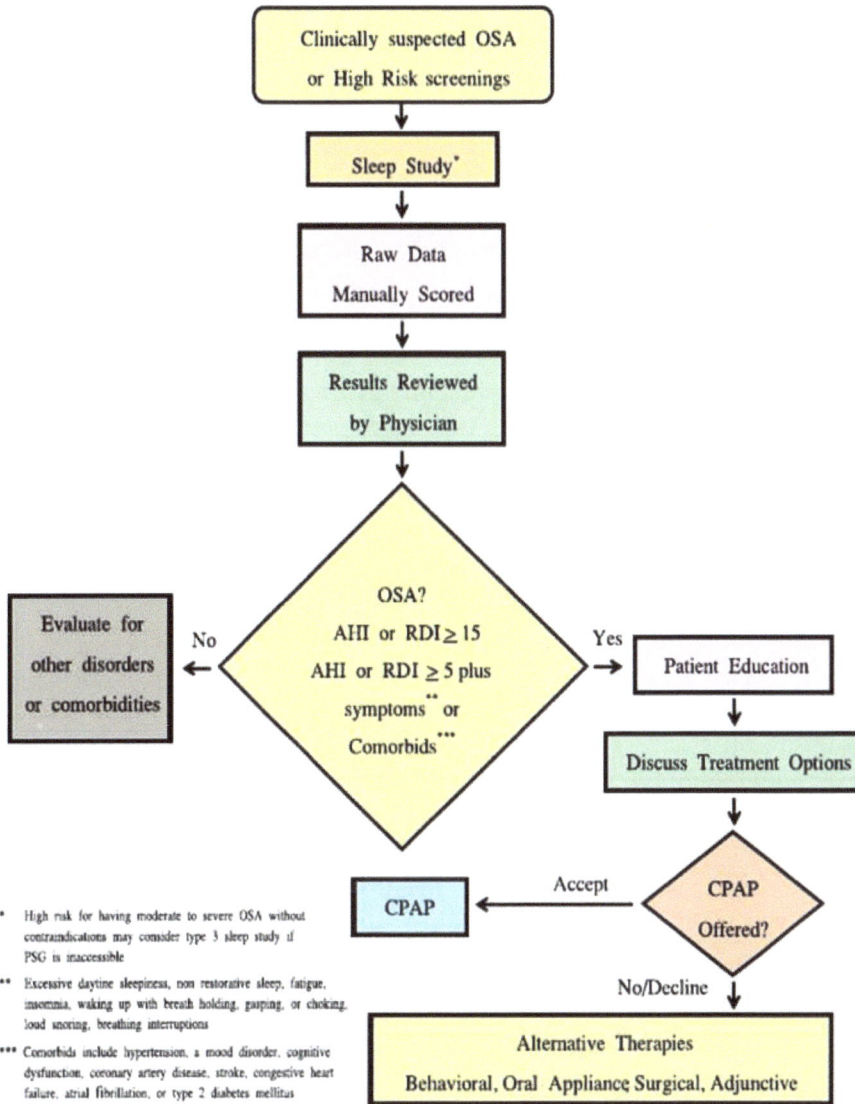

Fig. (2). Algorithm for management of adult obstructive sleep apnea.

To date, there are total of 66 level I sleep laboratories actively operating in Thailand. Approximately half of them are in Bangkok. There are 29 sleep laboratories in government hospitals and the rest are in private hospitals. Out of 73 provinces in Thailand, 19 provinces have at least one level I sleep laboratories. The rest of the provinces rely on level III or level IV (such as pulse continuous oximeter monitoring). To standardize sleep laboratory in Thailand, SST implemented standard international accreditation criteria to accredit sleep laboratory in Thailand. Total of 8 sleep laboratories are accredited by SST (7 sleep laboratories in government hospital and 1 sleep laboratory in private hospital). Fortunately, polysomnography conducted at a sleep laboratory in a government hospital is free of charge for most of the health care coverage programs including civil service welfare system (civil servants and their families). The cost of level I polysomnography is approximately 7,000-48,000 baht (230-1,600 USD) with an average cost of 10,000 baht (330 USD). However, the cost of continuous positive airway pressure (CPAP) is currently reimbursable only in the civil service welfare system, limited private health insurance, and certain state enterprise or government employees. The limit of 20,000 baht (660 USD) could be reimbursed for CPAP if there is the presence of obstructive sleep apnea using criteria of AHI > 15 events per hour or AHI 5-15 events per hour plus coronary artery disease, hypertension or stroke. The reimbursable value approximates the lowest cost of CPAP device available in Thailand. The CPAP device if malfunction and unable to be restored could be replaced by a new machine every 5 years up to 20,000 baht (660 USD) and the CPAP mask could be annually reimbursed up to 4,000 baht (130 USD). Surgical treatment for obstructive sleep apnea is generally reimbursable in government hospitals for the civil service welfare system (civil servants and their families), social security for private employees, and universal coverage scheme. However, an oral appliance is generally not reimbursable. For other treatments for sleep disorders such as cognitive behavior therapy for insomnia (CBT-i) is also not generally reimbursable.

CHALLENGES TO THE PRACTICE OF SLEEP MEDICINE IN THAILAND

Compared to other medical disciplines, sleep medicine is in a relatively early stage. A limited number of sleep medicine specialists are still an ongoing problem. However, a formal sleep medicine fellowship is in the hope to ease this problem. There is currently no medical practice regulation for sleep medicine practice. Practically, any actively licensed physician in Thailand could hold practice in sleep medicine including sleep disorders encounter, interpretation of polysomnography, or prescribe CPAP. These issues would likely discourage young medical practitioners to pursue this field.

Since most of the sleep laboratories are clustered in Bangkok, there is insufficient sleep laboratory in other provinces and oversaturated in Bangkok particularly in private hospitals/centers. However, even in Bangkok, there is still limited availability of sleep laboratory in government hospitals due to lower cost and reimbursability. The average waiting time for level I sleep study is from 3 months to 2 years in most of the government hospitals. As previously mentioned, CPAP is not reimbursable in most of the health care coverage programs including social security or universal coverage scheme. In 2020, an attempt was made by Health Systems Research Institute (HSRI) to study the cost-effectiveness of CPAP usage among obstructive sleep apnea patients [8]. This retrospective study was conducted in 8 centers throughout the nation and included a total of 681 patients. The study demonstrated improvement in quality of life with the use of CPAP. The major limitation of the study was the retrospective nature of the study, future prospective study is strongly recommended to study the cost-effectiveness of CPAP in terms of reduction in health care utilization and cost-related to comorbid conditions including stroke, hypertension, or coronary artery disease.

For other sleep disorders, there are some limitations in the availability of certain medications. For example, there is a lack of medication for the treatment of narcolepsy. The cornerstone treatment medication such as sodium oxybate which can treat hypersomnolence and cataplexy is not legally available in Thailand. Wakefulness promoting agent, armodafinil, which is indicated for narcolepsy as well as shift work disorder and CPAP-treated obstructive sleep apnea with residual excessive daytime sleepiness [9], had not been available until recently in December 2020. Stimulants such as methylphenidate have been prescribed for these conditions instead. On the other hand, for insomnia treatment, the only available z-drug in Thailand is zolpidem which could only be prescribed by neurologist, psychiatrist, or sleep medicine specialist. Benzodiazepines have long been the most prescribed hypnotics due to their lower cost and more availability. In 2022, the new hypnotics, lemborexant, the dual orexin receptor antagonist was recently approved by Thai FDA. This will give more options for the treatment of insomnia in Thailand. Besides pharmacological treatment, non-pharmacological treatment, particularly, cognitive behavioral therapy for insomnia (CBT-i) is crucial and should be considered as the first line treatment for insomnia due to more sustained efficacy and fewer side effect compared to pharmacological therapy [10]. Unfortunately, CBT-i is currently not reimbursable in Thailand.

UNIQUE NEEDS OF THE SLEEP FIELD IN THAILAND

As a relatively small country and in an early stage of sleep medicine, Thailand is honored to host many international sleep conferences. In chronological order, Thailand conducted the 3rd Asian Sleep Research Society Congress (ASRS) in December 2000, the 22nd International Physiology-Pathophysiology Symposia and Workshops in March 2004, the 2nd World Association of Sleep Medicine Congress (WASM) in February 2007, and the 2nd ASEAN Sleep Congress in August 2013. Thailand is honored to be recently selected to host the 4th Asian Society of Sleep Medicine (ASSM) Meeting in 2023. Furthermore, Thailand also received the

Distinguished Activity Award for World Sleep Day from the World Sleep Society for 3 consecutive years from 2017-2019 and also in 2021 and 2022. In 2020, Thailand received the Honorable Mention Award [11]. This World Sleep Day activity aims to raise public awareness of the importance of sleep and sleep disorders among Thai community. During each annual SST meeting, public education session has been conducted parallelly. SST has worked closely with the department of health and department of mental health to raise the importance of sleep disorders among executive officer/senior administration at national level. Sleep problems, tips for good sleep, and sleep in the elderly are the three books published by SST in cooperation with the department of health to educate the general public on sleep and sleep disorders. At international level, SST is a member and one of the founders of ASEAN Sleep Federation which was registered in 2020 and renamed as the Federation of South East Asian of Sleep Medicine (FSSM). SST is also an active member of the Asian Society of Sleep Medicine (ASSM). Continuous collaboration with these international sleep medicine societies has helped promote the visibility of Thailand in the region and globally.

Form research aspect of sleep medicine, there has been an increase in interest in sleep medicine research in Thailand. At the Sleep Society of Thailand Annual Meeting, a research contest has been conducted since 2017 to promote interest in research among sleep medicine researchers in Thailand. Furthermore, since 2016, Sleep Society of Thailand also provides up to 4 grants for research presentation at international conference worth 20,000 baht (660 USD) for a conference in the Asian continent and 40,000 baht (1320 USD) for other continents. The number of sleep research publications from Thailand has been increasing for the past years. Obstructive sleep apnea, insomnia, sleep duration & sleep timing, pediatric sleep medicine, and sleep and traffic accidents are among many categories published by Thai sleep medicine researchers and indexed in Scopus and PubMed databases. Nevertheless, there is still room for improvement. Thailand still lacks the national data in many aspects of sleep medicine. The data on the prevalence of obstructive sleep apnea was published in 2011 and there is a need for updated epidemiological data on this common sleep disorder. As mentioned earlier, there is also the need for well-conducted research on cost-effectiveness analysis of CPAP treatment in obstructive sleep apnea in order to put forward the universal national reimbursement for this gold standard treatment for all Thai citizens. Furthermore, screening for obstructive sleep apnea is not required by the department of Land Transport in order to obtain a driver license in Thailand. Even though, there are some preliminary studies including a cross-sectional design conducted on intercity bus drivers from 4 bus transportation companies which indicated that up to 18.1% of bus drivers were at high risk for OSA using the Thai Berlin Questionnaire to assess sleep apnea risk [12]. Only 19.7% of the drivers sleep more than 7 hours which is the recommended sleep duration by the National Sleep Foundation (7-9 hours) [13]. A self-answered questionnaire survey of 4331 commercial bus/truck drivers showed that 69% of the drivers reported accidents and one- third of these accidents was attributable to drowsiness, 17% was associated with chronic loud snoring with or without obesity [14]. Furthermore, the medical council of Thailand reported that 90% cause of death related to traffic accident in physicians between the age of 25-50 was insufficient sleep (2008-2017). A prospective cross-sectional study was performed among young doctors less than 40 years old working at King Chulalongkorn Memorial Hospital, Bangkok, Thailand, and Hospital Kuala Lumpur, Kuala Lumpur, Malaysia, using questionnaires and home sleep apnea testing among your physician less than 40 years of age. The study revealed the prevalence of OSA of 40.4% and OSAS of 5.8% [15]. There is a need to put forward routine screening for OSA and encourage adequate sleep duration among drivers to prevent the traffic accident. Future research studies on this important issue are needed.

Besides the Sleep Society of Thailand, many universities or professional societies also provide research grants. However, multicenter, multidisciplinary, longitudinal studies in the field of sleep medicine are still lacking at the moment and essential to compete for large local and global federal grants. Thailand also needs to implement knowledge in sleep medicine at an early stage of medical education such as in the medical school level. This will likely lead to growing interest in sleep medicine among young physicians which may encourage them to pursue this profession in the future. Improvement in the knowledge of sleep medicine for all physicians will also likely improve care and overall health of Thai population.

CONCLUSION

Sleep medicine is a growing field in Thailand and recognized as a medical specialty under the Medical Council of Thailand in 2018. The 2-year-formal fellowship training in sleep medicine was established in 2019. Currently, there is no national regulation for license to practice sleep medicine for physicians, sleep technologists, or dentists. There are limited numbers of sleep laboratories in the country particularly in government settings in which the cost is reimbursable. Few sleep centers are accredited at the society level. Polysomnography is reimbursable by most of the health insurance systems when conducted in government hospitals. However, CPAP reimbursement is limited only in civil welfare system and certain private insurances. There is progress in sleep medicine research in Thailand in recent years. Advancing sleep medicine in Thailand requires collaboration among various disciplines and public awareness of the importance of sleep and sleep disorders.

CONSENT FOR PUBLICATION

Not applicable.

CONFLICT OF INTEREST

The author declares no conflict of interest, financial or otherwise.

ACKNOWLEDGEMENT

Declared none.

REFERENCES

[1] Chirakalwasan N, Preutthipan A, Maranetra KN, Yongchaiyudh P, Kotchabhakdi N. Sleep medicine in Thailand. J Clin Sleep Med 2020; 16(3): 451-3.
[http://dx.doi.org/10.5664/jcsm.8228] [PMID: 31992423]

[2] http://sst.or.th/sleep/ Assessed January 13, 2022.

[3] Tantrakul V, Preutthipan A, Maranetra N. Sleep medicine in Thailand. Sleep Biol Rhythms 2016; 14(S1) (Suppl. 1): 31-5.
[http://dx.doi.org/10.1007/s41105-015-0010-1]

[4] http://www.thaipediatrics.org/Media/media-20170913112354.pdf Assessed January 13, 2022.

[5] http://sst.or.th/sleep/wp-content/uploads/2019/08/CPG-5-LOGO.pdf January 13, 2022.

[6] Neruntarat C, Chantapant S. Prevalence of sleep apnea in HRH Princess Maha Chakri Srinthorn Medical Center, Thailand. Sleep Breath 2011; 15(4): 641-8.
[http://dx.doi.org/10.1007/s11325-010-0412-x] [PMID: 20848319]

[7] Lappharat S, Taneepanichskul N, Reutrakul S, Chirakalwasan N. Effects of bedroom environmental conditions on the severity of obstructive sleep apnea. J Clin Sleep Med 2018; 14(4): 565-73.
[http://dx.doi.org/10.5664/jcsm.7046] [PMID: 29609708]

[8] https://kb.hsri.or.th/dspace/handle/11228/5174?locale-attribute=th Assessed January 13, 2022.

[9] Morgenthaler TI, Kapen S, Lee-Chiong T, *et al.* Standards of Practice Committee; American Academy of Sleep Medicine. Practice parameters for the medical therapy of obstructive sleep apnea. Sleep 2006; 29(8): 1031-5.
[http://dx.doi.org/10.1093/sleep/29.8.1031] [PMID: 16944671]

[10] Schutte-Rodin S, Broch L, Buysse D, Dorsey C, Sateia M. Clinical guideline for the evaluation and management of chronic insomnia in adults. J Clin Sleep Med 2008; 4(5): 487-504.
[http://dx.doi.org/10.5664/jcsm.27286] [PMID: 18853708]

[11] https://worldsleepday.org/activities/activity-awards Assessed January 13, 2022.

[12] Chaiard J, Deeluea J, Suksatit B, Songkham W. Factors associated with sleep quality of Thai intercity bus drivers. Ind Health 2019; 57(5): 596-603.
[http://dx.doi.org/10.2486/indhealth.2018-0168] [PMID: 30686814]

[13] https://www.sleepfoundation.org/press-release/national-sleep-foundation-recommends-new-sleep-times Assessed January 13, 2022.

[14] Leechawengwongs M, Leechawengwongs E, Sukying C, Udomsubpayakul U. Role of drowsy driving in traffic accidents: a questionnaire survey of Thai commercial bus/truck drivers. J Med Assoc Thai 2006; 89(11): 1845-50.
[PMID: 17205864]

[15]   Yasin R, Muntham D, Chirakalwasan N. Uncovering the sleep disorders among young doctors. Sleep Breath 2016; 20(4): 1137-44.
[http://dx.doi.org/10.1007/s11325-016-1380-6] [PMID: 27535070]

CHAPTER 13

Sleep Medicine in Iran: Current Practice, Challenges, and Future Direction

Arezu Najafi[1,2,*] and **Khosro Sadeghniiat-Haghighi**[1,2]

[1] *Occupational Sleep Research Center, Baharloo Hospital, Tehran University of Medical Sciences, Tehran, Iran*

[2] *Sleep Breathing Disorders Research Center, Tehran University of Medical Sciences, Tehran, Iran*

Abstract: The Iranian Sleep Medicine (ISM) Society, established in 2005, has worked to increase public knowledge of how important sleep is to maintain health in the community and safety on the roads. The ISM has also had a strong role in the implementation of sleep tests and laboratory standards in collaboration with the Ministry of Health, training sleep specialists to diagnose and treat sleep disorders, certifying sleep labs to ISM standards, and conducting much needed research to improve sleep amongst Iranians. In this chapter, we will first introduce the current healthcare system highlighting the practice of sleep medicine in Iran. Next, we identify three challenges in delivering sleep medicine to millions of Iranians with potential solutions. The challenges are: (1) a limited number of trained sleep medicine specialists unequally distributed across all districts; (2) a limited number of certified sleep labs; (3) the need for insurance to pay for the diagnosis and treatment of sleep disorders such as obstructive sleep apnea, narcolepsy, and insomnia. Lastly, we present future directions for Iranian sleep research including much needed population-based studies to assess the prevalence of sleep disorders. While much progress has been made since 2005 to improve sleep health in Iran, we still have much work to do to reach our goal of significantly reducing disparities and promoting sleep medicine all over Iran toward a healthier future.

Keywords: Accident, Cognitive Behavioral Therapy for insomnia, Commercial Drivers, CPAP, Insomnia, Iran, Iran University of Medical Sciences, Iranian Sleep Medicine Society, Isfahan University of Medical Sciences, Journal of Sleep Sciences, Mashhad University of Medical Sciences, Narcolepsy, Oral appliance, Qazvin University of Medical Sciences, Restless legs syndrome, Shahid Beheshti University Medical Sciences, Sleep apnea, Sleep medicine fellowship, Sleepiness, Tehran University of Medical Sciences.

* **Corresponding author Arezu Najafi:** Occupational Sleep Research Center, Baharloo Hospital, Tehran University of Medical Sciences, Tehran, Iran; BOX: 133 99 73 111, Tel: +98 21 55460184, Fax: +98 21 55648189, Emails: anajafee@sina.tums.ac.ir, najafeeaz@gmail.com

Hrayr P. Attarian, Marie-Louise M. Coussa-Koniski & Alain Michel Sabri (Eds.)

INTRODUCTION

Iran is a country home to one of the world's oldest civilizations located southwest of Asia and in the Middle East region. The United Nations estimated the population of Iran to be 83,992,949 (2020), making it the world's 17th most populous country. Iran is the second largest country in the Middle East spanning 1,648,195 km2 (636,372 sq mi) [1]. The population density is 49.15 people/km2 (2018 population census) with 74.9 percent in urban areas, most of which is concentrated in the north, north-west and west of the country [2]. Tehran, the capital and largest city, is the economic and cultural hub of Iran, and home to 15 million people that includes the metropolitan area.

Iranian society is ethnically diverse and includes Persians, Kurds, Lurs, Baloch, Azerbaijanis, Arabs, Turkmen and Turkic tribes, Armenians, Assyrians and Georgians [2]. Iran can be described as a young country, with 49 percent of the population below 30 years old, 24 percent below 15 years old, and only 6.1 percent aged 65 and over [2]. Males account for 51 percent of the total population [2]. Currently, the average annual middle-income worker salary is about 800-1600 million Iranian rials or US$ 4000-8000.

DESCRIPTION OF THE HEALTHCARE SYSTEM IN IRAN

Iran's health care system can be divided into three major healthcare systems: governmental healthcare, private healthcare and non-governmental healthcare such as charity organizations [3].

Governmental healthcare can be divided into primary care and hospital care. Primary care is delivered in both rural areas (*e.g.* health houses) and urban areas (*e.g.* health care centers). Hospital care is either academic or community based, offering general and/or specialized health care services. Governmental healthcare is mainly covered by a government insurance system available to all Iranians called "Social Welfare Insurance" affiliated with the Ministry of Welfare and Social Services. Another insurance, "Iranians' Health Insurance" which is affiliated with the Ministry of Health, is available. Hospitals affiliated with these two insurance systems provide health services to their members for little to no co-pay and cover basic healthcare and essential medicines listed on the World Health Organization Model List. Private health insurance can be purchased to supplement government insurance to cover additional health care services and specialized treatment.

Private healthcare includes clinics, offices, and hospitals which are located throughout the country. Individuals or companies may purchase one of several private and complementary insurance to cover health care services that include basic as well as additional healthcare services that include essential and specialized treatment including some newly approved medications and equipment such as continuous positive airway pressure (CPAP).

Non-governmental healthcare hospitals are funded by charitable donations for people who are unable to afford insurance and make up 20 percent of hospitals according to 2016 statistics. While these hospitals are located throughout the country, they are concentrated in the largest cities [4].

CURRENT PRACTICE OF SLEEP MEDICINE IN IRAN

The primary mission of the Iranian Sleep Medicine (ISM) Society, established in 2005 (ism-society.ir), is to train sleep medicine specialists using a multi-disciplinary approach, promote research in sleep medicine, and educate the community about sleep health. The ISM is represented by physicians from Anesthesiology, Ear, nose, throat surgery (ENT), Internal Medicine, Maxillofacial surgery, Neurology, Occupational Medicine, Pediatrics, Psychiatry, and Pulmonology. At the current time, the chief executive director of ISM is an ENT surgeon and the director is an occupational medicine specialist, both trained in sleep medicine. The ISM board members are currently represented by ENT, Maxillofacial surgery, Neurology, Occupational medicine, Pediatrics, Psychiatry, and Pulmonology. In addition to its primary mission, the ISM together with sleep research centers contribute and participate in international health congresses and events, and is a standing member of the World Sleep Society and participates in World Sleep Day. In 2017, the Occupational Sleep Research Center at Tehran University of Medical Sciences received an honorable mention award for their participation in World Sleep Day. Furthermore, the ISM works to increase public knowledge of sleep to maintain health and safety on the roads. The ISM has worked with the Ministry of Health to advise and implement and certify sleep testing and sleep lab standards as well as help train sleep specialists to diagnose and treat sleep disorders.

The Ministry of Health regulates sleep medicine in Iran in collaboration with the ISM. In 2020, the Ministry of Health implemented standards that trained Sleep Medicine specialists within only eight specialties (ENT, Anesthesiology, Internal Medicine, Neurology, Occupational Medicine, Pediatrics, Psychiatry, and Pulmonary Medicine) and physicians within only aforementioned eight specialties working at an academic sleep clinic are allowed to perform and interpret Polysomnography (PSG), PAP titration studies, Multiple Sleep Latency Test (MSLT), and Maintenance of Wakefulness test (MWT). In addition, they passed new regulations that only sleep labs that comply with the Ministry of Health standards for a sleep lab can perform sleep tests. As of Feb 2021, more than 40 physicians have been trained in sleep medicine and practice in over 30 accredited sleep clinics performing sleep studies and providing standard of care for sleep disorders. However, it is estimated that approximately 60 or more physicians are still practicing sleep medicine without completing a Sleep Medicine fellowship and practice in non-accredited sleep clinics and companies. The problem of sleep medicine practice by non-trained physicians is improving gradually after notification and implementation of standards for sleep clinics and sleep tests by the Ministry of Health [5].

Nurses, respiratory technicians, and sleep technicians are integral members of the team delivering sleep medicine practice and care. Currently, they are trained and certified in a special program instituted by the Ministry of Health in collaboration with Tehran University of Medical Sciences that was established in 2012. All health care professionals in Iran are involved in screening and referring patients with sleep problems. However, due to a lack of awareness of sleep disorders, lack of sleep testing, and lack of sleep specialists, the process of screening and referring patients is not yet well developed and is still a work in progress by the ISM. To rectify this, the ISM society makes a significant effort to increase public awareness of sleep disorders through programs *via* different media platforms including, TV, radio and other communication devices such as social media. Although the number of these programs is significant, there is still a lack of awareness on sleep disorders and problems among the public and health related professionals. Thus, more work is warranted to increase awareness.

PRACTICE GUIDELINES FOR COMMERCIAL DRIVING

Largely due to the efforts of the ISM society, several publications and practice guidelines have been implemented in regard to sleep medicine. Together with the Ministry of Health, there are now regulations to screen commercial drivers with validated Persian STOP-BANG and Epworth Sleepiness Scale (ESS) questionnaires within Occupational Medicine clinics for obstructive sleep apnea (OSA) and narcolepsy. And, in accordance with these regulations started from 2005, untreated OSA with abnormal MWT and drivers with narcolepsy will not be allowed to obtain a commercial driver's license. Iran also has a local ongoing pilot program to track commercial drivers involved in a fatal accident and listing the multiple injuries associated with the accident including traumatic brain injury, internal bleeding, spinal cord injury and broken bones. This tracking program will soon be nationalized in collaboration with traffic police, the Ministry of Health, and the Ministry of Road and Transportation.

Challenges to the Practice of Sleep Medicine in Iran

Number of Trained Sleep Medicine Specialists

The training programs in sleep medicine include two target populations: physicians and technicians. Sleep fellowships for physicians and separately, training programs for sleep technicians, are one year and three months programs, respectively, and acceptance into the program is based on oral and written examination scores. Tehran University of Medical Sciences was the first university to train sleep medicine fellows starting in 2011 followed by Shahid Beheshti University of Medical Sciences in 2013, and subsequently Qazvin University of Medical Sciences (devoted to pediatric sleep medicine), Iran University of Medical Sciences, Mashhad University of Medical Sciences, and Isfahan University of Medical Sciences. Tehran University of Medical Sciences was also the first university to train sleep medicine technicians starting in 2012.

The limited number of trained sleep medicine specialists is a current challenge that once solved can improve access to sleep medicine care for all Iranians. At the current time, there are only 15 Ministry of Health approved positions to train sleep medicine physicians every year. Currently there are many ongoing national sleep-related research projects and there is a need to dedicate more resources to promote a national network for sleep research that could be solved by training more sleep medicine specialists from different disciplines.

Solution: Increasing the number of approved positions to train sleep medicine specialists would be the first step. Perceived need for sleep medicine specialists because of limited knowledge of healthcare professionals about sleep disorders and their burden on the healthcare system is one of the barriers that could be resolved by the development of more national based programs. Another issue may be the financial problems for establishment of a standard sleep lab. Limited number of training facilities throughout the country also is an obstacle for increasing training centers. This could be overcome by planned virtual sleep medicine fellowship programs in combination with in-site training in accordance with current ministry's sleep medicine fellowship curriculum.

The ISM society together with universities that offer sleep medicine training programs sponsors continuous educational medical programs for both physicians and technicians. In addition, Tehran University of Medical Science and ISM publish an English sleep journal called "Journal of Sleep Sciences" (jss.tums.ac.ir) unique among Middle East countries. The primary mission of this journal is to promote high-quality sleep research in the region that takes into consideration the unique limitations of developing countries to provide sleep care services for their patients.

We welcome international collaboration to advise us on how to further develop practice guidelines for sleep medicine within the Middle East.

Number of Certified Sleep Labs

Iran has over 30 ISM-certified sleep labs with Tehran University of Medical Sciences being one of the first standardized academic sleep labs with 11 active beds. A standardized sleep lab is able to perform PSG, MSLT, MWT, Actigraphy, PAP titration studies, and Home Sleep Tests (HSTs). Patients have access to ISM certified sleep labs in the following cities: Ahvaz, Isfahan, Karaj, Kerman, Kermanshah, Mashhad, Orumia, Qazvin, Sari, Tabriz, Tehran, and Yazd.

Standard sleep tests cost more in private clinics and are less expensive in governmental clinics. Some insurance companies cover the cost of sleep tests but the main insurance companies do not cover sleep tests at the present time. Therefore, patients in lower socioeconomic levels with a monthly income of US$200-300 have financial barriers associated with the cost to diagnose and treat sleep disorders. (Prices for 2021: Sleep physician visit fee: US$2-3 in governmental centers and US$5-7 in private centers; Sleep Test Cost: US$40-60 in governmental hospitals where sleep tests are under coverage of health revolution program and US$100-200 in private center. Simple CPAP price is US$ 500-900 and the price of autoCPAP machine is US$ 700-1200.

Solution: Increasing the number of sleep-trained physicians and subsequently certified sleep labs will decrease the variability in the quality of sleep tests and treatment. Providing and sending available approved standards for sleep labs and also sleep tests to all active labs that are eligible according to the ministry's regulations will also reduce variability in the quality of sleep tests and managements. Continuous education programs by ISM would also be helpful in this regard. With more sleep physicians, we will also be able to work with all insurance companies to cover sleep tests and treatment. As much of the world is moving to utilize home sleep tests (HSTs) to keep costs down of running a sleep lab, currently, Iran does not yet have regulations for HSTs but one is in development. Lastly, in response to the COVID-19 pandemic, the technological infrastructure for telehealth sleep medicine has dramatically moved forward in some parts of the world, and while it is not yet available in Iran, this is also being evaluated to increase access to care.

Sleep Treatments Available and Reimbursement

Among treatment modalities available for obstructive sleep apnea (OSA), most insurance companies cover the cost of sleep surgeries of the upper airways and maxillofacial areas. One significant challenge is that non-invasive management of

OSA and central sleep apnea such as positive airway pressure (PAP) devices *e.g.* CPAP, BiPAP, and other advanced PAP devices, as well as Mandibular Advancement Devices, are currently not covered by governmental insurance. While some private and supplementary insurance companies pay for the cost of PAP, most of the Iranian population are not insured by these companies. Locally manufactured PAP devices are now available, but they are still not affordable for patients living on a minimum annual wage as the price of a simple PAP device is one to two times more than the monthly income of a middle-income worker. The cost of autoPAP devices is 30-50% more than the simple PAP device. Subsequently, patients are not motivated to be diagnosed with sleep disorders or undergo a PAP titration study because treatment is often times unaffordable.

Pharmacologic treatments such as anti-cataplectic and wake stimulating agents for narcolepsy and sleep promoting agents for insomnia are reimbursed by governmental insurance companies. Cognitive behavioral therapies for insomnia are available in Iran but currently are not widely available or covered by most insurances.

Solution: It would be very helpful and of great value for insurance companies to cover all management modalities to promote sleep health that is equally accessible to all Iranians. In parallel, local PAP manufacturing companies could work with the government to reduce the cost of each PAP device to make it more affordable to Iranians of all socioeconomic levels. Although mandibular advancement devices (MAD) are available in Iran, we need more dentists to be trained to fit and mold the different devices at an affordable price. Cognitive behavioral therapies for insomnia (CBTi) are also available in Iran, but not widely utilized. They require more attention from the ISM and related stakeholders to develop more trained professionals with an expertise in CBTi that are sensitive to the cultural ideals of Iran.

To increase the availability of pharmacologic treatments for sleep disorders, there needs to be recognition that sleep disorders are important by the World Health Organization (WHO) and the Iranian National health program. This will in turn increase the awareness of sleep disorders in health-related professions and the public to then develop a national program for sleep medicine in Iran. Collectively this will motivate insurance companies to partner with pharma companies to make new insomnia treatments (*e.g.*, sleep promoting medications like suvorexant, ramelteon, and lemborexant] and narcolepsy treatments (*e.g.*, wake promoting agents like armodafinil, sodium oxybate, and solriamfetol), available to the Iranian people.

FUTURE DIRECTIONS FOR SLEEP RESEARCH: NEED FOR MORE EPIDEMIOLOGICAL DATA OF SLEEP DISORDERS IN IRAN

There are several sleep centers in Iran devoted to sleep research. Some exclusively work on sleep related disorders which include Occupational Sleep Research Center at Tehran University of Medical Sciences and Sleep Research Center at Kermanshah University of Medical Sciences. Other centers that are involved in sleep research include: Bamdad Respiratory and Sleep Research Center at Isfahan University of Medical Sciences, Otolaryngology Research Center affiliated with Tehran University Sciences, Iran University of Medical Sciences, Shahid Beheshti University of Medical Sciences, Qazvin University of Medical Sciences, Mashhad University of Medical Sciences and Tabriz University of Medical Sciences. Collectively, we have several validated sleep related questionnaires such as STOP-BANG, Insomnia Severity Index (ISI), Epworth Sleepiness Scale (ESS), Pittsburgh Sleep Quality Index (PSQI), and Berlin questionnaire that have been translated to Persian and are used in epidemiological surveys related to sleep problems [6 - 9].

Although there are no current national data available on sleep quality, a meta-analysis has estimated an overall rate of 58% for sleep disturbances among Iranian medical and healthcare professional students which is highly prevalent and needs further investigation and intervention [10]. In a study on elderly's sleep quality, 74% had frequent awakenings during sleep and only 16% reported optimal sleep hygiene which also warrant more attention to sleep hygiene and sleep quality among this age group [11]. Insomnia, sleep apnea, restless legs syndrome, poor sleep quality, and narcolepsy are sleep disorders in Iran with the most published data. Using keywords "sleep" and "Iran", over 1000 publications can be found that are conducted by the Iranian scientific community with over 100 annual publications since 2013 according to the PubMed database in English language (Figs. **1** and **2**). This increasing trend of number of publications is promising in the field of sleep medicine in Iran. Here, we review several main studies, report on any ongoing studies and identify future research agendas.

Insomnia

In a large cross-sectional study among adults over 18 years, 59% of the population had insomnia with prevalence higher in people between the ages of 42-69 years old and females gender [12]. Another study on the elderly population reported the prevalence of insomnia to be 39% [13]. Qualitative research has indicated that reactions to insomnia among our people are dependent on their socio-cultural beliefs [14].

Future Direction

First, we need to establish sleep disorder specific (*e.g.* insomnia) committees for research within ISM and create a national sleep research network. These committees would conduct national surveys; for example, the committee for insomnia would set the inclusion of insomnia screening and treatment programs in national health programs with the Ministry of Health in collaboration with the WHO. In addition, surveys on the burden of insomnia on the healthcare system, peoples' performance and years lost due to insomnia could be studied which would ultimately lead to increased promotion of approaches to address insomnia. In parallel, national sleep awareness programs based on national statistics of insomnia and related action plans will be needed.

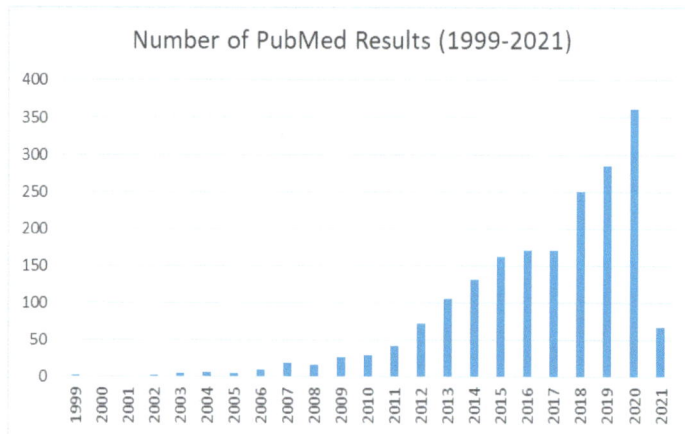

Fig. (1). Pub med results for the key words "Iran" and "Sleep" through the years.

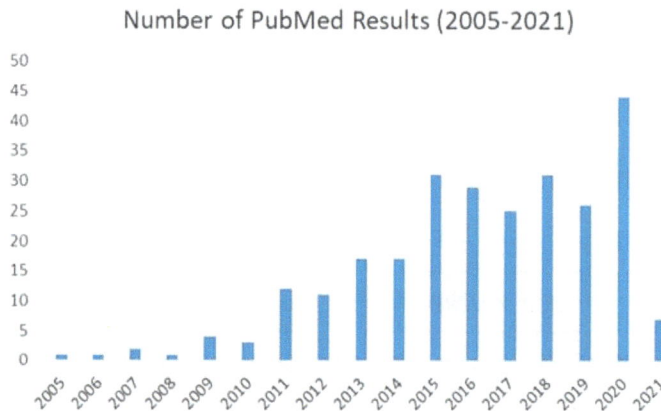

Fig. (2). Pub med results for the key words "Iran" and "Sleep apnea" through the years.

Sleep Apnea

"According to the latest WHO data published in 2018 Road Traffic Accidents Deaths in Iran reached 21,831 or 6.50% of total deaths. The age adjusted Death Rate is 29.37 per 100,000 of population ranks Iran #42 in the world [15]." Iran's informal police reports indicate that about 40% of traffic accidents are related to sleepiness in Iran, so it is noteworthy to screen for sleep disorders, particularly among commercial drivers. In a study that found a significant association between OSA and poor sleep quality with road traffic accidents, 19.6% of drivers had poor sleep quality and 23.8% had risk of OSA [16]. In a meta-analysis, 53.4% of drivers were found to have sleep quality disorder [17]. In another study, the best predictors of road traffic accidents were daytime sleepiness and sleep apnea [18]. A large study on 2200 commercial drivers revealed that about half of them suffer from poor sleep quality [19]. Furthermore, among train drivers, 59.9% had two or more risk factors of sleep apnea and this problem is overlooked among them up to now, although commercial drivers are screened for OSA [20]. A national project is ongoing to estimate the prevalence of OSA in Iran. However, several cross-sectional, regional population-based studies and also a meta-analysis are available in this regard. In a recent meta-analysis, the prevalence of Obstructive Sleep Apnea (OSA) in Iran is estimated to be about 44% [21]. Meanwhile, depending on the target population the prevalence may be different. For example, in a population of elderly people using STOP-BANG questionnaire, about 71% of the population were at high risk for OSA [22].

Future Direction

In addition to knowing the true prevalence of OSA as well as identifying the different OSA subtypes that may be unique to Iranians, we need to develop cost-effective diagnostic testing and management to decrease metabolic and cardiovascular events due to sleep apnea.

Restless Legs Syndrome

A systematic review on RLS in Iran, has revealed the prevalence of RLS as 32.9% with more frequency among women. The prevalence was estimated to be 13.8% among adults [23]. In another population-based study in north-east of Iran, RLS prevalence was 4.2% with higher frequency in the age range of 18-30 years [24].

Future Direction

More research on the prevalence of RLS in Iran is needed as there is a discrepancy in available statistics. Having national data on this subject would be very helpful in the implementation of preventive and also management strategies for promotion of sleep quality in Iran.

Narcolepsy

We have scarce data on patients with narcolepsy in Iran; however some studies are ongoing. In a study on 44 patients with narcolepsy, HLA DQB1*0602 was present in 78.9% of patients with narcolepsy and cataplexy [25].

Future Direction

Development of a national registry of patients with narcolepsy both for research and treatment issues would be very helpful. As the disease is almost unknown among the public and healthcare professionals, this also can increase their awareness and motivate them for further evaluation and treatment.

Pediatrics Sleep Medicine

It has also been the target of several studies although it is not as developed as adults' sleep medicine. We hope that with the addition of more sleep medicine fellows to the sleep medicine community this field will be more developed. In a study of 3-6 years old children from kindergartens of Qazvin city, children's average sleep duration was 10:54 minutes. The incidence of awakening during the night, sleep-disordered breathing and snoring was 13.9%, 1.2% and 2.7%, respectively. In the mentioned study, 87% of the children shared a room with their parents [26]. Another study revealed shorter sleep duration among preschool participants and a majority (85%) had sleep bedtime of 22:00 or later [27]. Regarding the prevalence of sleep disorders among children, the majority of children referred to the sleep clinic had sleep apnea which indicates that many cases of the disease remain unknown [28].

Future Direction The development of national screening programs for pediatric sleep problems and providing strategic preventive and management plans in this regard would be great directions for the future of pediatric sleep medicine in Iran as the children are future generations of this country.

FUTURE DIRECTION

Iranian sleep medicine practice and research are developing rapidly. While the number of trained sleep medicine physicians and technicians is not adequate to deliver sleep medicine to 84 million Iranians, by prioritizing sleep on the global and national level, we will have the support to train more sleep specialists, urge insurance to pay for PAP treatment as well as medications and behavioral therapies to treat narcolepsy and insomnia. The ISM in collaboration with the Ministry of Health has set standards for sleep labs including the use of appropriate equipment to diagnose sleep disorders but more certified sleep labs are needed and the use of novel, cutting-edge technology to diagnose the large numbers of patients with sleep disorders. More sleep research in Iran is needed including more epidemiological studies on the prevalence and incidence of sleep disorders at the national level and to run national projects on the management of sleep disorders, *e.g.*, in safety sensitive jobs such as commercial drivers. This research will facilitate the cost of diagnosis and management of sleep disorders being covered and will obtain the attention of authorities to put sleep in their national strategies and health budgets. This should save money by preventing potential adverse consequences of sleep disorders. We need to train more physicians and technicians to overcome disparity in different districts of the country. The ISM society with its team of dedicated trained sleep professionals will continue to work diligently to reduce disparities and promote sleep medicine throughout Iran to improve the health of its people.

CONSENT FOR PUBLICATION

Not applicable.

CONFLICT OF INTEREST

The authors declare no conflict of interest, financial or otherwise.

ACKNOWLEDGEMENTS

We would like to thank Dr. Mohammad Farhadi, the chief executive director of Iranian sleep medicine society, who with his bright scientific mind provided and supported a multidisciplinary background for the establishment and development of modern sleep medicine in Iran. Our thanks also go to Dr. Amin Amali, Dr. Babak Amra, Dr. Fariborz Rezaeitalab, Dr. Mirfarhad Ghalebandi, Dr. Mohammad Bayat, Dr. Shabnam Jalilolghadr, and Dr. ZahraBanafsheh Alemohammad, current board members of Iranian sleep medicine society. We would like to thank Dr. Alimohamad Asghari, Dr. Arezou Heshmati, Dr. Gholamreza Derakhshan Deilami, Dr. Hossein Mortazavi, and Dr. Mohammad Hossein Harirchian for their dedicated efforts in earlier years of ISM establishment. Without support of this multidisciplinary team, promotion of sleep medicine in Iran was impossible.

Our special thanks also go to the International Sleep Research Training Program (ISRTP) mentorship team of World Sleep Society for their great comments and edit of this chapter, Dr. Allan Pack, Brendan Keenan, Niusha Jafari from the

University of Pennsylvania, and Dr. Diane Lim from the University of Miami who dedicated her time and expertise in revising this chapter.

REFERENCES

[1]   https://en.wikipedia.org/wiki/Iran

[2]   https://fanack.com/iran/population/

[3]   Historical Background of the Ministry of Health in Iran. http://ird.behdasht.gov .ir/page/http-c-o-l-o-n-ird.behdasht.gov.irportalribbon.aspx

[4]   Iran Statistics' Center. https://www.amar.org.ir/news/ID/5564/%D8%AA%D8%B9%D8%AF%D8%A7%D8%AF-954-%D8%A8%DB%8C%D9%85%D8%   A7%D8%B1%D8%B3%D8%AA%D8%A7%D9%86-%D9%81%D8%B9%D8%A7%D9%84-%D8%AF%D8%-1-%DA%A9%D8%B4   D9%88%D8%B1-%D9%88%D8%AC%D9%88%D8%   AF-%D8%AF%D8%A7%D8%B1%D8%AF (In Persian)

[5]   Sleep   Medicine   Standards. http://vct.qums.ac.ir/Portal/home/?news/455295/836691/836706/%D8%A7%D8%B3%D8%AA%D8%A7%D9%86%D8%AF%D8%A7%D8%B1%D8%AF%D9%87%D8%A7%DB%8C-%D9%BE%D8%B2%D8%B4%DA%A9%DB%8C-%D8%AE%D9%88%D8%A7%D8%A8 (In Persian)

[6]   Sadeghniiat-Haghighi K, Montazeri A, Khajeh-Mehrizi A, *et al.* The STOP-BANG questionnaire: reliability and validity of the Persian version in sleep clinic population. Qual Life Res 2015; 24(8): 2025-30.
        [http://dx.doi.org/10.1007/s11136-015-0923-9] [PMID: 25613199]

[7]   Sadeghniiat Haghighi K, Montazeri A, Khajeh Mehrizi A, *et al.* The Epworth Sleepiness Scale: translation and validation study of the Iranian version. Sleep Breath 2013; 17(1): 419-26.
        [http://dx.doi.org/10.1007/s11325-012-0646-x] [PMID: 22327509]

[8]   Yazdi Z, Sadeghniiat-Haghighi K, Zohal MA, Elmizadeh K. Validity and reliability of the Iranian version of the insomnia severity index. Malays J Med Sci 2012; 19(4): 31-6.
        [PMID: 23613647]

[9]   Amra B, Nouranian E, Golshan M, Fietze I, Penzel T. Validation of the persian version of berlin sleep questionnaire for diagnosing obstructive sleep apnea. Int J Prev Med 2013; 4(3): 334-9.
        [PMID: 23626891]

[10]   Sepehrmanesh Z, Ahmadvand A, Ghoreishi F. PW01-111-Prevalence of insomnia in general population. Eur Psychiatry 2010; 25(S1): 1.

[11]   Mousavi F, Tavabi A, Iran-Pour E, Tabatabaei R, Golestan B. Prevalence and associated factors of insomnia syndrome in the elderly residing in kahrizak nursing home, tehran, iran. Iran J Public Health 2012; 41(1): 96-106.
        [PMID: 23113128]

[12]   Mazandarani AA, Aguilar-Vafaie ME, Esmaeilinasab M, Farahani H, Cheung JM. Perceptions of Insomnia among an Iranian Population: Causes and Responses. Journal of Sleep Sciences 2017; 2(1-2): 46-54.

[13]   Khaksarian M, Behzadifar M, Behzadifar M, *et al.* Sleep disturbances rate among medical and allied health professions students in Iran: Implications from a systematic review and meta-analysis of the literature. Int J Environ Res Public Health 2020; 17(3): 1011.
        [http://dx.doi.org/10.3390/ijerph17031011] [PMID: 32033482]

[14]   Bani S, Hasanpour S, Malakuti J, Abedi P, Ansari S. Sleep hygiene and its related factors among the elderly in Tabriz, Iran. Int J Women's Health Reprod Sci 2014; 2(3): 160-7.
        [http://dx.doi.org/10.15296/ijwhr.2014.24]

[15]   Sarokhani M, Goli M, Salarvand S, Ghanei Gheshlagh R. The prevalence of sleep apnea in Iran: a systematic review and meta-analysis. Tanaffos 2019; 18(1): 1-10.
[PMID: 31423134]

[16]   Baghi V, Shahbazi Hesabi P, Mohammadi H, Ghanei Gheshlagh R. The relationship between sleep apnea and quality of life of the elderly in Saqez-Iran. J Gerontol 2017; 2(2): 51-7.
[http://dx.doi.org/10.29252/joge.2.2.51]

[17]   World Health Rankings. https://www.worldlifeexpectancy.com/iran-road-traffic-accidents

[18]   Mozafari A, Zand N, Hoseini SA, *et al.* Relationship between road accidents with sleep apnea and sleep quality among truck drivers in Iran. European Respiratory Journal 44(Suppl 58)2014;

[19]   Tabrizi R, Moosazadeh M, Razzaghi A, *et al.* Prevalence of sleep quality disorder among Iranian drivers: a systematic review and meta-analysis. J Inj Violence Res 2018; 10(1): 53-9.
[PMID: 29362294]

[20]   Ebrahimi MH, Sadeghi M, Dehghani M, Niiat KS. Sleep habits and road traffic accident risk for Iranian occupational drivers. Int J Occup Med Environ Health 2015; 28(2): 305-12.
[http://dx.doi.org/10.13075/ijomeh.1896.00360] [PMID: 26182925]

[21]   Sadeghniiat-Haghighi K, Yazdi Z, Kazemifar AM. Sleep quality in long haul truck drivers: A study on Iranian national data. Chin J Traumatol 2016; 19(4): 225-8.
[http://dx.doi.org/10.1016/j.cjtee.2016.01.014] [PMID: 27578380]

[22]   Saraei M, Najafi A, Heidarbagi E. Risk factors for obstructive sleep apnea among train drivers. Work 2020; 65(1): 121-5.
[http://dx.doi.org/10.3233/WOR-193064] [PMID: 31868718]

[23]   Sorbi MH, Issazadegan A, Soleimani E, Mirhosseini SH. Prevalence of Restless Legs Syndrome in Iran: A Systematic Review and Meta-Analysis 2020.http://jhr.ssu.ac.ir/article-1-591-en.html
[http://dx.doi.org/10.18502/jchr.v9i3.4262]

[24]   Arshi S, Salmani M, Sadeghniiat-Haghighi K, Najafi A, Alavi S, Shamsipour M. Prevalence of obstructive sleep apnea among adults in north-west of Iran. Sleep Med 2017; 40: e18.
[http://dx.doi.org/10.1016/j.sleep.2017.11.046]

[25]   Geremew D, Rahimi-Golkhandan A, Sadeghniiat-Haghighi K, *et al.* Association study of HLA-DQB1* 0602 allele in Iranian patients with narcolepsy. Iran J Allergy Asthma Immunol 2017; 16(5): 452-6.
[PMID: 29149785]

[26]   Javadi M, Javadi A, Kalantari N, Jaliloghadr S, Mohamad H. Sleep problems among pre-school children in Qazvin, Iran. Malays J Med Sci 2014; 21(6): 52-6.
[PMID: 25897283]

[27]   Jalilolghadr S, Hashemi S, Javadi M, Esmailzadehha N, Jahanihashemi H, Afaghi A. Sleep habits of Iranian pre-school children in an urban area: Late sleeping and sleep debt in children. Sleep Biol Rhythms 2012; 10(2): 154-6.
[http://dx.doi.org/10.1111/j.1479-8425.2011.00516.x]

[28]   Jalilolghadr S, Saffari F, Mahram M, Sadeghi S, Yazdi Z. Obstructive sleep apnea syndrome in children referred to a sleep clinic. Journal of Sleep Sciences 2016; 1(2): 59-66.

CHAPTER 14

Current Practice of Sleep Medicine in India

Nitika Dang[1,*]

[1] *Consultant Sleep Medicine, Naõ Health, New Delhi, India (Fellow, American Academy of Sleep Medicine, World Sleep Federation - Indian Society of Sleep Research)*

Abstract: The history of sleep medicine dates back to millennia, carrying centuries of wisdom, decades of myths and challenges through the many years of struggle. Having been recognised as a body of knowledge in the last two decades and a formal branch of medicine in modern-day India. The burden of impending clinical practice, research and disproportionate health indices has allowed the tide of sleep medicine to be surfed by multiple specialties. With research interest dating back to 1965, the practice laid its formal beginning with the first sleep lab set up in New Delhi in 1995. The regulatory practices are thin on the ground that impedes the standardization of clinical research, labs or training of personnel in India. Initiatives at the behest of physicians have led to the setup of self-structured regulatory bodies, expanding the network of sleep labs in the country, albeit still very limited in comparison to the size of its populace. Increasing awareness about healthy sleep habits, bridging gaps in research, quality training and standards, improved regulatory frameworks, and translating knowledge from evidence-based medicine will drive the desired public health outcomes as well as the growth of standards and the future of sleep medicine practice in India.

Keywords: History, India, Regulation, Research, Sleep Medicine, Sleep technology, Training.

OVERVIEW

Sleep Medicine is not new to India, yet it is a growing arena of practice. The importance of sleep, sleep hygiene, and approach to sleep disturbances found a significant and detailed presence in ancient Indian texts, dating as far back as 1000 BC [1]. Ancient wisdom combined with a modern understanding of human neuro-physiology lends itself to effective targeted therapies through an integrated approach, which has yet to find impetus in this growing industry.

Research interest in modern sleep medicine dates back to 1965, with its epicenter at the All India Institute of Medical Sciences (AIIMS)[1], New Delhi [1]. AIIMS is

---

[*] **Corresponding author Nitika Dang:** Consultant Sleep Medicine, Naõ Health, New Delhi, India (Fellow, American Academy of Sleep Medicine, World Sleep Federation - Indian Society of Sleep Research); Tel: +91-98 736 20 858; E-mail: nitikadang@gmail.com

Hrayr P. Attarian, Marie-Louise M. Coussa-Koniski & Alain Michel Sabri (Eds.)

a premier, center-run tertiary medical institution in India, with the first one situated in New Delhi. Estd. in 1956, it continues in its leading role in fostering research, training and clinical practice in almost all medical specialties.

This is around the same time when medical research in sleep began in other parts of the world. The first polysomnography machine was installed in the Department of Pulmonary Medicine at Safdarjung Hospital[2], New Delhi in 1995 [2]. Safdarjung Hospital is a state-run tertiary medical institution, set up in pre-Independence India, in 1942, to serve as the base hospital for American and allied party soldiers during World War II. With three decades of continued development in the field, the practice has spread its wings across specialties but it has not yet penetrated the hearts of smaller towns, districts or villages in India. It is largely restricted to bigger medical centers in metropolitan cities. Outside of this, sleep medicine facilities are usually attached to a primary specialty. Sleep being a multi-disciplinary branch, has under its umbrella from primary care physicians, physiologists, internists, pediatricians, geriatricians, ENT specialists, anesthetists, psychiatrists, neurologists and pulmonologists. In a growing practice, dentists and surgeons, including bariatric surgeons also have a role to play. Despite the varied practice, sleep disorders go unattended, primarily due to lack of awareness, inadequate infrastructure, lack of trained sleep personnel and a low priority accorded to sleep related disorders. Adequate growth in this space is additionally hindered by a lack of treatment seeking behavior in low income and rural areas, socio-cultural beliefs, availability of over the counter tranquilizers and inadequacy of an effective supply chain management of sleep and related drugs. Bridging gaps in research, quality training, improved regulatory frameworks and translating knowledge from evidence based medicine will drive the desired public health outcomes as well as the growth of standards of sleep medicine practice in India.

EARLY DAYS OF SLEEP MEDICINE PAVING THE WAY FOR SLEEP LANDSCAPE IN INDIA TODAY

Sleep medicine has undertaken a significant journey since the launch of the first sleep lab in 1995, close to three decades ago, at the Safdarjung Hospital, a state-run tertiary hospital and medical institution in New Delhi, the capital city of India [2]. Research inquisitiveness, however, flamed up around 1965 with the team of neuro-physiologists at India's premier tertiary medical institute, All India of Medical Sciences (AIIMS), expanding their wings of knowledge in neural regulation of sleep [3 - 7].

Sleep-based research first started in neuro-physiology, moving to pulmonary medicine and later other specialties. The practice has now found its association with branches as distant as dentistry and surgery. This cross-pollination has ensured that sleep medicine has grown sufficiently albeit horizontally in the medical field; penetration to vast geographic areas with different socio-economic conditions, though, still remains a huge challenge. The first efforts for increasing awareness were made by the Indian Society of Sleep Research (ISSR) set up in September 1992, kicking off new beginnings in the country for the practice of sleep medicine through international symposia and conferences [8]. With the practice of sleep medicine evolving and spreading its wings, multiple societies and regulatory bodies emerged. Among them were the Indian Sleep Disorders Association (ISDA), which also started the first sleep medicine certification in the country and the Indian Association of Surgeons for Sleep Apnoea (IASSA), which offers sleep medicine courses, certifications and technician training. A recent addition is a two-year fellowship program for physicians by the Department of Psychiatry, AIIMS, Rishikesh[3]. Additionally, a bachelor's degree program has been introduced for sleep Technologists[4]. Privately run certificate courses have also come into the landscape, recently. However, this list is not exhaustive and is slowly expanding given the rise in the recognition of sleep practice in the country. The influence is growing with this network expanding to various parts of the country at the behest of more and more physicians following suit, whether they are based in private practice or in state-run teaching and research hospitals.

DISTRIBUTION BETWEEN STATE AND PRIVATE PROVIDERS

Emerging to be one of India's largest sectors owing to the population of the country, healthcare is growing at a brisk pace with increasing coverage and expenditure by both private and state providers. At the level of the government, healthcare in India is a "State" subject even though the recent Finance commission bench recommends putting it on the concurrent list - calling for a higher degree of shared responsibility between the National government and constituent state governments. Decision-making and policy implementation in the health sector are a shared responsibility between the union and state governments (in India's federal structure), though the final prerogative and implementation are managed at the "State level" [9]. Public health is a state matter as each state has the responsibility of ensuring primary and emergency healthcare services to all its people. Centrally, the Ministry of Health and Family Welfare (MoHFW) is entrusted with driving overall policy, and provisions in healthcare and national health programs.

Healthcare is widely distributed amongst public and private providers across the country. The bulk of the balance is tilted towards provision by private setups of varying degrees from hospitals, nursing homes to clinics, in tiered cities and districts across the country. Healthcare in urban cities is accessible but still remains a significant challenge in rural areas where traditional medicine, spiritual practices and superstitions continue to play a role [10].

Sleep medicine as a growing specialty faces similar challenges as do other practices. Provision of facilities like a sleep lab or home-based testing kits is made easy through private providers or the medical equipment companies like Respironics and ResMed, albeit at steep prices. There is a paucity of sleep beds as well as a lack of awareness among patients. This is the case even in the country's apex institutions like AIIMS which provide facilities at very low cost, thus furthering the challenge of coverage amongst a large segment of society.

The revised National health policy 2017, formulated to deliver affordable comprehensive primary health care for the well-being of all citizens without any financial burden, left increasing sleep complaints in the growing population unaddressed. In view of this, recommendations [11] were made for a national sleep policy in India to increase awareness, thus promoting treatment seeking behavior, understanding that timely interventions would have a large impact owing to India's magnitude of population and size.

TRADITIONAL MEDICINE IN INDIA AND EARLIEST ROOTS IN "AYURVEDA"

Though India's rich diversity and socio-cultural scenario allows traditional medicine systems like AYUSH (Ayurveda, Yoga & Naturopathy, Unani, Siddha and Homeopathy) to flourish alongside, modern medicine remains the unchallenged and preferred option of the privileged inhabiting the bigger metropolitans. Alternate therapy communities based on yoga and mindfulness are increasingly becoming popular. In fact, the advent of treatments related to sleep disorders has been recorded historically in Ayurveda, a traditional medicine system in India, through the Charka Samhita (encyclopedia) written in 1000 BC [12 - 15]. It alludes to excessive sleep and sleeplessness as related to an imbalance in basic factors or the three Dhatus which decide the health or ill-health of an individual. Ayurveda is state-recognized by practitioners receiving institutional training that is considered an equivalent [16] of western medicine in India. The Samhita also refers to medicinal preparations for curing insomnia [17]. The practice of Yoga as recorded in the Yoga Sutras by Patanjali almost 1000 years later (in 2nd century BC), holds information about the brain, consciousness and sleep [18]. Based on this, the current practices of inducing sleep using guided mindfulness-based practices of Yoga Nidra (Nidra translating to sleep) are being well accepted and practiced globally by health-based technology [19, 20]. Phone-based apps offer a variety of such courses and modules to a vast variety of consumers and influence their choice and understanding of sleep-related challenges, some of them being seemingly cured by such simple means. With such rich stronghold influencing socio-cultural beliefs of a population as well as national and international recognition and impetus provided to ancient systems of health and wellness such as Yoga and Ayurveda, their importance as systems of belief in approaching sleep related disorders cannot be entirely undermined. They continue to affect treatment seeking behavior in a significant way as far as the practice of sleep medicine is concerned.

Health is a fundamental right- a blessing in a democratic state like India. Being a state subject, healthcare in India rests on a phenomenal web of service provision by state organized and privately led practitioners across the country. The sheer size of the world's largest democracy and the 2nd most populous country in the world, brings with it the obvious challenges of adequacy and accessibility. With over 18% of the total world's population, India pegs an under 35 year population at 65% [21], according to the 2011 census, which is among the highest as compared to other countries in the world [22]. Although most districts across the country have public health facilities and major cities have tertiary care centers run and managed by the governments in the federal structure.

SLEEP-TECH INFLUENCING SLEEP MEDICINE IN INDIA

Sleep technology startups in India have seen a sudden boom with sleep disturbances on a steep rise. With erratic daily routines and a stressful "work from home" culture, where the office hours are stretched by virtue of physically being at home, the burden of work, screen time, anxiety, mental health issues and poor sleep hygiene in residents of metro cities has shot up exponentially. Sleep health has found its fascination for technology at the intersection of the wellness block with much happening on the awareness, sleep hygiene and monitoring fronts outside of mindfulness and meditation apps for managing stress and anxiety levels with guided mindfulness techniques and Yoga Nidra [23].

Indians are being awakened to the realization of the importance of sleep health and hygiene, more pronounced by the recent COVID-19 pandemic that redefined work culture while one was confined to home. This has been a trigger in initiating innovative products from pillows to mattresses that boast of significantly better sleep quality.

Technology brings with it the inevitable sea of changes in practices in diagnostics more than therapeutic sleep medicine. The advent of "smartness" of gadgets translates directly to the smartness of diagnostic and supportive sleep medicine through apps supporting recording and collection of data of vital parameters such as the cardiac rhythm, breathing and others like time in bed, position while in bed, snoring and supportive that support sleep hygiene and healthy lifestyle practices promoting sleep, *etc.*

With the internet and data entering the farthest of households in India, technology and its effect are not far for the lower income groups living in remote villages, smaller towns or tier-three cities. Other than this physical penetration of devices, there is also growing discourse on enabling healthier sleep through mindfulness-based phone apps (in most of which Sleep appears to be a prominent section). India seems to be following the same trend as the rest of the world in this regard. There is increasing recognition of terms like Yoga-Nidra or body scan and guided meditations to support better sleep hygiene. Modern-day technology enables reporting over mobile apps offering to consolidate and analyze data on one's sleep. Sleep health related apps are now being spoken about by the young, more aware and technology friendly socio-economic classes. More apps promoting sleep hygiene through multi-pronged approaches such as diet, yoga and mindfulness, being unveiled across the globe are also finding their footing in India. With the influx of affordable smart bands and similar devices, awareness about one's sleep and its effects on health have increased in the general population using these devices.

The advent of mHealth has proven to be a turning point in medical history globally with eHealth as a new specialty seen with newer apps and technologies flocking the health sector across ages and geographical zones. However, it has yet to influence the lower-middle income and developing countries when compared to the higher-income or developed nations [24 - 26]. Although amounting to a drop in the ocean, sleep apps and technologies are being used in a small percentage of urban high-income groups in metropolitan cities where access and affordability are not the least of constraints.

THE PRACTICE OF SLEEP MEDICINE DURING THE COVID-19 PANDEMIC

The COVID-19 pandemic strengthened human abilities beyond expectations and far ahead of the pre-conditions even in the distant and smallest of zones in each nation across the globe. The far-reaching effects have encompassed all bereaved in some way or another. The pandemic has been a major setback for Sleep practitioners in India. With the countrywide lockdown starting in March 2019, the practice of sleep medicine suffered profoundly and unexpectedly as it came in the category of non-essential services. Sleep, being vital for the well-being and optimal functioning of human beings, guidelines [27] for safer practices were published keeping the safety of all as a priority, with teleconsultations being widely accepted in practice. About 72% of physicians surveyed responded that they had closed the sleep lab during the pandemic, with 24% reporting that they had shifted to home-based testing for sleep apnoea [38]. The government regulation came down heavily on the general masses, although for their own well-being. The far-reaching effects on mental well-being which beget sleep disturbances [28 - 30] leading to a vicious cycle of sleep disturbances and fear, anxiety and depression were profound.

A major challenge in developing nations is the rising trend of Sleep disturbance triggered further by the COVID-19 pandemic owing to the lockdowns and work from home culture and personal losses of dear ones during these difficult times. Studies over the last few decades suggested about 17% of patients surveyed across Asian and African countries with established complications from various sleep disorders, which have now peaked to a pooled prevalence of around 54% in children and adolescents in covid times. Whereas in samples of the population between 45-60 years, the prevalence of sleep disturbance was reported to be over 30% [31 - 36]. Further research may provide better clarity on sleep hygiene, patterns and disturbances in patients of COVID-19, health workers, the general population and the post covid infected population.

REGULATORY PRACTICES

India's diverse and mixed healthcare system allows governing agencies, regulatory bodies and/or accreditation agencies, either established through legislation in the parliament having statutory authority or self-governing structures established by groups of private individuals. In the overall landscape of medicine in India, some of these bodies include the Medical Council of India which governs and regulates licenses for physicians. For healthcare providers like hospitals and small format clinics or 'nursing homes' (with overnight admission facilities) there is a separate body for accreditation. The national Accreditation Board of Hospitals and Healthcare Providers (NABH), is an initiative of the Government of India through its arm Quality Council of India. NABH ensures quality in standards of practice through accreditation. Similarly, National Accreditation Board for Testing and Calibration Laboratories or NABL ensures quality through accreditation of pathological laboratories. The latest addition to this space is the National Commission for Allied and Healthcare Professions Act, 2021 [37] legislated by the Government of India, on 28, March, 2021 to provide for regulation and maintenance of standards by sleep technologists amongst others. The other (non-medical) aspects of healthcare facilities like labor, insurance, *etc.* are all governed and regulated separately by independent regulations governing these domains. A healthcare facility thus relies on various permissions from the government to run and operate by ensuring standards in all these areas. Over the years, different bodies based on voluntary intent to steer the quality and standards in the health sector have grown and some like Indian Medical Association have become significant enough to impact public opinion by supporting the Governments in framing various guidelines, as was the case recently, during the coronavirus pandemic in 2019.

For Sleep Medicine, a government driven regulatory framework exclusively governing the practice of sleep medicine in India, is yet to be formulated. Self-regulation by professional groups/bodies/councils may be legally or voluntarily mandated such as the Indian Society of Sleep Research (ISSR) which puts forth voluntary recognition and accreditation of sleep labs. Sleep professionals in the sleep arena are accredited by the mother body, the World Association of Sleep Medicine (WASM) *via* the national regulatory bodies, in this case the ISSR, is trying to maintain quality standards. ISSR, although well placed in the practice with its initiation at the All India Institute of Medical Sciences, New Delhi, is not independently empowered as a regulator to ensure standards of practice. In such cases, a specific regulatory framework setup as a legal statute may be looked at as a potential response to address problems especially in a developing and growing field of sleep medicine.

The landscape of Sleep regulation in India is a self-organized one with ISSR and ISDA at the forefront of licensing. From standardization of training of medical and paramedical personnel to standards of practice and lab setup, these voluntary bodies have been spearheading the practice. Fellowships offered by both of these bodies entail clearing of an exam for physicians that standardizes the knowledge front, thereby minimizing knowledge gaps in the varied specialties physicians come from to practice sleep medicine. Similarly for technicians, clinical hands-on training in an established sleep setup under a specified number of hours has been paving way for certification of sleep techs in India, with the scenario now changing. Sleep labs may receive accreditation following a check by specialists with established practice ensuring basic standards for practice.

Limited and varied regulations with respect to patient care and monitoring of sleep labs in India allow the standards of practice to vary. In most cases, the appropriate choice of sleep equipment and the level of study is entirely at the discretion of the treating physician. Thus, there is naturally a skepticism on sleep reporting as the inclination of the physician and the technologist does not always lie with the manual scouring of epochs but with the automated reporting of the overnight polysomnograms. In private sector hospitals, this may find preference given that automated reporting is more time-efficient and human resource efficient. This is usually not the case in government run teaching hospitals.

THE PRACTICE OF SLEEP MEDICINE AND LAB ECOSYSTEMS

Sleep Medicine ecosystem in India has grown multifold over the last few years in three broad categories: physicians exclusively practicing sleep medicine, physicians practicing sleep medicine as a limited part of their primary specialty (pulmonology, neurology, psychiatry, dentistry, pediatrics); and sleep researchers from basic science disciplines [38].

A sleep lab usually has a trained sleep technologist carrying out the PSG on the orders of a physician. Levels of study may vary according to the clinical indication and readiness of the patient. Since sleep is a secondary specialty, standalone sleep clinics and labs are fewer in India. Information on these setups is available with the ISSR and ISDA but given the voluntary nature of these organizations and its members, it is hard to establish a comprehensive database of sleep facilities in the country.

A Sleep Lab facility in India is usually affiliated with a primary specialty or affiliated with one or more labs. For instance, the sleep lab affiliated with Neurology, usually shares space with the Neuro-electrophysiology lab. Labs affiliated with Pulmonary Medicine may also offer Level 2 and Level 3 studies which for instance may also be supportive in the diagnosis or prognosis of restrictive lung diseases.

Expensive PSG equipment, burden of out-of-pocket expenditure for diagnosis and treatment of sleep ailments and lack of awareness have continued to hinder access, even in metropolitans where sleep labs are limited to one or two beds in a particular setup. Given the vast socio-economic disparity in the population, widespread geography and lack of adequate medical facilities in most towns and cities, sleep disorders still figure at the bottom of recognizable ailments. This increases the burden of treatable non-communicable diseases in India as labs are only visited by the privileged few.

Sleep labs require adequate sleep personnel to carry out PSGs which is a visible gap in the practice. Multiple courses have been introduced in the recent past for sleep technicians by private as well as state-run institutions. Most of these are on the job training certificate or diploma courses requiring a high school certificate, enabling one to pursue a career in sleep.

CHALLENGES, GAPS AND WAY FORWARD

India, like every country, has her own set of challenges; one being the unmet need for quality healthcare for all her citizens. A rich cultural heritage, accumulated beliefs, myths and mythologies passed on as traditions, have influenced the mindsets of people and continue to do so even today, especially in smaller towns and rural areas. Snoring, for instance, is still considered a sign of sound and healthy sleep. On the other hand, REM behavior disorders and NREM parasomnias may be passed off as karmic burdens or manifestations. Lacunae in sleep hygiene across ages in the general population are dismally low. The percentage of primary care or family physicians addressing sleep in clinical routines, remains dissatisfactory. If sleep is considered an integral part of wellbeing, red flags must be raised at the primary level of health screening as research has enough evidence to substantiate deleterious consequences of sleep deprivation [39]. Shortcomings in India's evolving healthcare system go untended as the population grows, further outgalloping the existing gaps, by virtue of the basic needs yet unmet.

In a country like India where basic survival in the weakest sections continues to wobble the national demographics with low function literacy rates, and limited access to healthcare, strengthening deficiencies of the public health system like lack of infrastructure, trained and efficient health personnel, strengthening regulatory and standardizing bodies will help bridge the gaps faster [40].

Since Sleep medicine continues to be a growing specialty in India, with the population growing exponentially, healthy sleep and sleep hygiene are a growing concern, especially, after the pandemic has put urban metropolitan dwellers in a circadian disarray with extended work hours in the work from home culture and increasing stress levels. Mental health and sleep have crossed paths only to become parallels with the pandemic sparing no household of vagaries. The gaps in planning and governance in special situations like these end up in public health chaos that further triggers the vicious cycle of anxiety and insomnia, for instance, highlighting an urgent need for preventive, pro-motive, rehabilitative and public health measures for healthy sleeping hygiene.

The field of sleep medicine in India is fraught with major gaps and challenges that have only deepened and taken a complex shape over the last couple of decades of its growth in the country. In the space of medicine, it is still finding its stronghold amongst other advanced specialties. The space is also evolving rapidly being influenced as much by economics as it is by socio-cultural knowledge, attitudes and practices - a case with any nascent field of medicine. This is clearly evidenced by the fact that sleep medicine does not find its due in the medicine curriculum at the graduate level. Public Health view of sleep related disorders is also missing from the larger public perspective. There are no specific policies for public health safety where sleep disorders may affect industrial/shift workers or commercial vehicle drivers. There is a lack of adequate facilities in state-led institutions affecting coverage in a hugely populous country such as India. Insurance, another driver of coverage, is not clear and direct about the inclusion of sleep unless referred by physicians for in-patients.

Transformation in the perspectives, awareness and scientific application of what has already been learnt by research and practice the world over can be brought about by first incorporating sleep medicine as a domain of learning medical curriculum. The latest initiative of creating a bachelor's degree and a formal two-year post-doctoral fellowship program at AIIMS, Rishikesh is a welcome move. Creating a space for research and practice of sleep medicine, even across different specializations, will support the cause of awareness as well as the development of the scientific basis of practice. Inclusion in insurance (reimbursable claims for overnight PSGs); transport policy especially for commercial vehicle driving (restrictions in driving time, awareness modules for drowsy driving, screening for daytime sleepiness); and amendments in labor laws (restrictions in the number of working hours for adequate sleep) are some of the key changes that would significantly change the public health aspects related to sleep in India, directly translating into positive outcomes. Supply chain management making quality sleep related drugs available in cities of all tiers would enable satisfactory and timely treatment-seeking behavior in people. Setting up of periodic sleep boards or regulatory bodies would standardize the approach to treatment and update physicians on the global advances in the practice. A National Sleep Policy, independent of the National Health Policy of India (published from time to time, the last one being in 2017) will lead to an integrated approach to solve challenges in this arena. With the incorporation of recommendations given by ISSR [11], a shift in knowledge, attitudes and practices would pave the way for Indians experience better sleep hygiene and health.

CONCLUSION

India is a large country, only second to China in terms of population. It promises great opportunity and significant contribution to the sleep arena provided unmet needs and gaps in the sector are satisfied. Specific research interests, interventions and regulations will bring about the requisite leap for India as quality research and data would help contribute to the global body of knowledge in Sleep Medicine.

CONSENT FOR PUBLICATION

Not applicable.

CONFLICT OF INTEREST

The authors declare no conflict of interest, financial or otherwise.

ACKNOWLEDGEMENT

Declared none.

NOTES

[1]All India Institute of Medical Sciences (AIIMS), a premier, center-run tertiary medical institution in India, with the first one situated in New Delhi. Estd. in 1956, it continues in its leading role fostering research, training and clinical practice in almost all medical specialties.

[2]Safdarjung Hospital is a state run tertiary medical institution, setup in pre-Independence India, 1942, to serve as base hospital for American and allied party soldiers during World War II.

[3]All India Institute of Medical Sciences, a tertiary level government institution of the central government located at Rishikesh, a foothill town in the northern Indian state of Uttarakhand setup as part of regionally expanding the reach of AIIMS, New Delhi.

[4]B.Sc. (Sleep Technology and Electrical Neurophysiology) at AIIMS, Rishikesh (https://aiimsrishikesh.edu.in).

REFERENCES

[1]   Kumar VM, Mallick HN, Shrivastava D. The history of Indian Society for Sleep Research (ISSR) from its inception to the launching of the journal "sleep and vigilance.". Sleep Vigil 2017; 1(1): 3-5.
       [http://dx.doi.org/10.1007/s41782-016-0002-5]

[2]   Kumar VM, Mallick HN. Early History of Sleep Research and Sleep Medicine in India. Sleep Vigil 2021; 5(1): 3-4.
       [http://dx.doi.org/10.1007/s41782-021-00140-w]

[3]   Desiraju T. Stimulus-response relationship in the production of after-discharges and their spread from intact cerebral gyri to neuronally isolated slabs. Electroencephalogr Clin Neurophysiol 1966; 21(4): 345-54.
       [http://dx.doi.org/10.1016/0013-4694(66)90040-X] [PMID: 4162428]

[4]   Singh B, Desiraju T, Anand BK. Electrical activity of the ventral hippocampus during sleep. Neurol India 1966; 14(3): 154-6.
       [PMID: 5924723]

[5]   Desiraju T. Effect of intraventricularly administered prostaglandin E1 on the electrical activity of cerebral cortex and behavior in the unanesthetized monkey. Prostaglandins 1973; 3(6): 859-70.
       [http://dx.doi.org/10.1016/0090-6980(73)90010-5] [PMID: 4199677]

[6]   Desiraju T. Neural integrations in the substrate for sleep and vigilance. Biosystems 1971; 4(1): 1-11.
       [http://dx.doi.org/10.1016/0303-2647(71)90002-5] [PMID: 4325204]

[7]   Desiraju T, Anand BK, Singh B. Responses of oculomotor nucleus and marginal gyrus in sleep. Experientia 1968; 24(6): 565-6.
       [http://dx.doi.org/10.1007/BF02153774] [PMID: 4301538]

[8]   ISSR-Indian Society for Sleep Research https://issr.in

[9]   Chokshi M, Patil B, Khanna R, *et al.* Health systems in India. J Perinatol 2016; 36(S3): S9-S12.
[http://dx.doi.org/10.1038/jp.2016.184] [PMID: 27924110]

[10]   Amin A, Dutta M, Brahmawar Mohan S, Mohan P. Pathways to Enable Primary Healthcare Nurses in
Providing Comprehensive Primary Healthcare to Rural, Tribal Communities in Rajasthan, India. Front
Public Health 2020; 8: 583821.
[http://dx.doi.org/10.3389/fpubh.2020.583821] [PMID: 33330325]

[11]   Akhtar N, Mallick H. Recommendations for a National Sleep Policy in India. Natl Med J India 2019;
32(1): 59-60.
[http://dx.doi.org/10.4103/0970-258X.272131] [PMID: 31823948]

[12]   Kumar, V. Sleep Medicine in Ancient and Traditional India. In: Chokroverty, S., Billiard, M. (eds)
Sleep Medicine. Springer, New York, NY. 2015; pp. 25-28.
[http://dx.doi.org/10.1007/978-1-4939-2089-1_4]

[13]   Sharma RK, Dash VB. Agnivesa's Charak Samhita. Varanasi: Chowkhamba Sanskrit Series Office
1976; p. 619.

[14]   Bhishagratna KKL. The Sushruta Samhita-an English translation based on original texts. Calcutta:
Kaviraj Kunjalal Bhishagratna; 1916. (Year printed by M. Bhattacharyya, At the Bharat Mihir Press,
25, Roy Bag An Street) 1916.

[15]   Pooja S, Sonali E, Yogesh P.A scientific ayurvedic exploration of concept of sleep (NIDRA). 2018.

[16]   https://www.hopkinsmedicine.org/health/wellness-and-prevention/ayurveda

[17]   Keswani NH. Medical heritage of India.The science of medicine and physiological concepts in ancient
and medieval India. New Delhi: National Book Trust 1974; pp. 3-52.

[18]   Wood E. Practical yoga, ancient and modern Being a new, independent translation of Patanjali's yoga
aphorisms, interpreted in the light of ancient and modern psychological knowledge and practical
experience. London: Rider 1951.

[19]   Telles S, Gupta RK, Verma S, Kala N, Balkrishna A. Changes in vigilance, self rated sleep and state
anxiety in military personnel in India following yoga. BMC Res Notes. 2018; 11(1): 518.
[http://dx.doi.org/10.1186/s13104-018-3624-y]

[20]   Panjwani U, Dudani S, Wadhwa M. Sleep, cognition, and yoga. Int J Yoga 2021; 14(2): 100-8.
[http://dx.doi.org/10.4103/ijoy.IJOY_110_20] [PMID: 34188381]

[21]   Nagarathna R, Bali P, Anand A, *et al.* Prevalence of Diabetes and Its Determinants in the Young
Adults Indian Population-Call for Yoga Intervention. Front Endocrinol (Lausanne). 2020; 11: 507064.
[http://dx.doi.org/10.3389/fendo.2020.507064]

[22]   Division UP. The impact of population momentum on future population growth United Nations,
Department of Economic and Social Affairs Population Division; (2017) Available at:
https://esa.un.org/unpd/wpp/publications/Files/PopFacts_2017-4_Population-Momentum.pdf

[23]   Rao M, Metri KG, Raghuram N, Hongasandra NR. Effects of Mind Sound Resonance Technique
(Yogic Relaxation) on Psychological States, Sleep Quality, and Cognitive Functions in Female
Teachers: A Randomized, Controlled Trial. Adv Mind Body Med. 2017 Winter;. 2017; 31(1): 4-9.
[PMID: 28183071]

[24]   Abaza H, Marschollek M. mHealth Application Areas and Technology Combinations*. A Comparison
of Literature from High and Low/Middle Income Countries. Methods Inf Med. 2017;56(7):e105-e122.
[http://dx.doi.org/10.3414/ME17-05-0003]

[25]   Bassi A, John O, Praveen D, *et al.* Current status and future directions of m-Health interventions for
health system strengthening in India: systematic review JMIR Mhealth Uhealth 2018;6 .
[http://dx.doi.org/10.2196/11440]

[26]   Madanian S, Parry DT, Airehrour D, Cherrington M. mHealth and big-data integration: promises for healthcare system in India. BMJ Health Care Inform 2019; 26(1): e100071.
       [http://dx.doi.org/10.1136/bmjhci-2019-100071] [PMID: 31488497]

[27]   Gupta R, Kumar VM, Tripathi M, *et al.* Guidelines of the Indian Society for Sleep Research (ISSR) for Practice of Sleep Medicine during COVID-19. Sleep Vigil 2020; 4(2): 61-72.
       [http://dx.doi.org/10.1007/s41782-020-00097-2] [PMID: 32838116]

[28]   Jahrami H, BaHammam AS, Bragazzi NL, Saif Z, Faris M, Vitiello MV. Sleep problems during the COVID-19 pandemic by population: a systematic review and meta-analysis. J Clin Sleep Med 2021; 17(2): 299-313.
       [http://dx.doi.org/10.5664/jcsm.8930] [PMID: 33108269]

[29]   Bhat S, Chokroverty S. Sleep disorders and COVID-19 [published online ahead of print, 2021 Jul 18]. Sleep Med. 2021; S1389-9457(21): 00403-2.
       [http://dx.doi.org/10.1016/j.sleep.2021.07.021]

[30]   Alimoradi Z, Broström A, Tsang HWH, *et al.* Sleep problems during COVID-19 pandemic and its' association to psychological distress A systematic review and meta-analysis. EClinicalMedicine 2021; 36: 100916.
       [http://dx.doi.org/10.1016/j.eclinm.2021.100916]

[31]   Krishnamoorthy Y, Rajaa S, Murali S, Rehman T, Sahoo J, Kar SS. Prevalence of metabolic syndrome among adult population in India. A systematic review and meta-analysis 2021; 15(10): e0240971.
       [http://dx.doi.org/10.1371/journal.pone.0240971]

[32]   Gupta R, Das S, Gujar K, Mishra KK, Gaur N, Majid A. Clinical Practice Guidelines for Sleep Disorders. Indian J Psychiatry 2017; 59(5) (Suppl. 1): 116.
       [http://dx.doi.org/10.4103/0019-5545.196978] [PMID: 28216789]

[33]   Kumar N, Gupta R, Kumar H, *et al.* Impact of home confinement during COVID-19 pandemic on sleep parameters in Parkinson's disease. Sleep Med 2021; 77: 15-22.
       [http://dx.doi.org/10.1016/j.sleep.2020.11.021] [PMID: 33302094]

[34]   Maity K, Nagarathna R, Anand A, *et al.* Sleep Disorders in Individuals With High Risk for Diabetes in Indian Population. Ann Neurosci 2020; 27(3-4): 183-9.
       [http://dx.doi.org/10.1177/0972753121998470] [PMID: 34556958]

[35]   Sharma M, Aggarwal S, Madaan P, Saini L, Bhutani M. Impact of COVID-19 pandemic on sleep in children and adolescents: a systematic review and meta-analysis. Sleep Med 2021; 84: 259-67.
       [http://dx.doi.org/10.1016/j.sleep.2021.06.002] [PMID: 34182354]

[36]   Gupta B, Sharma V, Kumar N, Mahajan A. Anxiety and Sleep Disturbances Among Health Care Workers During the COVID-19 Pandemic in India: Cross-Sectional Online Survey. JMIR Public Health Surveill 2020; 6(4): e24206.
       [http://dx.doi.org/10.2196/24206] [PMID: 33284784]

[37]   https://egazette.nic.in/WriteReadData/2021/226213.pdf

[38]   Kanchan S, Saini LK, Daga R, Arora P, Gupta R. Status of the practice of sleep medicine in India during the COVID-19 pandemic. J Clin Sleep Med 2021; 17(6): 1229-35.
       [http://dx.doi.org/10.5664/jcsm.9172] [PMID: 33612159]

[39]   Liew SC, Aung T. Sleep deprivation and its association with diseases- a review. Sleep Med 2021; 77: 192-204.
       [http://dx.doi.org/10.1016/j.sleep.2020.07.048] [PMID: 32951993]

[40]   Kasthuri A. Challenges to Healthcare in India - The Five A's. Indian J Community Med 2018; 43(3): 141-3.
       [http://dx.doi.org/10.4103/ijcm.IJCM_194_18] [PMID: 30294075]

CHAPTER 15

Sleep Medicine in Nepal: Practice Differences, Resources and Gaps in Knowledge

Narendra Bhatta[1,*], **Deebya Raj Mishra**[1], **Avatar Verma**[1], **Rejina Shahi**[1], **Sion Hangma Limbu**[1], **Srijan Katwal**[1] and **Nishad Bhatta**[1]

[1] *Department of Pulmonary, Critical Care & Sleep Medicine, B.P. Koirala Institute of Health Sciences (BPKIHS), Dharan, Nepal*

Abstract: The Federal Democratic Republic of Nepal is one of the most beautiful and stunning Himalayan countries in the world where health care needs of the majority of the population are delivered by a hybrid system of public and private sectors. Public does not perceive sleep disorders to be as critical as other health problems because they remain unaware of the serious consequences of sleep deprivation and sleep disorders. Multiple segments of the Nepalese population are awake across all hours of the 24-hour day because of the large proportions of people working as migrant workforce across the globe in different time zones. Current data reveals a high public health burden of sleep loss and sleep disorders are among them yet these disorders are frequently ignored, readily treatable, and unrecognized health problems in Nepal.

Sleep medicine remains an interdisciplinary field crossing different specialties but in Nepal, it has become almost a subspecialty of pulmonary medicine in the past few years. Nepal does not have sufficient healthcare resources to deliver the appropriate care to patients with sleep-related disorders because of an inadequate number of physicians trained in sleep medicine. Sleep disorders and sleep medicine as a specialty are under-recognized by both the public and health professionals. The government should rethink policies and redesign the programs to address the evolving syndemic of sleep disorders, metabolic syndrome, and tobacco smoking in Nepal and incorporate sleep medicine in undergraduate and postgraduate medical curricula to address the gap in the clinical care of patients with sleep disorders in Nepal.

Keywords: Medical Curriculum, Nepal, Sleep Disorders, Sleep Medicine, Syndemic.

INTRODUCTION

"Sleep health" is explicitly defined and measured; five dimensions of sleep have been identified. Four measures of quality: satisfaction, alertness, timing,efficiency

* **Corresponding author Narendra Bhatta:** Department of Pulmonary, Critical Care and Sleep Medicine, B. P. Koirala Institute of Health Sciences (BPKIHS), Dharan, Nepal; Email: bhattanarendra@hotmail.com

Hrayr P. Attarian, Marie-Louise M. Coussa-Koniski & Alain Michel Sabri (Eds.)

and one duration. The quality and quantity of sleep and/or their association with health and quality of life at the population level are affected by technological, demographic, cultural and geographical disparities [1]. The public health burden of sleep loss is immense and sleep disorders are among the most common yet frequently overlooked, readily treatable and frequently unrecognized health problems in low-income countries like Nepal [2, 3]. Surprisingly, there is a lack of high-quality national data about sleep health, and sleep medicine. With reference to locally published data, this review aims to discuss the unmet healthcare needs, the potential causes of treatment gaps from the perspective of pulmonary medicine and the present position of sleep medicine as a specialty in a low-income country like Nepal. To address this information gap, the present review was guided by the following research questions: what is Nepal's geopolitical profile (health care system, age and income distribution)? What is the socio-ecology of Sleep in Nepal? What are the local epidemiological data, what are the existing facilities for providing care to patients with sleep disorders, what about access, barriers and disparity? What is the current status of Sleep Medicine? What type of practitioners is involved in sleep medicine? Are there any practice guidelines, professional societies, or regulatory bodies? What is the research situation? What are the challenges and unique needs of sleep medicine in Nepal?

NEPAL: COUNTRY PROFILE (INCLUDING A BRIEF DESCRIPTION OF GEOPOLITICAL DATA AND HEALTH CARE SYSTEM)

The Federal Democratic Republic of Nepal is one of the most beautiful and stunning Himalayan countries in the world. It has a population of 30 million and a surface of 147,516 km^2 distributed between three regions: the capital of Nepal is Kathmandu. The country consists of three topographic regions: the Himalayan Mountains in the north the middle hills (Mid-hills), and the Terai plains in the south. Its elevation ranges from 60 meters (m) above the sea level in the southeastern Terai to the highest point on earth, Mount Everest at 8,848.86 m. It has eight of the world's ten tallest mountains and contains more than 240 peaks over 6,096 m above sea level. Most Nepalese live either on the country's fertile plains or in the hills, only less than 7% of the population lives in the remote mountainous regions. Nepal is home to people from more than 100 ethnic groups, most of whom share the official Nepali language [4].

Nepal is one of the Low Middle Income Country (LMIC), Nepal's gross domestic product (GDP) per capita for 2016 was $729 in US dollars (USD) and ranks 197/229 countries by its GDP per capita (purchasing power parity adjusted). Agriculture accounts for 34 percent of GDP despite employing 70 percent of the population. Life expectancy at birth in 2016 was 70 years (68 years for males, 71 years for females) according to the World Bank. Nepal's steady increases in GDP as well as the healthcare resources were strained after the 2015 earthquake [5].

In Nepal, healthcare is delivered by a hybrid system of public and private sectors and includes predominantly modern healthcare with some traditional Ayurveda health care and other alternative medicines. The healthcare needs of the majority of the Nepalese population are covered by the public healthcare system which includes hospitals, primary healthcare centers and health posts in the rural area. Recent political reforms in Nepal have decentralized power to federal, state and local to facilitate access to health services. The private health care system consists of private clinics in suburban areas and some huge state-of-the-art super specialty hospitals in urban areas [5, 6]. However patients need to pay nearly 100% of the health care costs out of pocket irrespective of what health care system they access. Social Health Security coverage started to be implemented since 2015, nevertheless, Nepal does not have an organized national public health insurance system.

Nepal's life expectancy for both males and females combined is 70.9 (95% UI: 69.8–72.1) years. Life expectancy increased from 59 to 73 years for females, and 58 to 69 years for males, between 1990 and 2017. Ischemic heart disease (16.4% of total deaths), chronic obstructive pulmonary disease (COPD) (9.8% of total deaths), diarrheal diseases (5.6% of total deaths), lower respiratory infections (5.1% of total deaths) and intracerebral hemorrhage (3.8% of total deaths), were the top five causes of death in 2017. The rise of NCDs is partly due to the changing age structure and lifestyle changes such as increased sedentary behavior, tobacco use, changes in eating habits, and harmful use of alcohol [5 - 7].

Despite these considerable challenges and with limited resources, Nepal has made remarkable progress in reducing poverty, increasing access to education and improving the health status of its people, and achieved many of the Millennium Development Goals (MDGs) by 2015. While the country is making progress towards federalism, the COVID-19 pandemic has deeply affected the economy in diverse ways, including the overall management of the health sector and its functionality [8].

Social-ecology of Sleep in Nepal

Human sleep is remarkably social in nature and sleep health is a complex product of cultural and social influences independently of diseases. Sleep in real world is driven by many of the same factors that drive health-related behaviors, such as diet and exercise [9]. For example co-sleeping defined as sharing the bed, is influenced by maternal attitudes: sleeping with a child is considered to increase the probability of his/her survival. The advent of globalization, competition (24/7 society), social networking and cultural belief have, also, significantly impacted the sleep health.

KNOWLEDGE AND ATTITUDE OF HEALTH PROFESSIONALS AND THE GENERAL PUBLIC TOWARD SLEEP DISORDERS AND SLEEP MEDICINE

The health system in Nepal relies on the referral system, where the patient's first exposure is usually to the PHC physician, who assesses and decides the patient's plan of management.

Sleep disorders and sleep medicine as a specialty are under-recognized by both the public and the medical community. Sleep medicine is not included in the curriculum of the schools of medicine nor of the post graduate training programs,

All these limitations are responsible of a low awareness about the importance of sleep pathology, its consequences and comorbidities at all levels including the health care authorities (public and private) who are not interested by investing into the sleep diseases field. Finally, this low awareness is responsible of under diagnosis and mismanagement and lack of creation of accessible sleep centers and as is the case in developed countries.

Magnitude of the Problems Sleep Disorders in Nepal

Prevalence of sleep disorders data is limited.

The low availability of sleep health resources is mainly reflected in 2 dimensions [1, 2]: the sleep health facilities and specialized physicians are concentrated in urban areas.

Low awareness among the public and the medical community, represents a public health issue especially older people and women.

Bhatta *et al* in 2018 explored both behaviorally and culturally based sleep habits and patterns in a cross-sectional, questionnaire-based, observational study in Nepal and reported that majority of people in Nepal slept for 7-8 hours. The biggest sleepers are younger with an average of 8 hours of sleep. Men tend to go to bed earlier than women. 14% of people smoked some form of tobacco before sleep while 44% of people consumed beverages before sleeping. It was also revealed in their study that 7% of subjects <40 yrs. and 15% of people > 40 yrs. had snoring while sleeping [10]. Sleep-Related Breathing Disorders (SRBD) are common in Nepalese patients with Chronic Obstructive Pulmonary Disease (COPD). Presence of Sleep-Related Breathing Disorders (SRBD) results in non-restorative sleep, daytime sleepiness and fatigue, increases the odds of several other adverse health outcomes and worsening the already diminished quality of life in patients with COPD.

Koirala *et al* in 2018 studied the Sleep Patterns and Disorders in patients with Chronic Obstructive Pulmonary Disease (COPD) in Nepal and reported that 62.5% patients with COPD had evidence of various forms of Sleep Related Breathing Disorder (SRBD.) Loud Snoring, Higher BMI, and current smoking status were associated with severe SRBD in COPD. The Presence of SRBD had a significant impact on the clinical outcome of COPD patients in their study. The authors recommended regular screening of COPD patients regarding sleep pathology and treatment of associated sleep disorders [11].

In another study related to Sleep Related Breathing Disorders (SRBD) & Bronchial Asthma in Nepal Bhatta *et al* in 2018 reported evidence of various forms of Sleep Related Breathing Disorder (SRBD) in 60% of patients presenting with bronchial asthma and concluded that Presence of SRBD was an independent risk factor of severity for patients with severe bronchial Asthma [12].

Bhatta *et al* in 2020 conducted a study to determine prevalence of Obstructive Sleep Apnea (OSA) in Metabolic Syndrome (MetS) and explored its clinical correlates with tobacco smoking incorporating the concept a "Syndemic" in developing countries and reported that 70% of patients with Metabolic Syndrome (MetS) had Obstructive Sleep Apnea (OSA) [13, 14]. In addition, hospital based observational studies have suggested a more than 10-year delay between symptom onset and referral to sleep disorder clinical care center which supports the belief that sleep disorders are under-recognized and under-diagnosed, resulting in a significant delay in diagnosis and treatment.

Current Position of Sleep Medicine in Nepal

Sleep medicine remains an interdisciplinary field crossing different specialties but in Nepal it has become almost a subspecialty of pulmonary medicine in the past few years. The use of proper "type I" full polysomnography in Nepal started relatively recently; the service is still in its early stages and faces many challenges. There are only few clinical facilities that provide clinical diagnostic and therapeutic services for patients with different sleep disorders.

Current Obstacles Facing of the Practice of Sleep Medicine in Nepal

The major obstacles facing the Practice of Sleep Medicine in Nepal can be categorized as follows:

• Inadequate number of qualified specialists: The number of trained qualified sleep medicine specialists in Nepal is reportedly 10 physicians located in a few hospitals in three major cities. Some non-specialists with no adequate training practice sleep medicine also, essentially in the private sector, Moreover, the majority of sleep medicine specialists deal with sleep disorders as a small part of a larger pulmonology medical practice. Establishing a good sleep medicine service requires a dedicated specialist who has protected time for practicing sleep medicine.

• A lack of trained sleep technologists who can perform polysomnography is another major obstacle that prevented the establishment of a sleep medicine service. This obstacle can be overcome by organizing workshops or a program for sleep technologists in academic medical centers. The data acquisition, scoring and interpretation of a sleep test require expertise.

• Another major obstacle that faces practitioners in developing countries is the after-sale service of diagnostic equipment related to sleep medicine. Local agents of sleep-diagnostic systems promote their machines but do not provide efficient after-sale service because of a lack of adequate training and knowledge of the product sold.

• In general, most physicians receive no or minimal education about sleep medicine during medical school or residency training, the number of sleep specialists in the country is very low and does not meet the increasing demand for service. We need also to increase awareness of other specialties such as internal medicine, to be able to diagnose and refer patients to sleep specialists. B .P. Koirala Institute of Health Sciences (BPKIHS) has made a major step forward by initiating post-doctoral subspecialty training doctorate of medicine (DM) in Pulmonary, Critical Care & Sleep Medicine (PCCSM) but still more training academic programs are needed to meet the increasing demand.

• It is obvious that more sleep research is needed, academic centers, in collaboration with internationally renowned research centers, should develop research that addresses the prevalence of different sleep disorders in Nepal in order to convince healthcare providers and decision-makers of the size of the problem and to stimulate them to apply appropriate solutions.

• Use of media channels and/or new technologies and also through the NRS to educate and increase awareness of the public about the serious consequences of sleep disorders, sleep deprivation and disturbances of biological rhythms.

Need to Incorporate Sleep Medicine in Medical School Curriculum and why Pulmonary Medicine Should Lead the Effort

Sleep medicine is a dynamic and rapidly growing multidisciplinary field that crosses all domains of medicine. Pulmonary medicine has made important contributions to the field of sleep medicine for many years. Pulmonary specialists have always had an important role in the recognition, management, and research in regard to sleep-related breathing disorders. On the other hand, sleep disorders constitute a significant health problem and, all physicians, regardless of their specialty, should have the knowledge and awareness to diagnose them.

Incorporating sleep medicine contents in the medical school curriculum and initiating early exposure to sleep medicine clinical training will raise sleep health awareness to improve patient care and expose future clinicians to the importance of good sleep hygiene for themselves. Understanding sleep is critical for medical students, residents, and physicians because they are among those at greatest risk for sleep loss due to their educational and professional obligations. The main obstacle to implementing adequate sleep medicine education in the curriculum of medical schools is curriculum overload and time constraints. A viable alternative approach is to integrate sleep medicine into the existing curriculum and create post-graduate training programs in the academic centers.

CONCLUSION

Sleep medicine in Nepal is still in the early phases of development. Currently, it remains primarily in the domain of pulmonary medicine. However, interdisciplinary efforts are well on the way. The limitations remain primarily in the integration of sleep medicine into the medical school curricula and expansion of sleep-related public health education. Integration of sleep in pulmonary medicine education can be the first step in mitigating these factors.

CONSENT FOR PUBLICATION

Not applicable.

CONFLICT OF INTEREST

The author declares no conflict of interest, financial or otherwise.

ACKNOWLEDGEMENT

Declared none.

REFERENCES

[1]   Saverio Stranges MD. An Emerging Global Epidemic? Findings from the INDEPTH WHO-SAGE Study among More Than 40,000 Older Adults from 8 Countries across Africa and Asia Sleep 2012; 35(8): 1173-81.

[2]   KK. The burden and determinants of non-communicable diseases risk factors in Nepal: Findings from a nationwide STEPS surveyKirchmair R, ed PLoS ONE. 2015; 10.(8).

[3]   Dhimal M, Karki KB, Sharma SK, *et al.* Prevalence of selected chronic non-communicable diseases in Nepal. J Nepal Health Res Counc 2019; 17(3): 394-401.
[http://dx.doi.org/10.33314/jnhrc.v17i3.2327] [PMID: 31735938]

[4]   Thapa R, Bam K, Tiwari P, Sinha TK, Dahal S. R, Bam K, Tiwari P, Sinha TK, Dahal S. Implementing federalism in the health system of Nepal: opportunities and challenges. Int J Health Policy Manag 2018; 8(4): 195-8.
[http://dx.doi.org/10.15171/ijhpm.2018.121] [PMID: 31050964]

[5]   Pandey AR, Chalise B, Shrestha N, *et al.* Mortality and risk factors of disease in Nepal: Trend and projections from 1990 to 2040. PLoS One 2020; 15(12): e0243055.
[http://dx.doi.org/10.1371/journal.pone.0243055] [PMID: 33270728]

[6]   Yadav UN, Lloyd J, Hosseinzadeh H, Baral KP, Bhatta N, Harris MF. Self-management practice, associated factors and its relationship with health literacy and patient activation among multi-morbid COPD patients from rural Nepal. BMC Public Health 2020; 20(1): 300.
[http://dx.doi.org/10.1186/s12889-020-8404-7] [PMID: 32143673]

[7]   Yadav UN, Lloyd J, Baral KP, Bhatta N, Mehta S, Harris MF. Using a co-design process to develop an integrated model of care for delivering self-management intervention to multi-morbid COPD people in rural Nepal. Health Res Policy Syst 2021; 19(1): 17.
[http://dx.doi.org/10.1186/s12961-020-00664-z] [PMID: 33568139]

[8]   Nepal Health Research Council (NHRC), Ministry of Health and Population (MoHP) and Monitoring Evaluation and Operational Research (MEOR). Nepal Burden of Disease 2017:A Country Report based on the Global Burden of Disease 2017 Study. Kathmandu, Nepal: NHRC, MoHP, and MEOR; 2019.

[9]   Knutson KL. Sociodemographic and cultural determinants of sleep deficiency: Implications for cardiometabolic disease risk. Soc Sci Med 2013; 79: 7-15.
[http://dx.doi.org/10.1016/j.socscimed.2012.05.002] [PMID: 22682665]

[10]   N.Bhatta V. Kattel. N. Bhatta. Study of Sleep Habits and Patterns Across Various Age Groups: An Exploratory Study from Developing Country Am J Respir Crit Care 2018; 197: A7294.

[11]   P. Koirala R.H. Ghimire D. Mishra B. Bista B. Shah N. Bhatta; Sleep Patterns and Disorders in Patients with Chronic Obstructive Pulmonary Disease (COPD) in Nepal. A J Respir. Crit Care Med 2018; 197: A2418.

[12]   Bhatta N. P. Koirala RH Ghimire D. Mishra B. Bista, R Chetry; Study of Sleep Related Breathing Disorders (SRBD) and Bronchial Asthma in Developing Countries; Connecting the Dots Between Nocturnal Awakenings and Breathlessness. Am J Respir Crit Care Med 2017; 195: A6982.

[13]   Bhatta N, Arjun O, Maskey R, *et al.* Obstructive Sleep Apnea, Metabolic Syndrome and Tobacco Smoking: A Wakeup Call for Evolving Syndemic in Developing Countries Am J Respir. Crit Care Med 2020; 201: A4711.

[14]   Benjafield AV, Ayas NT, Eastwood PR, *et al.* Estimation of the global prevalence and burden of obstructive sleep apnoea: a literature-based analysis. Lancet Respir Med 2019; 7(8): 687-98.
[http://dx.doi.org/10.1016/S2213-2600(19)30198-5] [PMID: 31300334]

CHAPTER 16

Sleep Disorders in Syria

Mohammed Zaher Sahloul[1,*] and **Abdul Ghani Sankari**[2]

[1] *University of Illinois, Chicago, IL, USA*

[2] *Wayne State University, Detroit, Michigan, USA*

Abstract: Although there is no data on the prevalence of sleep disorders in the Syrian population, extrapolating from neighboring countries like Lebanon, Jordan, Iraq, and other Arab and Mediterranean countries, sleep disorders including sleep-disordered breathing are common. Non-Communicable diseases account for two-thirds of deaths. Hypertension, obesity, diabetes, and tobacco smoking are among the highest in the region. There is a strong association between NCDs and sleep-disordered breathing. Most sleep disorders in Syria are undiagnosed and untreated due to the absence of or very low access to sleep specialists and sleep testing, the absence of national policies, and low awareness within the medical community and among the public. The long conflict in Syria, which began in 2011, has resulted in a complex humanitarian emergency, with 6.7 million internally displaced people and 6.5 million refugees out of a total estimated population of 22.5 million. The conflict and the resultant destruction of the health infrastructure have led to a severe public health crisis, which has further impacted the health of the population. There is low access to sleep education, testing, and treatment, mostly in major urban centers, although the demands are increasing. There are ample opportunities to improve the practice of sleep medicine, in spite of the long conflict and war, if local champions, NGOs, national authorities, and medical societies adopted already-available resources, guidelines, and regulations, incorporated creative means and telehealth, and followed the recommendations of the World Health Organization on Sleep and Health.

Keywords: Syria, Sleep medicine, SDB, Insomnia, The Syrian crisis, Conflict, Displacement, Attacks on healthcare, Human resources, War, Post-crisis recovery, NCDs, Telehealth, Online training, Psychological trauma, PTSD, Refugee health, COVID-19, Operation Breathe.

AN OVERWHELMING CRISIS

The Syrian conflict that started in 2011 has resulted in a complex humanitarian emergency. The Syrian crisis, now in its eleventh year, has created an unprecedented strain on health services and systems due to the protracted nature

*** Corresponding author Mohammed Zaher Sahloul:** University of Illinois, Chicago, IL, USA; Tel: 1-708-935-6723; Email: sahloul@medglobal.org

Hrayr P. Attarian, Marie-Louise M. Coussa-Koniski & Alain Michel Sabri (Eds.)

of the warfare [1], the targeting of medics and health care infrastructure, the exodus of physicians and nurses, the shortage of medical supplies and medications, the unprecedented and enormous displacement of populations internally and externally, and the disruption of medical education and training.

The movement which was a part of the Arab Spring in 2011, turned into the biggest refugee crisis of the modern world, with millions of Syrian fleeing their neighborhoods and cities and becoming refugees in other countries, and over six million internally displaced, and enormous destruction to the infrastructure, healthcare system, social status of the population, economic crisis, and an increasing need for humanitarian support from the international community.

BEFORE THE CONFLICT

Before the current war, Health indicators improved consistently in the Syrian Arab Republic over the past three decades before the war [2] according to data from the Syrian Ministry of Health with life expectancy at birth increasing from 56 years in 1970 to 73.1 years in 2009; infant mortality dropped from 132 per 1000 live births in 1970 to 17.9 per 1000 in 2009; under-five mortality dropped significantly from 164 to 21.4 per 1000 live births, and maternal mortality fell from 482 per 100 000 live births in 1970 to 52 in 2009 [2].

The Syrian Arab Republic was in an epidemiological transition from communicable to non-communicable diseases with the latest data showing that 77% of deaths were caused by non-communicable diseases [2]. Total government expenditure on health as a percentage of Gross Domestic Product was 2.9 in 2009 [2]. Despite such a low public investment, access to health services has increased dramatically since the 1980s, with rural populations achieving better equity than before [2].

Despite the apparently improved capacity of the health system, a number of challenges persisted including inequities in access to health care between urban and rural areas, between the poor population and the wealthy, between refugees and displaced population and host communities, between loyal populations to the regime and populations that were perceived as opposing to the regime, and between the capital and other cities.

Other problems include poor quality of care, lack of health insurance for most of the population, inadequate national policies, lack of medical research, corruption and nepotism, the brain drain that was exacerbated due to a decade of war and economic deterioration, worsening economy, lack of vetted data, lack of transparency, inadequate utilization of capacity, inadequate coordination between providers of health services, uneven distribution of human resources, high turnover of skilled staff and leadership, inadequate number of qualified nurses and allied health professionals. In the past two decades, there has been an uncontrolled and largely unregulated expansion of private providers, resulting in uneven distribution of health and medical services among geographical regions. Standardized care and quality assurance and accreditation are major issues. A study done during the last pandemic revealed that mortality rates among critically ill patients admitted to the intensive care units with severe 2009 H1N1 influenza A was 51% in Damascus compared to an APACHE II-predicted mortality rate of 21% [2].

At the start of the civil war in 2011, NCDs represented nearly two-thirds of the burden of death and disability in Syria.

THE IMPACT OF THE WAR ON THE HEALTHCARE SECTOR

Prior to the conflict, Syria's health system was comparable with that of other middle-income countries; however, the prolonged conflict has led to a significant destruction of the health infrastructure. The lack of security and the direct targeting of health workers and health facilities have led to an exodus of trained staff leaving junior health workers to work beyond their capabilities in increasingly difficult circumstances. This exodus together with the destruction of the health infrastructure has contributed to the increase in communicable and non-communicable diseases and the rising morbidity and mortality of the Syrian population [3]. Strengthening the health system in the current and post-conflict phase requires the retention of the remaining health workers, incentives for health workers who have left to return as well as engagement with the expatriate Syrian and international medical communities.

The health sector was hit hard by this war [4], up to 50% of the health facilities have been destroyed and up to 70% of the healthcare providers fled the country seeking safety, which increased the workload and mental pressure for the remaining medical staff [5]. The international community failed to prevent the destruction of the health infrastructure [4], which resulted in the collapse of Syria's healthcare system and left millions of internally displaced people [IDPs] in desperate need of medical assistance.

Within a decade, the life expectancy of resident Syrians has declined by 11 years. Over the first 11 years of the conflict, at least 350,200 civilians died from injuries incurred in the violence from March 2011 to March 2021 according to the United Nations although other estimates put the number around 650,000 deaths due to injuries [6]. One in 13 of those who died in the conflict was a woman and about 1 in 13 was a child. Although there is no exact data, it is estimated that more than twice as many civilians, including many women and children, have probably died prematurely of infectious and noncommunicable chronic diseases (NCDs) due to a shortage of adequate health care [1]. Doctors, local administrators, and nongovernmental organizations are struggling to manage the consequences of the conflict under substandard conditions, often using unorthodox methods of healthcare delivery in field hospitals and remotely by telehealth communication. Much-needed medical supplies are channeled through dangerous routes across the borders from Lebanon, Jordan, Iraq, Turkey, and European countries.

With the war came economic hardship and collapse. Nine out of 10 Syrians live below the poverty line according to the United Nations [7]. Spending on health became a lower priority for most families struggling to sustain basic necessities including shelter and food. Most families can't afford to spend on medications, expensive treatments, elective surgeries, cancer treatment, dialysis, or medical devices especially with the lack of health insurance.

A CRISIS OF REFUGEES AND DISPLACEMENT

The crisis created the worst refugee crisis since WW2. According to the United Nations Refugees Agency (UNHCR), half of pre-war Syria's population is displaced internally or externally. Syria had a population of 22 million before the crisis. One out of four refugees and one out of five displaced persons in the world are from Syria. Currently, there are 6.6 million Syrian refugees, residing mostly in neighboring countries including Turkey (3.7 million), Lebanon (851,000), Jordan (672,000), Iraq (252,500), Egypt (136,000) [8].

Syrian refugees have been resettled through UNHCR resettlement programs in many European and Western countries. There are 674,000 Syrian refugees in Germany and 128,000 in Sweden. About 23,000 Syrian refugees were resettled in the US [9] and 44,600 in Canada [10]. Syrians fleeing the war took refuge in 125 countries including the Gaza strip and Somalia. Currently, Syria is the first country in terms of the origin of refugees for the past 6 years. Most Syrian refugees are non-camped. 75% of Syrian refugees are women and children. Syrian refugees don't have consistent or adequate access to primary, secondary or tertiary healthcare, including diagnosis and treatment of Sleep disorders, especially in Lebanon, Jordan, and Iraq. Many of the governments hosting the most refugees spend relatively little on health and are already struggling with a fast rise in NCDs in their native populations. The majority of Syrian refugees reside in Jordan, Lebanon, and Turkey, where NCDs already account for more than three-quarters of the deaths in each of these countries.

Neighboring countries have responded to the influx of Syrian refugees with different approaches to the organization and financing of health services for NCDs [11]. Until 2014, the Jordanian Ministry of Health provided access to primary and secondary care for Syrian refugees free of charge. Since then, the government has required refugees to register with the Ministry of the Interior and obtain an identification card to become eligible to pay a subsidized rate for care that is approximately 80 percent of what uninsured Jordanians pay. In August 2016, more than a quarter of the refugees in Jordan's camps had not received identification cards.

In Turkey, the host government bears the burden of providing free health services to only registered refugees; non-registered people have to pay out of pocket. With no national health insurance schemes to finance treatment costs, nearly all Syrian refugees—registered or unregistered—in Lebanon rely almost exclusively on humanitarian organizations for health care.

In Lebanon, refugees who have registered with UNHCR can access primary care services at public primary healthcare centers at a subsidized cost and can be referred to a secondary or tertiary health center if they meet specific criteria established by UNHCR, which takes into account the necessity of the treatment, financial need, disease prognosis, and overall cost. UNHCR considers care for chronic illnesses, such as cancer, on a case-by-case basis. If a case is deemed life-threatening, then UNHCR covers 75 percent of the treatment cost. The protracted nature of the Syrian crisis and limited funding from humanitarian organizations and donors have left UNHCR with an 83 percent deficit in overall funding for its budget.

Inside Syria, the United Nations Refugee Agency registered about 6.7 million internally displaced persons in 2021, more than the previous year [12]. The 2021 Syria Humanitarian Needs Overview (HNO) puts the number of people in need of assistance inside Syria at over 13.4 million. Of that number, approximately 5.9 million are in acute need of humanitarian assistance.

A cross-sectional study of Syrian refugees in the United States of America found that almost one-third (32.3%) of the sample had post-traumatic stress disorder (PTSD) prevalence, not due to a previous diagnosis [13]. A recent study reported a strong relationship between PTSD and sleep disturbances in Syrian refugees fleeing the war between 2013 and 2019. The study reported that increased experiences of current living difficulties and past trauma are associated with PTSD symptomology [14].

FOUR HEALTHCARE SYSTEMS

After a decade of unrest and war between different warring parties and involvement of different countries including Russia, Iran, the USA, Turkey, and others, Syria is divided administratively into at least four different areas. Each has its own political and military authority. And each has its own healthcare system, administration, priorities, funding, and statistics. There is minimal or no coordination among the four areas.

The government-controlled area includes major urban centers including the capital Damascus, and Rif Dimashq, Daraa, Sweida, Qunaitera, Homs, Hamah, Aleppo, Tartous, and Latakia. It has a population of 13.6 million living in 60% of the country [15]. Damascus has the only two sleep centers in the country in Al-Basel University Hospital and Tishrin Veterans hospital. Damascus has the most specialists and subspecialists in the country. There are eight public universities and 22 private universities in government-controlled areas including 6 medical schools.

The Northwest is controlled by the opposition group HTS. It is supported by Turkey. It depends mostly on cross-border humanitarian aid from the Bab-Alhawa border crossing that was established by the UNSC in 2015. It has a population of 3.4 million, half of them are IDPs. 1.4 million live in IDP camps. There are no sleep centers or specialists in that region. The main cities are Idlib, Ariha, Al-Dana, Salkeen, Kafr Takahreem, Jisr Shughour, Darkush, Harem, Alatarib, and Sarmada. There are two public universities- Idlib and Aleppo, 3 private universities, and 2 branches of Turkish universities. It has two medical schools.

The Turkish-administered region is controlled by Turkey and the "Syrian National Army", an opposition group. It is further divided into three administered areas: Euphrate Shield, Olive Branch, and Peace Spring. It has an estimated population of 1.7 million [16]. There are no sleep centers or specialists in that region. The main cities are Azaz, Efrin, Al-Bab, Jrablus, Tal Abyad, and Raas Al-Ein.

The Northeast is controlled by the "Syrian Democratic Front", a group of Kurdish-Arab Syrians that aspires for a self-autonomous region. It is supported by small American troops. This region was controlled by ISIS until it was defeated in 2017-2018. It has an estimated population of 1.8 million. There are no sleep centers or specialists in that region. The main cities are Raqqa, Deir Alzour, Hasaka, and Kamoshli.

Healthcare services in the opposition-controlled areas are limited and hard to access, some attempts to rebuild the healthcare system have already begun, however, no significant change has been made until now. There is no sleep testing, specialists, centers, or treatments available in these areas. For the refugees in the neighboring countries, access to healthcare services is different according to the host country, financial problems, and limited access to healthcare, and the outbreaks of many diseases were the major problems.

THE PREVALENCE OF SLEEP DISORDERS IN SYRIA

The estimated risk for OSA in the US general population is 5–15% [17]. The prevalence of sleep disorders in the Syrian population is unknown due to the absence of national data and statistics. Extrapolating from neighboring countries like Lebanon, Jordan, Iraq, and other Arab and Mediterranean countries, sleep disorders including sleep-disordered breathing are common.

There is significant evidence of the correlation between Metabolic Syndrome and Obstructive Sleep Apnea [18]. The presence of Metabolic Syndrome may be the trigger to the development of OSA. Metabolic abnormalities increase the chance of upper airway collapsibility. Hypertension, obesity, cardiovascular disorders, Dyslipidemia, and diabetes are all common in Syria, which are associated with sleep-disordered breathing.

Also, there is a high level of PTSD and other psychological trauma due to the war which increases the risk of obstructive sleep apnea and other sleep disorders, especially insomnia [19].

Most sleep disorders in Syria are undiagnosed and untreated due to the absence of or very low access to sleep specialists and sleep testing, the absence of national policies, and low awareness within the medical community and among the public.

Epidemiological studies have shown a strong association between OSA and hypertension and metabolic syndrome as major risk factors for CAD. Moderate-to-severe OSA has been shown to increase the risk and mortality from cardiovascular diseases (CVD), including fatal and non-fatal CAD. The Eastern Mediterranean Region (EMR) is recognized as a hotspot for CVD [20], where projections of its burden exceed those of other regions, yet local data to inform health policy is inadequate. Hypertension is common in Syria. 47.4% of adult men and 34.9% of adult women have reported hypertension [21].

Despite the high importance of providing health services for NCDs, very limited research articles and resources have been found covering this issue [4]. The World health organization (WHO) published a report in 2016 regarding the prevalence of NCDs for the population living inside Syria. Cardiovascular diseases had the highest percentage of NCDs with almost 25% of all the cases, 9% were cancer, 2% chronic respiratory diseases, 1% diabetes, 5% had communicable maternal or perinatal and nutritional conditions, and 8% for other NCDs, while war-related injuries had a significantly high percentage for about 50% [4]. In 2016, cross-sectional research studied the prevalence of non-communicable diseases in Lebanon among Syrian refugees and compared the results to the host community. Over half of the Syrian refugees reported at least one of the five main NCDs which are (hypertension, cardiovascular disease, diabetes, chronic respiratory diseases, and arthritis) [4]. Among the refugees, arthritis had the highest prevalence (60%), followed by hypertension (47%), chronic respiratory diseases (38%), cardiovascular disease (3.3%), and diabetes (3.3%) [4].

In a study by Maziak *et al.* about the cardiovascular health among adults in Syria, he found that Coronary artery disease (CAD) is the leading cause of mortality in adults in Aleppo, Syria. Coronary Vascular disease was responsible for 45% of overall mortality reported in 5 years and 49% of CVD deaths occurred before the age of 65 years [21].

In the same study, the prevalence of detected hypertension was 40.6%, compared to 11.8% who reported physician-diagnosed hypertension, and 8.6% who were taking antihypertensive treatment at the time of the survey. The prevalence of obesity was 38.2%, and the prevalence of smoking (cigarettes or waterpipe) was 38.7%. In men, 51.4% were daily cigarette smokers who consumed on average 20.8 ± 14.0 cig/day.

Hypertension, smoking, and obesity were widely spread among adults, affecting about three-quarters of adults in the studied population. Hypertension and smoking were more common among men, while obesity was more a problem for women, affecting almost half of them. Hypertension estimates were comparable to those reported from other Arab countries as well as from developed countries affecting about a third of adults. However, the fact that most hypertension cases in our population were not diagnosed or treated is alarming and requires the attention of health authorities to this major treatable CVD risk factor.

An excess in weight is more crucial for OSA than either age or gender [18]. For every percent in weight reduction, there is a 3% reduction in the AHI [18]. Increased waist diameter correlates with an increased incidence of OSA [18]. Obesity is an important factor, more importantly, central obesity. Central obesity is linked to higher leptin production with resistance to said hormone and leads to an increased probability of developing OSA.

The prevalence of obesity, especially among Syrian women, is high. A study showed a prevalence of 28.8% among men and 46.4% among women [21], which is higher than those reported in other Arab countries, including the affluent societies of the Arabian Peninsula [22]. Other Mediterranean countries, which share many climatic and nutritional patterns with Syria, have less prevalence of obesity among women such as Spain (15.2%), Greece (15%), and Turkey (29.4%) [23, 24].

A strong association between smoking and OSA has been demonstrated in observational studies. Cigarette smoking may increase the severity of OSA through alterations in sleep architecture, upper airway neuromuscular function, arousal mechanisms, and upper airway inflammation [25]. Conversely, some evidence links untreated OSA with smoking addiction. Current smokers had a greater odds of moderate or severe OSA compared with nonsmokers [26].

The rate of smoking among Syrian men is the highest among other Arab countries. 51.3% of Syrian men smoke, compared to, 39.7% in Palestine, and 42.1% in Lebanon; among women, prevalence is 8.4% in Syria, although increasing quickly especially with waterpipes, 10.9% in Jordan, and 24.3% Lebanon [27]. Another study found that about 63.6% of Syrian men smoke compared to 19.2% of women [21].

One in two Syrian refugee households had a member with NCDs [28]. Such a significant prevalence was also noted by the Disaster and Emergency Management Survey, which showed that 10.0% of Syrian refugees reported a form of NCDs. This finding adds further evidence to existing knowledge that refugees from middle-income countries such as Syria present a different demographic and disease profile burden than the classical profile of refugees fleeing conflicts in Africa where diseases of poverty (such as diarrhea, cholera, or malaria) are more prevalent [29]. Examination of reported prevalence rates of specific NCDs among Syrian refugees showed that the most commonly reported NCD was hypertension (7.4–9.7%), followed by Type 2 Diabetes (3.3–5.3%), which is in line with the results of the Disaster and Emergency Management Survey which showed that hypertension and diabetes were the most common NCDs among Syrian refugees [30].

Among the Jordanian population, 16.8% of individuals attending primary care were at high risk for OSA, 28.7% reported having snoring, and 34% had daytime sleepiness [31]. The prevalence of OSA is higher among patients with CAD (26–69%) [32].

Similarly, a regional study from Saudi Arabia showed a high prevalence of OSA among patients with CAD, with 82% of their patients at risk of OSA and 56.4% having polysomnography confirmed OSA [33].

A study from Lebanon assessed the prevalence of insomnia and sleep apnea risk and examined their relationship with sociodemographic, lifestyle, and health characteristics in a sample from Greater Beirut. A total of 44.5% of participants reported insomnia symptoms > 15 nights/mo and 34.5% reported insomnia. 31% of participants were at high risk for sleep apnea, but only 5% received the diagnosis from a physician. Increased sleep apnea risk was associated with unemployment, high body mass index, snoring, hypertension, arthritis, and other medical comorbidities [34].

A study from neighboring Iraq assessed the risk of obstructive sleep apnea among Iraqi people in 2019 by using the STOP-BANG assessment model. It involved 4027 in all 18 Governorates of Iraq. The age mean was 33.50 years, and the standard deviation was 12,735. The participants were 52.1% males and 47.9% females. Sixty-two percent of participants had low OSA risk, 14.8% had moderate OSA risk, and 23.2% had a high OSA risk [35].

In a pilot study done in 2006, the number of sleep tests increased over the period of the study after several campaigns of awareness. Sleep studies were performed on 197 patients who were referred for a sleep study after they presented with sleep complaints to a local Pulmonologist in Damascus who had the only in-clinic sleep center at the time of the study [36].

Mean age was 45.6 years (singles: 12%, married: 88%). The male/ female ratio was 86/14%. There was no correlation between OSA and type of profession, socioeconomic status, smoking status, and residence. The mean BMI was 35.5 kg/m². For patients 40-50 years, the mean BMI was 43.6 kg/m² and mean BP was 132/84. Most common associated diseases were HTN (39%), nasal pathology (24%), arthropathy (12%), DM (9%), CAD (7%), hypothyroidism (3%), CVA (3%), Hypercholesterolemia (3%). Mean TST (total sleep time was 5.6 hours. Mean REM periods were 44.1 minutes, mean REM/TST was 0.13). Snoring was detected in 88% of patients. OSA was the main diagnosis, accounting for 72% of patients. Respiratory disturbance index (RDI) ranged from mild (5-10/h) to very high (>35/h). Meantime of Oxygen desaturation below 90% was 49 min, and below 80% was 16 minutes. Non-OSA included normal (11%), upper airway resistance syndrome (4%). Mean CPAP pressure needed to alleviate snoring and apnea was 6.8 cm H_2O, which is a very low level compared to the level of CPAP used in other countries [36].

The above data, and extrapolation from neighboring countries, indicate a high prevalence of sleep disorders especially sleep-disordered breathing among the Syrian population.

THE CURRENT PRACTICE OF SLEEP MEDICINE IN SYRIA

In spite of the challenges, there are some available resources for Sleep patients, especially in major urban areas.

Although sleep studies were introduced in Damascus by private practitioners in 2000, they are still being used at a very limited capacity. There are no laws or requirements for sleep testing for driver licensing for truck drivers or other jobs with occupational hazards due to hypersomnia. There are no national sleep societies, sleep guidelines, mandatory screening for patients, sleep education, sleep curriculum in medical schools, or separate sleep board or specialty. There are no sleep foundations or funding opportunities for research. Patients have to pay mostly out of pocket for sleep testing, sleep devices, or other treatments. Health insurance is limited for government employees and veterans and does not cover testing and treatment of sleep disorders.

There are several pulmonologists, cardiologists, ENT specialists, and neurologists who diagnose and manage sleep disorders with the limited resources available. There are at least two Sleep Lab centers in Damascus. One performs daytime napping studies (Al-Basel hospital), and another one located in Tishreen Military hospital, also performs sleep studies.

Most sleep studies are performed at home using three or four-channel portable sleep testing devices. Home Sleep Apnea Test does not measure EEG, EMG, EOG, and ECG but it measures 3 or 4 parameters including airflow, pulse oximetry, respiratory effort, heart rate, and microphone for snoring. It is conducted outside of the hospital, at the patient's home, which is more convenient than in-lab sleep study and costs less. These are important advantages in the setting of a low-income country in the midst of war and economic crises. They are usually interpreted by the referring physician.

A Portable Sleep study costs about 100,000 Syrian Lira, the equivalent of $28 in today's currency, which is a little higher than the average monthly salary in Syria. Most patients can't afford to pay for it. And even if they did, most will not be able to afford to buy CPAP or BIPAP machines. An average CPAP costs about 1,750,000 Syrian Lira, the equivalent of $500. Health insurance does not provide coverage to sleep treatment or devices.

Because of the cost, most CPAP and BIPAP machines are provided or rented to patients at discounted prices by charities and medical non-profits. Several home health companies provide home Oxygen, CPAP, BIPAP machines, and supplies. Most home health companies have trained and resourceful technicians who perform the setup, patient education, maintenance, and trouble-shooting of sleep devices.

In spite of the prohibited cost, a busy Pulmonologist in Damascus performs an average of 2 portable sleep studies per week. The demand for sleep testing and treatment is increasing in spite of the limited resources.

Rare patients undergo UPPP either in Syria or in neighboring Lebanon, Jordan, or Turkey. Oral appliances and Inspire devices are not available in Syria. Tracheostomy is not accepted culturally in general even for severe Obesity Hypoventilation Syndrome or very severe obstructive sleep apneas.

There is no availability of MSLT or MWT studies. There are a few pediatricians who diagnose and treat sleep disorders among children in spite of its common prevalence based on studies in neighboring countries. A recent study showed 19% of Children In Lebanon experienced sleep disorders [37]. A similar study showed a 21% prevalence of sleep-disordered breathing in Saudi Arabia [38].

Narcolepsy, Insomnias, RLS, and parasomnias are diagnosed clinically and treated by primary practitioners or neurologists. Basic medications are available.

Over-counter hypnotics and sleeping pills are available and usually are provided by pharmacists without prescriptions.

Underlying psychiatric disorders that affect sleep and cause insomnia are underdiagnosed due to the shortage of psychiatrists and social stigma. Patients, in general, are reluctant to take antidepressants, anxiolytics, and antipsychotic medications even if they are diagnosed with mental illness.

PTSD disrupts sleep and causes insomnia. It is very common due to war, violence, trauma, displacement, and uncertainty and it goes underdiagnosed and untreated. Several studies showed a high prevalence of PTSD and psychological trauma among Syrians, Syrian refugees, and internally displaced persons. In a study of mental disorders and PTSD among Syrians in wartime, 44% had a likely severe mental disorder, 27% had both likely severe mental disorder and full PTSD symptoms, 36.9% had full PTSD symptoms, and only 10.8% had neither positive PTSD symptoms nor mental disorder on the K10 scale. Around 23% had low overall support. Half of the responders were internally displaced, and 27.6% were forced to change places of living three times or more due to war. Around 86.6% of the respondents believed that the war was the main reason for their mental distress [39].

Refugees and asylum seekers are susceptible to developing common mental disorders due to their exposure to stressful experiences before, during, and after their flight. The Syrian Civil War, which started in 2011, has led to a massive number of Syrians seeking refuge and asylum in European countries.

Symptoms of mental disorders and feelings of uncertainty, frustration, and injustice were the most common psychological problems and were mentioned by more than one-third of the participants in one of the studies. The finding that almost half of the participants reported typical symptoms of mental health disorders suggests that a considerable number of Syrian refugees and asylum seekers might need mental healthcare [4].

A longitudinal investigation has shown a significant relationship between trauma exposure, post-migration stress, sleep disturbance, and mental health in Syrian refugees [40].

THE CHALLENGES FOR SLEEP MEDICINE IN SYRIA

The state of medicine in Syria, in general, has deteriorated significantly since the war started in 2011. Before 2011 there were efforts to assess the prevalence of sleep disorders in the general population in Syria, like neighboring countries. For example, it was estimated that the prevalence of sleep-disordered breathing (SDB) is ~20%, especially with the increase in obesity and expected to be more prevalent in individuals with chronic illnesses such as diabetes, stroke, or heart disease. However, to date, there is no data specifically on the prevalence of SDB or other sleep disorders in Syria due to the lack of adequate clinical and research resources and awareness from the public and physicians alike. These challenges have magnified several folds since the war started in 2011.

The list of challenges can be summarized as follows:

1. The paucity of data and research about the prevalence and incidence of different sleep disorders. There is no national registry or statistics on different sleep disorders. Medical research in general is very weak even before the war [41].

2. Absence of clear policies about sleep disorders from the Ministries of Health, Higher Education, Labor, Veterans Affairs, Transportation, and Information.

3. Lack of safety regulations and policies related to sleep disorders in factories, truck companies, and other industries and businesses.

4. Lack of sleep specializations or licensing by the Ministry of Health or Higher Education. There is no recognized Sleep board in Syria until now.

5. Lack of training for sleep technicians.

6. Lack of expertise of physicians and adequate training in sleep medicine for both children and adults.

7. Insufficient awareness of sleep hygiene, disorder, treatment, and health in the general public and among healthcare professionals.

8. Poverty is a major challenge. As mentioned Nine out of ten Syrians are below the poverty line according to the UN which impedes treatment with CPAP machines for patients with SDBs

9. Significant and unpredictable shortage of electricity that prevents the use of electrically operated CPAP or BIPAP machines.

10. Spotty, slow, and expensive internet services. On the other hand, the usage of smartphones is very high, which creates opportunities for telehealth and public awareness programs. According to the Kepios Digital 2020 report, the percentage of mobile connections is 83% in 2020.

11. Attacks on healthcare that led to a critical shortage of medical subspecialists, even in major urban centers [5]. Many have fled the country to seek better opportunities in other countries due to the war and economic collapse.

12. The concentration of sleep centers and sleep specialists mostly within the capital, Damascus, or in a few urban areas prevents patients who live in smaller cities or rural areas from access. The inequity between major urban areas and rural areas was a major problem before the war but it was further exacerbated by the war, displacement, and economic downturn.

13. The deterioration of the economy and high inflation rate with rapid loss of the buying power of the Syrian Lira. An average salary is about 25 dollars/month which is barely enough for basic foods. Spending on healthcare has suffered in general as families prioritized food, shelter, and other basic needs. The high inflation in Syria leads to difficulty purchasing imported devices like positive airway pressure (PAP) devices.

14. The large displacement of the population inside and outside Syria led to a large number of internally displaced people living in camps. More than 1.2 million IDPs live in camps that are deprived of basic services including electricity, access to primary, secondary, and tertiary healthcare.

15. The COVID pandemic led to reprioritizing of health needs. Sleep disorders became less important compared to the threat of infection, hospitalization, and death from COVI19. This is exacerbated by low rates of vaccination. Syrians got their COVID-19 vaccines through the COVAX platform. Less than 7% of the population were vaccinated as of the date of this report.

16. The direct effect of war on the public, particularly those in hot zones areas where bombing and shelling occurred, leading to trauma. Most of the medical resources were directed toward the treatment of victims of snipers, bombs,

chemical weapons, and shelling, and the ensuing long-term physical and mental disabilities [42].

17. The increased risk of sleep disturbances is associated with post-traumatic stress disorders related to war and conflict in adults and children.

18. The inability of patients to travel to seek medical attention within the country due to safety concerns.

19. The presence of cultural, social, and economic barriers that prevent the acceptance and adherence to various treatments of sleep disorders, such as the acceptance of mechanical devices for treatment of SDB. Barriers to testing and treatment in higher among rural *versus* urban patients, the less educated and illiterate, the displaced populations, patients who live in areas of war and under siege, patients who live in opposition-controlled areas, and patients with low socioeconomic status. Patients may be reluctant to use CPAP due to the fear of suffocating, claustrophobia, disruption of electricity, concerns of increased risk of infections and pneumonia, and other stigmata.

20. Cultural barriers to the use of PAP for SDBs were found in neighboring stable Arab countries. Studies have shown that there is low compliance with CPAP treatment even in patients with severe OSA among other Arab patients [43]. After 12 months of study among Saudi patients, only 49.3% of the women and 33.3% of the men were still using PAP therapy even though that all Saudi patients have free access to government-funded healthcare services and PAP devices. Other studies found a higher compliance rate (80%) among Saudi patients after intensive educational interventions [43]. Compliance studies showed a 68-76% compliance rate among Western patients [43].

21. The stigma surrounding mental health disorders and sleep is still widespread in Syria and neighboring countries, which creates a significant barrier in efficiently managing sleep disturbances and addressing root causes of these common comorbid conditions (including insomnia and circadian rhythm disorders).

22. The presence of 4 disconnected administrative healthcare systems with minimal or no coordination.

23. The ongoing war and conflict, its chronicity, and lack of a political solution that will guarantee the safe and dignified return of the displaced and the refugees and focus on recovery.

Post Crisis Recovery and Reconstruction

A number of measures are required to address the population health needs both inside Syria and for refugees outside the country, and a concerted effort must be made to retain and train health workers in both the current and post-conflict period. The ongoing and complex nature of the conflict further undermines the health of the population and delays the rebuilding of the health infrastructure. As long as it is unsafe for refugees and IDPs to return to their homes, it will be difficult to persuade health workers to remain in Syria or to return. As such, efforts to end the conflict, protect civilians and enforce medical neutrality will have the greatest impact on the health of IDPs and refugees. All these factors are affected by the uncertain security situation inside Syria.

Re-establishing the health infrastructure in the current and post-conflict period could be a way of establishing peaceful co-existence and promoting the rights of marginalized groups, allowing for civil society participation and government accountability [3]. As such, the health system could enhance the legitimacy of the emerging government, particularly if based on principles of equity of access, non-discrimination, and transparency. This can be seen as an opportunity to build a strong health system that serves the current and future needs of the population.

The recovery and post-conflict period will present numerous challenges but also opportunities to establish health systems that can reduce excess mortality and mortality. The aim should be to establish community-based, integrated basic health services to reach areas in need. Maintaining a supply chain for medical equipment, and medication is essential.

Rebuilding Syria's shattered health system is a must [3]. The priorities for the rebuilding process include:

1. A harmonized approach to the collection and sharing of data should be actively sought, as health information systems [HIS] are required for real-time assessments of disease prevalence and population health needs. A functioning HIS would help identify new health needs as they arise [44].

2. Increased utilization of "m-technology," mobile devices to collect epidemiological data in focused efforts by individuals trained in collecting epidemiological data, or indeed by healthcare providers themselves, may prove increasingly important for real-time data [3].

3. Focusing on the retention of health workers, by providing competitive salaries, support, and training.

4. Address the epidemic of burnout and psychological trauma among healthcare workers.

5. Establishing incentives for those who have left to return.

6. Supporting those who remain and identifying the barriers preventing those who have left to return are key to the development of a successful health service.

7. Identifying the most needed specialties and providing training and salaries are important.

8. Encouraging innovative approaches including the harnessing of technology will aid the remaining health workers, and task shifting will allow for the training of enough health workers to support the health needs of the population.

9. Engagement with the expatriate Syrian and international medical and humanitarian organizations is key in supporting the health needs of the Syrians both inside and outside of Syria. An example of such a response is the work of medical relief organizations like Medglobal [45] and others have done in response to the current COIVD19 pandemic in Syria. MedGlobal launched "Operation Breathe" to provide Oxygen concentrators, CPAP, and BIPAP machines to patients treated at home with mobile health teams and in partnership with a network of local Non-Governmental health Organizations in different cities, in addition to providing training on management of COVID-19 to Syrian doctors and nurses using online platforms and building sustainable Oxygen generators in several hospitals. "Operation Breathe" was funded by individual donors from the Syrian diaspora community in the US and grants from other foundations. That can be set as a model to follow in the post-crisis and recovery phase [45].

10. Given that there is likely to be an ongoing shortage of healthcare workers in the current and post-conflict period, innovative ways to support and build the capacity of the current health workers, volunteers, and community members, will be increasingly important. This may be a part of telemedicine programs that have been successfully established or through the training of community health workers [46].

11. Rebuild and empower the non-profit health sector and encourage sustainable approaches to healthcare using the successful experiences of local non-profits that survived the conflict and expanded their services in spite of the strain on the system.

12. Embrace the humanitarian principles of humanity, medical neutrality, impartiality, and independence, and address the laws and legislations that conflict

with these principles. Such essential reforms will provide protection for healthcare workers during protracted conflicts.

13. Expand health insurance to provide coverage to Syrians with low income and to prevent catastrophic healthcare expenses.

Clinical Opportunities

Rebuilding Syria's shattered health system requires a holistic approach that addresses a number of issues [3]. Among the most important are focusing on the retention of health workers, providing support and training, and establishing incentives for those who have left to return. Encouraging innovative approaches including the harnessing of technology will aid the remaining health workers, and task shifting will allow for the training of enough health workers to support the health needs of the population. Policies that uphold medical neutrality and the safety of medical workers and prohibit attacks on medical facilities are key to protecting the remaining health workers. Given the protracted nature of the conflict and the funding shortage, engagement with the expatriate Syrian and international medical communities is key in supporting the health needs of the Syrians both inside and outside of Syria.

Sleep medicine in Syria lags behind its counterpart not only in developed countries, but also in the neighboring countries with more advanced healthcare systems like Jordan, Lebanon, Turkey, and the Gulf States. Furthermore sleep practice lags behind other medical specialties that incorporate testing and procedures, like cardiology, gastroenterology, neurology, renal, and surgery. Due to the high prevalence of Sleep Disorders in Syria especially SDB and in light of the shortage of clinical resources, there are ample opportunities to improve the access to sleep education, testing, and treatment.

It is essential to improve the public's safety from an untreated condition such as SDB associated with hypersomnia. If not recognized and treated, these conditions have been linked to severe consequences such as motor vehicle accidents and work-related accidents with their socio-economic and legal implications [47]. Following are some of the steps to improve the clinical aspects:

1. Adopting guidelines from other countries and the World Health Organization (WHO) is highly recommended to allow sharing of information and implementing best practices related to sleep health.

2. Addressing sleep-related health issues such as cardiovascular disorders and sleep cognitive function and sleep, and mental and sleep health.

3. Adopt and expand online training for health professionals and potential sleep technicians. A model of remote training for Portable Ultrasound (POCUS) in disaster regions like Yemen and Bangladesh [48] to enhance clinical decision making, improve resource utilization and optimize patient health outcomes can be followed.

4. Expand portable home sleep apnea testing and home virtual monitoring.

5. Establish medical training program for Syrian physicians in sleep medicine and provide adequate resources for testing and treatment.

6. Use Auto-adjusting and smart PAP devices with battery backup.

7. Address the sleep health needs of individuals living in Syria, including internally displaced individuals, at risk of psychological trauma and sleep disturbances.

8. Use alternative therapies such as oral appliances, positional therapy, and surgical treatment when PAP fails or is not tolerated.

9. Adopt national policies and legislation to reduce tobacco smoking.

10. Adopt national campaigns to control weight, improve wellness, and combat obesity, and,

11. Incorporating telemedicine [49] for the diagnosis and treatment of sleep disorders [50] especially in difficult-to-reach regions [46], rural areas, small cities, and other remote areas or under siege can be connected to nearby referral centers [49].

RESEARCH OPPORTUNITIES

The infrastructure of medical research in Syria is limited, but recent individual efforts by Syrian physicians have been noticed, particularly in areas related to the impact of conflict on public health [1], communicable diseases like Tuberculosis [49], the use of Telehealth [49], and other solutions like field hospitals [51] to improve access of healthcare to populations in war zones or under-siege, and COVID-19 [52]. To address gaps and barriers for sleep medicine in Syria, the development of infrastructures for medical research are critical. WHO emphasized the need to address sleep health in Syria over two decades ago in their report (Worldwide Project on Sleep and Health) published in collaboration with World Federation on Sleep Research Societies. The report highlighted the grave consequences of sleep disorders on the health of individuals and society. Thus, addressing these sleep health priorities requires several steps:

1. Funding availability to academic centers to assess the accurate prevalence of sleep disorders and the basic epidemiology of sleep disorders in Syria is vital.

2. Participation in international studies related to sleep health is also essential.

3. Conducting need assessment studies to address research priorities specific to Syrian patients (both under government and outside government-controlled areas).

4. Collaboration with neighboring countries on sleep-related population studies is beneficial, especially between health ministries and/or academic institutions.

5. Use validated tools (such as questionnaires) for sleep research translated to local language (Arabic) to ensure accurate results and feasibility of implementation in the near future in clinical settings. Some of these tools are already available in Arabic [53] and can be accessed freely by researchers like the Validation of the Arabic Version of Epworth Sleepiness Scale [54].

6. Junior researchers can apply to international organizations such as the American Thoracic Society and the American Academy of Sleep Medicine mentoring programs to build capacity and learn the longitudinal methodology of sleep-related research [55].

7. Partnering with WHO members and international educational institutions to provide necessary tools for research and education to the public and physicians.

Public Awareness Opportunities

Several initiatives could be explored using clinical and research innovations and increasing public awareness. Many of these initiatives have been adopted by other countries to overcome these challenges and barriers. These challenges interact and overlap; therefore, any proposed solution should be comprehensive and holistic.

The presence of several barriers and significant challenges requires collaboration and partnership with the public. Like other countries around the world, this can be achieved in several ways, such as establishing organizations that can raise awareness of sleep issues and are culturally and lingually sensitive.

There are several systemic gaps that need to be addressed by legislators, Ministries of planning, health, higher education, interior, transportation, and information, national medical associations, national and regional doctors unions, and medical schools and universities.

Some of the opportunities to improve the public awareness and embracement of diagnosis and treatments of different sleep disorders include:

1. The establishment of Syrian Sleep Society, and Syrian Sleep Foundation.

2. Introducing national policies for safe driving and sleep.

3. Mandating sleep testing for truck drivers and workers in heavy machinery.

4. Introducing sleep medicine into medical school curriculum.

5. Establishing a separate sleep specialty.

6. Introducing sleep practice guidelines especially through primary care, pulmonary, cardiology, ENT, neurology, anesthesia, and pediatrics medical societies.

7. Mandating sleep screening for patients requiring outpatient or inpatient moderate or deep sedation or Anesthesia.

8. Introducing sleep training in allied health programs.

9. Raising funds to provide financial assistance for patients who are unable to pay for diagnostic tests, Oxygen, or CPAP/BIPAP machines.

10. Partnering with other foundations on education and research.

11. Supporting NGOs that are providing assistance for home health sleep devices, and,

12. Introducing public awareness campaigns using medical influencers and celebrities to educate the public on sleep hygiene, different sleep disorders, treatment of sleep disorders, and impact of treatment on health and well-being using traditional and social media platforms.

CONCLUSION

Sleep disorders, especially SDBs and Insomnia, are common in Syria. NCDs are common among Syrians with their association with SDBs. The long conflict has placed a huge strain on the public healthcare system. There is low access to sleep education, testing, and treatment, mostly in major urban centers, although the demands are increasing. There are ample opportunities to improve the practice of sleep medicine, in spite of the long conflict and war, if local champions, NGOs, national authorities, and medical societies adopted already-available resources, guidelines, and regulations, incorporated creative means and telehealth, and followed the recommendations of the WHO on Sleep and Health.

The recovery and post-conflict period will present numerous challenges but also opportunities to establish health systems that can reduce excess mortality and mortality. The aim should be to establish community-based, integrated basic health services to reach areas in need. Maintaining a supply chain for medical equipment, and medication is essential.

DISCLOSURE

"Part of this chapter has previously been published in The Effect of the Conflict on Syria's Health System and Human Resources for Health, in World Health & Population, vol 16, no. 1, in 2015, pg 87-95."

CONSENT FOR PUBLICATION

Not applicable.

CONFLICT OF INTEREST

The authors declare no conflict of interest, financial or otherwise.

ACKNOWLEDGEMENT

Declared none.

REFERENCES

[1] Sahloul MZ, Monla-Hassan J, Sankari A, *et al.* War is the Enemy of Health. Pulmonary, Critical Care, and Sleep Medicine in War-Torn Syria. Ann Am Thorac Soc 2016; 13(2): 147-55.
[http://dx.doi.org/10.1513/AnnalsATS.201510-661PS] [PMID: 26784922]

[2] Kherallah M, Alahfez T, Sahloul Z, Eddin KD, Jamil G. Health care in Syria before and during the crisis. Avicenna J Med 2012; 2(3): 51-3.
[http://dx.doi.org/10.4103/2231-0770.102275] [PMID: 23826546]

[3] Abbara A, Blanchet K, Sahloul Z, Fouad F, Coutts A, Maziak W. The Effect of the Conflict on Syria's Health System and Human Resources for Health. World Health Popul 2015; 16(1): 87-95.
[http://dx.doi.org/10.12927/whp.2015.24318]

[4] Alhaffar MHDBA, Janos S. Public health consequences after ten years of the Syrian crisis: a literature review. Global Health 2021; 17(1): 111.
[http://dx.doi.org/10.1186/s12992-021-00762-9] [PMID: 34538248]

[5] Sahloul MZ. What They Don't Teach You In Medical School. New Line Magazine July 9 2021.
https://newlinesmag.com/first-person/what-they-dont-teach-you-in-medical-school/ accessed December 30th 2021

[6] United Nations. Syria: 10 years of war has left at least 350,000 dead. UN News. 24 September 2021.
https://news.un.org/en/story/2021/09/1101162 accessed December 30th 2021

[7] United Nations. As Plight of Syrians Worsens, Hunger Reaches Record High, International Community Must Fully Commit to Ending Decade-Old War, Secretary-General Tells General Assembly. UN Press Release 30 MARCH 2021.
https://www.un.org/press/en/2021/sgsm20664.doc.htm accessed December 30th 2021.

[8]   NHCR. Syria Emergency. UNHCR website. March 15th 2021. https://www.unhcr.org/en-us/syri-
        -emergency.html accessed December 30th 2021.

[9]   Refugee Processing Center. Admissions and Arrivals. RPC website.November 30th 2021.
        https://www.wrapsnet.org/admissions-and-arrivals/ accessed December 30th 2021.

[10]   Government of Canada. #Welcome Refugees. Canada website. November 1st 2021..
        https://www.canada.ca/en/immigration-refugees-citizenship/services   /refugees/welcome-syria-
        -refugees/key-figures.html accessed December 30th 2021.

[11]   Alawa J, Bollyky T. A Silent Crisis. Council on Foreig Relations. https://www.cfr.org/report/silent-
        crisis accessed December 30th 2021.

[12]   UNHCR. Syria: UNHCR Operational Update, June 2021.reliefweb. July 18th 2021.
        https://reliefweb.int/report/syrian-arab-republic/syria-unhcr-operational-update-june- 2021 accessed
        December 30th 2021.

[13]   Javanbakht A, Amirsadri A, Abu Suhaiban H, *et al.* Prevalence of Possible Mental Disorders in Syrian
        Refugees Resettling in the United States Screened at Primary Care. J Immigr Minor Health 2019;
        21(3): 664-7.
        [http://dx.doi.org/10.1007/s10903-018-0797-3] [PMID: 30066059]

[14]   Sankari S. The Relationship Between Sleep Quality and PTSD Symptoms in Syrian Refugees in
        Michigan   University   of   Michigan   Website   August   14th   2019
        https://deepblue.lib.umich.edu/handle/2027.42/150626 accessed December 30th 2021.

[15]   Aydıntaşbaş A. A new Gaza: Turkey's border policy in northern Syria. The European Council on
        Foreign   Relations   May   8th   2020..
        https://ecfr.eu/publication/a_new_gaza_turkeys_border_policy_in_northern_syria/ accessed December
        30th 2021.

[16]   Hoffman M, Makovsky A. Northern Syria Security Dynamics and the Refugee Crisis. American
        Progress. May 6th 2021.. https://www.americanprogress.org/article/northern-syria-security-dynam-
        cs-refugee-crisis/ accessed December 30th 2021

[17]   Young T, Palta M, Dempsey J, Peppard PE, Nieto FJ, Hla KM. Burden of sleep apnea: rationale,
        design, and major findings of the Wisconsin Sleep Cohort study. WMJ 2009; 108(5): 246-9.
        [PMID: 19743755]

[18]   Castaneda A, Jauregui-Maldonado E, Ratnani I, Varon J, Surani S. Correlation between metabolic
        syndrome and sleep apnea. World J Diabetes 2018; 9(4): 66-71.
        [http://dx.doi.org/10.4239/wjd.v9.i4.66] [PMID: 29765510]

[19]   Colvonen PJ, Masino T, Drummond SPA, Myers US, Angkaw AC, Norman SB. Obstructive sleep
        apnea and posttraumatic stress disorder among OEF/OIF/OND veterans. J Clin Sleep Med 2015;
        11(5): 513-8.
        [http://dx.doi.org/10.5664/jcsm.4692] [PMID: 25665698]

[20]   Sadeghi M, Simani M, Mohammadifard N, *et al.* Longitudinal association of dietary fat intake with
        cardiovascular events in a prospective cohort study in Eastern Mediterranean region. Int J Food Sci
        Nutr 2021; 72(8): 1095-1104.
        [http://dx.doi.org/10.1080/09637486.2021.1895725]

[21]   Maziak W, Rastam S, Mzayek F, Ward KD, Eissenberg T, Keil U. Cardiovascular health among adults
        in Syria: a model from developing countries. Ann Epidemiol 2007; 17(9): 713-20.
        [http://dx.doi.org/10.1016/j.annepidem.2007.03.016] [PMID: 17553700]

[22]   Al-Nuaim AA, Bamgboye EA, Al-Rubeaan KA, Al-Mazrou Y. Overweight and obesity in Saudi
        Arabian adult population, role of socio-demographic variables. J Community Health 1997; 22(3): 211-
        23.
        [http://dx.doi.org/10.1023/A:1025177108996] [PMID: 9178120]

[23] Bartrina A. J. Prevalencia de obesidad en los países desarrollados: situación actual y perspectivas. Nutr Hosp 2002; 17 (Suppl. 1): 34-41.

[24] Erem C, Arslan C, Hacihasanoglu A, *et al.* Prevalence of obesity and associated risk factors in a Turkish population (trabzon city, Turkey). Obes Res 2004; 12(7): 1117-27.
[http://dx.doi.org/10.1038/oby.2004.140] [PMID: 15292476]

[25] Krishnan V, Dixon-Williams S, Thornton JD. Where there is smoke…there is sleep apnea: exploring the relationship between smoking and sleep apnea. Chest 2014; 146(6): 1673-80.
[http://dx.doi.org/10.1378/chest.14-0772] [PMID: 25451354]

[26] Wetter DW, Young TB, Bidwell TR, Badr MS, Palta M. Smoking as a risk factor for sleep-disordered breathing. Arch Intern Med 1994; 154(19): 2219-24.
[http://dx.doi.org/10.1001/archinte.1994.00420190121014] [PMID: 7944843]

[27] Abdulrahim S, Jawad M. Socioeconomic differences in smoking in Jordan, Lebanon, Syria, and Palestine: A cross-sectional analysis of national surveys. PLoS One 2018; 13(1): e0189829.
[http://dx.doi.org/10.1371/journal.pone.0189829] [PMID: 29381734]

[28] Naja F, Shatila H, El Koussa M, Meho L, Ghandour L, Saleh S. Burden of non-communicable diseases among Syrian refugees: a scoping review. BMC Public Health 2019; 19(1): 637.
[http://dx.doi.org/10.1186/s12889-019-6977-9] [PMID: 31126261]

[29] Karaki FM, Alani O, Tannoury M, *et al.* Noncommunicable Disease and Health Care-Seeking Behavior Among Urban Camp-Dwelling Syrian Refugees in Lebanon: A Preliminary Investigation. Health Equity 2021; 5(1): 261-9.
[http://dx.doi.org/10.1089/heq.2020.0106] [PMID: 34095705]

[30] Aziz IA, Hutchinson CV, Maltby J. Quality of life of Syrian refugees living in camps in the Kurdistan Region of Iraq. PeerJ 2014; 2: e670.
[http://dx.doi.org/10.7717/peerj.670] [PMID: 25401057]

[31] Khassawneh B, Ghazzawi M, Khader Y, *et al.* Symptoms and risk of obstructive sleep apnea in primary care patients in Jordan. Sleep Breath 2009; 13(3): 227-32.
[http://dx.doi.org/10.1007/s11325-008-0240-4] [PMID: 19082647]

[32] De Torres-Alba F, Gemma D, Armada-Romero E, Rey-Blas JR, López-de-Sá E, López-Sendon JL. Obstructive sleep apnea and coronary artery disease: from pathophysiology to clinical implications. Pulm Med 2013; 2013: 1-9.
[http://dx.doi.org/10.1155/2013/768064] [PMID: 23691310]

[33] Wali SO, Alsharif MA, Albanji MH, *et al.* Prevalence of obstructive sleep apnea among patients with coronary artery disease in Saudi Arabia. J Saudi Heart Assoc 2015; 27(4): 227-33.
[http://dx.doi.org/10.1016/j.jsha.2015.03.004] [PMID: 26557740]

[34] Chami HA, Bechnak A, Isma'eel H, *et al.* Sleepless in Beirut: Sleep Difficulties in an Urban Environment With Chronic Psychosocial Stress. J Clin Sleep Med 2019; 15(4): 603-14.
[http://dx.doi.org/10.5664/jcsm.7724] [PMID: 30952222]

[35] Hashim HT. Assessment of Obstructive Sleep Apnea Among Iraqi People in 2019 by Using (STOP-BANG) Model. SN Compr Clin Med 2020; 2(11): 2260-4. [STOP-BANG].
[http://dx.doi.org/10.1007/s42399-020-00572-x]

[36] Shahrour N. Pilot study on sleep disorders in Syria. Rev Mal Respir 2006; 23(4-C2): 146.
[http://dx.doi.org/10.1016/S0761-8425(06)71689-8]

[37] Sfeir E, Haddad C, Akel M, Hallit S, Obeid S. Sleep disorders in a sample of Lebanese children: the role of parental mental health and child nutrition and activity. BMC Pediatr 2021; 21(1): 324.
[http://dx.doi.org/10.1186/s12887-021-02795-w] [PMID: 34301219]

[38] Baidas L, Al-Jobair A, Al-Kawari H, AlShehri A, Al-Madani S, Al-Balbeesi H. Prevalence of sleep-disordered breathing and associations with orofacial symptoms among Saudi primary school children.

BMC Oral Health 2019; 19(1): 43.
[http://dx.doi.org/10.1186/s12903-019-0735-3] [PMID: 30866906]

[39]   Kakaje A, Al Zohbi R, Hosam Aldeen O, Makki L, Alyousbashi A, Alhaffar MBA. Mental disorder and PTSD in Syria during wartime: a nationwide crisis. BMC Psychiatry 2021; 21(1): 2.
[http://dx.doi.org/10.1186/s12888-020-03002-3] [PMID: 33388026]

[40]   Lies J, Drummond SPA, Jobson L. Longitudinal investigation of the relationships between trauma exposure, post-migration stress, sleep disturbance, and mental health in Syrian refugees. Eur J Psychotraumatol 2020; 11(1): 1825166.
[http://dx.doi.org/10.1080/20008198.2020.1825166] [PMID: 33425241]

[41]   Saadi TA, Abbas F, Turk T, Alkhatib M, Hanafi I, Alahdab F. Medical research in war-torn Syria: medical students' perspective. Lancet 2018; 391(10139): 2497-8.
[http://dx.doi.org/10.1016/S0140-6736(18)31207-8] [PMID: 29976463]

[42]   Footer KHA, Clouse E, Rayes D, Sahloul Z, Rubenstein LS. Qualitative accounts from Syrian health professionals regarding violations of the right to health, including the use of chemical weapons, in opposition-held Syria. BMJ Open 2018; 8(8): e021096.
[http://dx.doi.org/10.1136/bmjopen-2017-021096] [PMID: 30082351]

[43]   Almeneessier AS, Aleissi S, Olaish AH, BaHammam AS. Long-Term Adherence to Positive Airway Pressure Therapy in Saudi Ambulatory Patients with Obesity Hypoventilation Syndrome and Severe Obstructive Sleep Apnea: A One-Year Follow-Up Prospective Observational Study. Nat Sci Sleep 2021; 13: 63-74.
[http://dx.doi.org/10.2147/NSS.S290349] [PMID: 33469401]

[44]   Taleb ZB, Bahelah R, Fouad FM, Coutts A, Wilcox M, Maziak W. Syria: health in a country undergoing tragic transition. Int J Public Health 2015; 60(S1) (Suppl. 1): 63-72.
[http://dx.doi.org/10.1007/s00038-014-0586-2] [PMID: 25023995]

[45]   MedGlobal. Operation Breathe March 2021.. https://medglobal.org/wp-content/uploads/2021/03/Operation-Breathe-PDF-Report.pdf accessed December 30th 2021.

[46]   Belayashi D. An app to help treat patients in Syria, 10,000 km away. The Observers 28th of July 2016.. https://observers.france24.com/en/20160728-app-doctors-syria-hospitals- telemedecine accessed December 30th 2021.

[47]   Tregear S, Reston J, Schoelles K, Phillips B. Obstructive sleep apnea and risk of motor vehicle crash: systematic review and meta-analysis. J Clin Sleep Med 2009; 5(6): 573-81.
[http://dx.doi.org/10.5664/jcsm.27662] [PMID: 20465027]

[48]   Inteleos PRM Newswire website May 26 2021. https://www.prnewswire.com/news-releases/inteleo--announces-medglobal-and-global-ultrasound-institute-as-missionpocus-selecti-n-for-2021-301300035.html accessed December 30th 2021.

[49]   Moughrabieh A, Weinert C. Rapid Deployment of International Tele–Intensive Care Unit Services in War-Torn Syria. Ann Am Thorac Soc 2016; 13(2): 165-72.
[http://dx.doi.org/10.1513/AnnalsATS.201509-589OT] [PMID: 26788827]

[50]   Shamim-Uzzaman QA, Bae CJ, Ehsan Z, *et al.* The use of telemedicine for the diagnosis and treatment of sleep disorders: an American Academy of Sleep Medicine update. J Clin Sleep Med 2021; 17(5): 1103-7.
[http://dx.doi.org/10.5664/jcsm.9194] [PMID: 33599202]

[51]   Sankari A, Atassi B, Sahloul MZ. Syrian field hospitals: A creative solution in urban military conflict combat in Syria. Avicenna J Med 2013; 3(3): 84-6.
[http://dx.doi.org/10.4103/2231-0770.118467] [PMID: 24251237]

[52]   Mohsen F, Bakkar B, Armashi H, Aldaher N. Crisis within a crisis, COVID-19 knowledge and awareness among the Syrian population: a cross-sectional study. BMJ Open 11(4): e043305.

[53]   Suleiman KH, Yates BC. Translating the insomnia severity index into Arabic. J Nurs Scholarsh 43(1):

49-53.

[54] Ahmed AE, Fatani A, Al-Harbi A, *et al.* Validation of the Arabic version of the Epworth sleepiness scale. J Epidemiol Glob Health 2014; 4(4): 297-302.
[http://dx.doi.org/10.1016/j.jegh.2014.04.004] [PMID: 25455647]

[55] Al Maqbali M, Hughes C, Gracey J, Rankin J, Dunwoody L, Hacker E. Validation of the Pittsburgh Sleep Quality Index (PSQI) with Arabic cancer patients. Sleep Biol Rhythms 2020; 18(3): 217-23.
[http://dx.doi.org/10.1007/s41105-020-00258-w]

CHAPTER 17

Current Practice of Sleep Medicine in Nigeria

Morenikeji Adeyoyin KOMOLAFE[1], Oluwatosin Eunice OLORUNMOTENI[2,*], Kikelomo Adebanke KOLAWOLE[3], Olufemi K. OGUNDIPE[4], Michael Bimbola FAWALE[1], Akintunde Adeolu ADEBOWALE[1], Ahmed Omokayode IDOWU[5], Ahmad Abefe SANUSI[5], Josephine Eniola A. EZIYI[6] and Kolawole Samuel MOSAKU[7]

[1] *Department of Medicine, Obafemi Awolowo University, Ile-Ife, Osun State, Nigeria*

[2] *Department of Paediatrics and Child Health, Obafemi Awolowo University, Ile-Ife, Osun State, Nigeria*

[3] *Department of Child Dental Health, Faculty of Dentistry, Obafemi Awolowo University, Ile-Ife, Osun State, Nigeria*

[4] *Department of Oral Maxillofacial Surgery, Obafemi Awolowo University Ile-Ife, Osun State, Nigeria*

[5] *Department of Medicine, Obafemi Awolowo University Teaching Hospitals Complex, Ile-Ife, Osun State, Nigeria*

[6] *Department of Otorhinolaryngology, Obafemi Awolowo University, Ile-Ife, Osun State, Nigeria*

[7] *Department of Mental Health, Obafemi Awolowo University, Ile-Ife, Osun state, Nigeria*

Abstract: Sleep is an important physiological function that contributes significantly to the health and well-being of people worldwide. In Nigeria, the most populous country in Africa, sleep problems have been reported across various age groups from childhood to the elderly population. It is therefore noteworthy to access and report the state of sleep medicine practice in Nigeria as well as the strengths, weaknesses, opportunities, and threats to the establishment of a successful sleep medicine program in the country.

Sleep problems appear to be on the rise in the Nigerian population. This may be due to an increase in the prevalence of some risk factors for sleep disorders. It can also be attributed to the growing interest in sleep research and clinical sleep medicine practice by a wide range of specialists. However, the practice of sleep medicine in Nigeria appears to be significantly limited by the poor manpower development, lack of sleep societies/organizations, lack of training programs, lack of equipment and sleep laboratories, limited treatment options, inadequate funding, poor national awareness, and political will. The increasing political unrest and brain drain of health professionals constitute a major threat to the availability of human resources.

* **Corresponding author Oluwatosin Eunice OLORUNMOTENI:** Department of Paediatrics and Child Health, Obafemi Awolowo University, Ile – Ife, Osun State, Nigeria; Tel: +234803 941 3535; Email: oeolorunmoteni@oauife.edu.ng

Hrayr P. Attarian, Marie-Louise M. Coussa-Koniski & Alain Michel Sabri (Eds.)

The practice of sleep medicine in Nigeria is faced with challenges as well as diverse opportunities. Thus, sleep medicine practice in Nigeria has the potential to grow rapidly and contribute significantly to the global picture if given attention. The growing interest of Nigerian researchers in Sleep medicine, especially in the last decade, as well as the large population of Nigerians, many of whom have risk factors for sleep disorders, suggest that Nigeria may be a significant contributor to the global burden of sleep disorders. Therefore, we suggest concerted and coordinated efforts to enhance the strengths and opportunities highlighted while minimising or eliminating the challenges to improve the practice of sleep medicine in Nigeria.

Keywords: Nigeria, Sleep disorders, Sleep medicine program, Sleep practice, Sleep training.

INTRODUCTION

Nigeria has a land area of 923,768 km (356,669 mi), making it the world's 33rd-largest country [1, 2]. It is the most populous country in Africa and the seventh most populous country in the world with an estimated 206 million inhabitants [3]. The majority of the population is young, with 42.5% between the ages of 0–14 years [4]. Sleep disturbance, especially in the adolescent, may be associated with excessive daytime sleepiness, impaired neurocognitive function, and a host of others leading to suboptimal performance. Sleep disturbances also increase with age such that up to 50% of elderly individuals report at least one form of sleep disturbance [5].

Sleep is a basic biologic function that is essential for life and occupies one-third of people's lives [6]. It has been shown that adequate sleep helps to improve memory and learning, increase attention and creativity, enhance healing and repair of cells, clear out toxins that accumulate in the brain, and improve the proper functioning of the immune system [7 - 9]. Modern medicine has demonstrated that sleep has essential physiological functions, and sleep disorders have deleterious effects on many bodily functions [10, 11]. Cardio-metabolic disorders such as hypertension, diabetes, obesity, and coronary artery disease are among the deleterious effects associated with these sleep disorders and can have a bidirectional relationship [12, 13]. Although sleep medicine is considered a relatively new specialty, interest in sleep and sleep disorders has existed since the beginning of mankind. The specialty has grown, and the number of sleep specialists is on the increase in Nigeria. Nevertheless, sleep medicine is still underdeveloped, particularly in the areas of clinical service, education, training, and research. This is due to factors such as the limited number of well-trained sleep specialists and other specialists like neurologists or pulmonologists; unavailability of accredited sleep labs in the country; lack of awareness of and the trivialization of sleep disorders; unavailability of sleep societies in Nigeria; no authorized body for sleep medicine training and certification; and lack of motivation even among medical practitioners. There are only about 4 well-established sleep laboratories in Nigeria that are privately owned and run. The sleep laboratories are only in one state (Lagos) and the Federal capital territory (Abuja) out of the 36 states in Nigeria serving more than 200 million inhabitants. This is grossly inadequate and reflects the level of underdevelopment in the field of sleep medicine in Nigeria. There are no sleep societies, no government-owned sleep laboratories, and no sleep medicine-related courses offered in any of the tertiary institutions in Nigeria.

From previous studies [14 - 17], it appears that sleep disorders are common among Nigerians, and the demand for sleep medicine services is currently rising with an expected exponential increase in the nearest future. It is surprising though that awareness about sleep disorders and their serious consequences is low even among health care workers, health care authorities, and the general public in developing countries like Nigeria. The growth and the recognition of sleep medicine in developed countries can be attributed to many factors, including the recognition of an increasing number of sleep disorders, the increasing evidence linking sleep disorders to serious medical problems, the availability of training programs for sleep medicine, and the increased awareness of the general public about sleep disorders and their consequences [18].

Sleep Disorders in Nigeria

A review of the literature revealed insomnia to be the most common sleep disorder in Nigerian adults presenting to the outpatient clinic and in women attending antenatal care clinic with a prevalence rate of 27.3% and 47.3%, respectively [19, 20]. Komolafe *et al.* (2015) also reported the prevalence of sleep disorders in people living with epilepsy (PWE) to be as high as 82% with parasomnias being the most common disorder among them [21]. Parasomnias are quite common among adolescents with a lifetime prevalence of 725 per 1,000 for the occurrence of any parasomnia and an incidence of 211 per 1,000 [22]. Incidence estimates show that all parasomnias persist into adulthood at reduced rates. Alcohol intake and long duration of night sleep predisposed subjects to a higher occurrence of parasomnias. A systematic review by Mume (2010) to identify studies that reported the epidemiology of sleepwalking disorders revealed the estimated lifetime prevalence of somnambulism to be 6.9% [14]. Recent studies that assessed obstructive sleep apnea (OSA) revealed the prevalence of OSA among Nigerian adults to be 23.2% [23, 24], 19% [25], and 18% [26] which were strongly associated with moderate to severe obesity. None of these studies utilized polysomnography to objectively assess and confirm OSA. Anyanwu *et al.* (2015) also reported that the prevalence of sleep-disordered nocturnal enuresis among Nigerian children was 37% and was significantly associated with behavioural problems and poor sleep hygiene [27]. This was similar to the finding by Sebanjo *et al.* who reported the prevalence of sleep-disordered nocturnal enuresis as 42% and concluded the aforementioned to be the most common sleep disorder in children less than 12 years [28]. The use of modern technological devices has also significantly impacted sleep habits among Nigerian adolescents. Olorunmoteni *et al.* reported that the majority of school-attending Nigerian adolescents use one or more electronic devices mainly cell phones at bedtime and a high proportion of them have insufficient sleep on weekdays and significantly sleep less during weekdays compared to weekends [15]. Even among Nigerian undergraduates, the presence of psychological distress and symptoms of depression were significantly associated with poor quality of sleep which underscores the benefit of advocating for habits that can improve optimal mental health and sleep quality among undergraduate students [29]. Likewise, the academic performance of students with good sleep quality was significantly better than those with poor sleep quality [30].

The practice of sleep medicine in Nigeria is still rudimentary and a lot still has to be done vis-a-vis creating more awareness about the field even among students, health care professionals, and the general public; creating a well-established sleep society platform; introducing sleep-related courses in Nigerian tertiary institutions; and establishing more well-equipped sleep laboratories, among others.

Evaluation and Treatment of Sleep Disorders in Nigeria

Sleep problems and disorders appear to exist in the entire Nigerian population. Various types of sleep problems have been reported among children adolescents, adults, and the elderly population [31 - 33]. However, the evaluation of sleep disorders appears to be largely based on the use of sleep questionnaires and screening guides [15]. The majority of the studies did not use objective methods or instruments for sleep evaluation. For example, none of the epidemiological studies that have attempted to describe the pattern and determinants of sleep disorders in children and adolescents utilised objective measures like polysomnography or actigraphy. Furthermore, the sleep questionnaires used were largely adapted from sleep questionnaires validated in developed countries. These questionnaires may not put into consideration, the cultural nuances involved in the description of sleep problems in the Nigerian context. Recently, Igbokwe *et al.*, developed the Sleep Disorders in Nigeria Questionnaire (SDINQ), a culturally relevant instrument for assessing sleep disorders among Nigerian adolescents [34]. Hopefully, this will trigger the development of more culturally relevant instruments for the evaluation of sleep disorders in other categories of the population.

The type of clinicians involved in the care of people with sleep disorders is mainly specialists. While there is no nationwide study or publication on sleep practitioners in Nigeria, the type of specialists involved in clinical research on sleep can be used to derive the nature of specialists involved in sleep practice and research. These specialists include Neurologists, Pulmonologists, Psychiatrists, Psychologists, Dentists, and Ear, Nose, and Throat (ENT) Surgeons, among others. However, Nigeria does not have a society for sleep medicine, just like many other African countries [35]. The absence of a Sleep society in Nigeria has made it difficult to have a coordinated and goal-directed workforce focused on sleep medicine in Nigeria. Also, the lack of regulatory professional societies that can regulate sleep practice in the country limits the development and coordination of nationwide practice guidelines [35]. Consequently, it is difficult to create a national registry of sleep disorders and coordinate nationwide epidemiological surveys on sleep and sleep disorders in the Nigerian population.

Furthermore, the practice of sleep medicine in Nigeria is limited by the non-availability of medications required to treat sleep disorders. While sleep medications such as melatonin, an important drug for treating insomnia and shift-work-related sleep disorders are becoming overused as an over-the-counter medication in many developed countries, it remains scarce in developing countries like Nigeria. Other medications for treating hypersomnia like narcolepsy are largely unavailable. Conversely, sedative hypnotics like benzodiazepines are wrongly purchased and used in the self-treatment of some sleep disorders. These benzodiazepines are often purchased over-the-counter, without a prescription, from poorly regulated pharmacy shops. Therefore, the non-availability of appropriate medications and the abuse of inappropriate medications due to poor regulatory efforts limit the success of pharmacological treatment of sleep disorders in Nigeria.

It has been established that obstructive sleep apnoea (OSA) is quite common in Nigeria, from questionnaire-based studies [32, 33, 36]. However, the use of CPAP in managing people with OSA is very difficult. This is partly due to the scarcity of sleep laboratories as well as the lack of CPAP machines and masks. As a result, many patients live with untreated OSAS with resultant worsened morbidities and mortalities. Furthermore, the limitation in providing adequate treatment for OSA may be due to insufficient knowledge of doctors about OSA. Kuti *et al.* [37], reported a poor level of knowledge about childhood OSA among 204 newly graduated Nigerian doctors. Their knowledge of the recognition and management of children with OSA was assessed using the validated OSAKA-KIDS questionnaire [38]. He reported that seventy-two (35.3%) of the doctors had never heard of OSA and fifteen (7.4%) doctors felt OSA was not an important clinical disorder. Therefore, improved exposure of medical students to OSA and other forms of sleep disorders may be necessary to improve the capacity and interest of young Nigerian doctors in Sleep Medicine. This can be achieved through an improved emphasis on sleep medicine in the medical curriculum.

The Practice of Paediatric Sleep in Nigeria

The practice of sleep medicine in Nigeria is evolving. Whereas there are very few clinicians and laboratories where sleep studies and management are being conducted, these services are mainly for adults in urban communities. There is no Paediatric sleep laboratory in Nigeria. Sleep laboratories dedicated to children have been advocated for the evaluation of Paediatric sleep disorders [38, 39]. These laboratories are better equipped with the human resources and tools for diagnosing and management in children. Sleep problems have been reported to be prevalent in Nigerian children just like their counterparts all over the world [28, 32, 40]. The burden of their sleep problems may even be worse than what is obtained in developed countries [28]. Unfortunately, there is a lack of dedicated Paediatric sleep practices to meet this need. Thus, there is a need to further explore the needs and opportunities for Paediatric Sleep in Nigeria.

CHALLENGES

Challenges of Awareness and Diagnosis

Although the criteria for diagnosis have been reviewed and revised to be as sensitive as possible, hazy areas still exist.

Low Awareness: The diagnostic challenge associated with sleep disorders was identified by Desalu *et al.* (2017) which may also be related to the poor level of awareness and under-reporting of sleep symptoms in Nigeria [26]. Low awareness about sleep disorders and their serious consequences among patients, the general public as well as health care workers constitute a major challenge to the practice of sleep medicine in Nigeria. Many patients are unaware of over 90 different types of sleep disorders and treatment options. There is a need to boost patient education about sleep disorders by providing information about these diseases and treatment options so that patients can make more informed health care decisions. Increasing awareness among healthcare workers can result in better communication between patients, referring primary care physicians, sleep specialists, and allied health professionals so that providers can better assist patients in achieving their preferred outcomes.

Non-Availability of Manpower: The main challenge to having an accurate diagnosis of sleep disorders in Nigeria appears to be the availability of manpower. This problem is multifaceted, there are very few specialists in sleep medicine, and other specialists interested in sleep medicine are few and concentrated in tertiary institutions located mainly in major cities across the country. The majority of practitioners interested in sleep medicine are domiciled in the urban areas of the country leading to limited access to sleep care. In addition, there is a lack of trained technicians and specialists.

Competence/ Training: Beyond manpower availability, competence in sleep medicine requires an understanding of a plethora of very diverse disorders, many of which present with similar symptoms such as excessive daytime sleepiness and insomnia. Successful management however requires accurate diagnosis because of differences in treatment modalities. The spectrum of treatment options ranges from medication/medical therapy (sleep specialist), cognitive-behavioral treatments (sleep nurses/technologist), PAP (sleep specialist), oral appliances (orthodontist), upper airway surgery (ENT), to orthognathic/ jaw surgery (maxillofacial surgeon). These have implications for treatment efficacy, determining the suitability of each method, and titrating treatment to the outcome. Early identification of affected individuals and subsequent referral to a sleep specialist are important.

Community of Sleep Specialists: Whereas in the developed nations, many sleep societies exist for research and management of sleep disorders, not many of them exist in the African continent. Sleep societies exist only in four countries namely Egypt, Algeria, Morocco, and South Africa. The South African Society of Sleep Medicine (SASSM) was launched in the last decade [35]. In addition, there are currently few patient advocacy/support groups and leadership from professional organizations and industries relevant to sleep medicine.

Undergraduate Training: Undergraduate training in sleep medicine appears grossly inadequate as currently obtains in the University curricula. Ozoh *et al.*, (2015) demonstrated a need to formally incorporate the evaluation of sleep disorders into the undergraduate medical curriculum with the clear objective of enabling recognition of clinical features of common sleep disorders [41]. The inadequate undergraduate training is compounded by the fact that there is currently no structured training for sleep physicians and laboratory technicians in Nigeria. A study among a population of doctors showed that the practice and care of patients with obstructive sleep apnea OSA are suboptimal [42]. Also, there is currently insufficient professional content of sleep medicine to justify the recognition of sleep medicine as an independent specialty by relevant government, accrediting agencies in Nigeria.

Diagnosis/ History Taking: Management of individuals with sleep disorders often begins with a thorough history and examination. Obtaining accurate and adequate history can also be quite challenging considering the state of altered consciousness and reduced interaction with surroundings that occurs during sleep. The reports of a bed partner or family member, therefore, become very important and useful. There are also cultural inhibitions encountered with history taking in Nigeria, Nigerians are generally not generous with volunteering information including medical information. Patients often fail to give information about medical conditions and drug use. Superstitious beliefs also appear to blur the thinking of many in Nigeria. Ohaeri (1992) Reported that the popular view associated with sleep paralysis in Nigeria is that it is caused by witchcraft [43].

Obtaining a sleep log or diary which is also necessary for diagnosis may also be challenging. In a country like Nigeria, where constant and continuous power supply is a rarity, the effect of the incessant power outage on obtaining an accurate sleep log may be greater than imagined. Societies without electric light have been reported to sleep in a variety of patterns that seldom resemble the habit of sleeping in a single eight-hour bout [44].

The degree of disturbance to sleep necessary in an individual to be of significance may sometimes not be clear making subjective judgments the necessary alternative. This has necessitated the use of sleep questionnaires such as the Epworth sleepiness Scale (ESS) and other scales for standardization. While these scales have been of tremendous benefit in the assessment of sleep disorders, reading and comprehension of these questionnaires may be sometimes problematic among the illiterate population in Nigeria.

Challenges of Investigation

Some laboratory studies required to make an accurate diagnosis of sleep disorders are unavailable in many parts of Nigeria. Most of the tertiary hospitals, research centers, and private clinics where patients are managed do not have sleep laboratories. Only four sleep laboratories are available to the Nigerian population of about a 200million individuals, moreover, these laboratories are mainly located in urban cities. Appropriate equipment for investigations such as polysomnography is therefore unavailable to the majority of affected Nigerians. This is largely due to poor funding and limited resources available in the health sector in Nigeria.

Actigraphy which can give a gross picture of sleep-wake cycles and is often used to verify the sleep diary is not readily available. It is cost-efficient when full polysomnography is not required. Tests like the Multiple sleep latency test (MSLT) and Maintenance of wakefulness test (MWT) used to assess improved alertness following therapeutic interventions are also not readily available. Sometimes obtaining imaging studies which may be required if a patient is to be evaluated for the neurodegenerative disease may also be challenging. Surgical management of conditions such as OSAS entails the identification of the site of obstruction. This requires investigations like Endoscopy, Pressure catheter, Fluoroscopy, CT scan, and MRI which are not readily available in many Nigerian practices. Genetic markers which are known to help with early detection are presently not available for use in Nigeria.

Challenges of Management

Pharmacological management appears to be the mainstay of management in sleep medicine. However, the availability of drugs in the appropriate and required dosage can also be challenging. This is coupled with the challenge of the provision of low-quality generic alternatives to some drugs from some Asian countries. Short and long-term treatment of disorders with medications is also not devoid of the challenge of side effects. Management of disorders like Restless Legs Syndrome (RLS) involves the use of dopaminergic agents. Treatment with dopaminergic agents is complicated by rebound worsening of symptoms and augmentation. This could restrict the duration of drug use even in the absence of complete resolution of symptoms.

Non-pharmacological treatments for conditions such as chronic insomnia include stimulus control therapy, sleep restriction, sleep hygiene education, cognitive therapy, paradoxical intention, relaxation therapy, and multicomponent therapy. Behavioral changes and light therapy may be beneficial for circadian rhythm disorders. Appropriate personnel and facilities for these interventions are also unavailable in Nigeria.

Shift work sleep disorders are not uncommon in the population due to the high number of health care workers and other professionals who practice work shifts. While these may exist, occupational medicine and workers' compensation programs appear non-existent in Nigeria.

The appropriate light environment is essential for such a category of workers which involves exposure to light during the first portion of the shift and protection from bright light after work may not be available [45].

Disorders of excessive somnolence such as Sleep apnea, hypopnea Upper airway resistance syndrome (UARS) may require surgical and non-surgical management. Non-surgical treatment encompasses behavioural measures, such as weight loss, body position during sleep, and mechanical measures, which include continuous positive airway pressure (CPAP) or bilevel positive airway pressure (BIPAP) and oral appliances. While behaviour modifications are easy to advocate, maintaining weight loss may be challenging because of the heavy calories typical of Nigerian meals.

Professional involvement of Orthodontists and oral and maxillofacial surgeons with sleep medicine in Nigeria is minimal. Orthodontists and orthodontic dental technologists can collaborate with other specialists for the provision of oral appliances required for mandibular displacements for the management of sleep-related breathing disorders, bruxism, and clenching. However, this option appears not to have been adequately explored in Nigeria. This may be due to the relatively few numbers of Orthodontists and Orthodontic Dental Technologists available compared to the Nigerian population.

The management of patients with sleep disorders sometimes requires surgery. There is however a general apathy towards surgery in Nigeria, partly because of lack of awareness and also because of the poor state of facilities at our teaching hospitals. While phase I surgeries involve palatal and lingual surgeries which are readily accessible, Phase II surgeries may involve maxillofacial surgery including maxilla mandibular osteotomies and distraction procedures which are not readily available in Nigerian hospitals.

Lack of Interdisciplinary Platform: The lack of an interdisciplinary platform for sleep specialists and allied health professionals (sleep medicine-trained nurses and sleep technologists) is a major challenge to the practice of sleep medicine in Nigeria. Overwhelming evidence suggests that interdisciplinary care results in more timely and more efficient care ensures adherence to treatment protocols and reduces the risk of the patient being under-treated or over-treated.

Poor Treatment Monitoring: Monitoring of treatment adherence and adverse effects which have implications for relapse is grossly inadequate in Nigeria. Illiteracy, poverty, inadequate patient database, bad housing layouts, and poor communication networks make patient follow-up difficult.

Low utilization of Emerging Patient-driven Healthcare Technology: Technologies such as electronic self-tracking, social networking methods, mobile technology, cloud services, and telemedicine are effective in automating scoring sleep and information sharing between the patient and providers. Technology can also be used to obtain more accurate patient-specific information to make evidence-based treatment recommendations, personalized treatment plans and prompt/rapid identification of treatment failure.

Poor Funding: The healthcare sector in Nigeria which is heavily dependent on budgetary allocations from the Federal or State Government suffers greatly from inadequate funding. The limited resources available are insufficient for the deployment of available software and equipment for procedures such as automated sleep staging. These require the Government's commitment to a large initial investment of funds for the acquisition of facilities and training of personnel.

UNIQUE NEEDS

As clearly pointed out earlier in this chapter, the practice of sleep medicine in Nigeria is still rudimentary and faced with many challenges. Below are a few of the unique needs which we believe can improve the practice of sleep medicine in the country.

1. Manpower Development: Nigeria is blessed with a young population, with most youths ready to learn and explore new things but is often held back by lack of opportunity. Sleep medicine is an area that can be further developed if training facilities for middle-level practitioners become available. Both senior and middle-level manpower (Sleep technologists etc) in the area of sleep medicine is acutely short, or even non-existent a situation that can be remedied if there are training facilities or organizations.

2. Sleep societies/organizations: At the moment, no National or local organization can bring practitioners of sleep medicine together in the country to share ideas, compare notes and chart a path for the future of the practice of sleep medicine in the country. While it is true that in a few tertiary institutions, practitioners interested in research in the area of sleep medicine come together such as the team in the University College Hospital (UCH) Ibadan and that in Obafemi Awolowo University Teaching Hospitals Complex, Ile-Ife (OAUTHC) and others in other tertiary institutions each team does its separate research guided and driven only by the interest of members. A National Sleep Society can galvanize more interest in the practice of sleep medicine, provide guidelines, and set agenda for future development in this area. An organization like the American Academy of Sleep Medicine dedicated exclusively to the practice of sleep medicine, setting standards, and promoting excellence in education, practice, and research in the area of sleep medicine has contributed positively to the development of sleep medicine in America and all over the world. Having a Local or National organization in Nigeria will make a lot of difference in the practice of sleep medicine in the country.

3. Training Programs: While there are few sleep specialists in the country presently, there is enough evidence to show that interest in sleep medicine is strong from the quantum of research in this area. What needs to be done is to improve the training of interested specialists to improve their practice. Such

training may be organized as CME programs at the moment, however, the curriculum can be expanded and improved upon to make it a certificate program.

4. Equipment: Very few clinics in Nigeria have a polysomnography machine for sleep studies. This has affected the quality of research, diagnosis, and treatment of patients with sleep disorders. There is a need for international support to get more equipment in recognized sleep clinics in public tertiary hospitals where it can easily be accessed by practitioners and researchers.

5. National awareness: There is a need to improve awareness for sleep disorders nationally. While research has shown that sleep disorders are relatively common (ref) very few people seek help, many rather go for self-medication or complain of other conditions without making problems with sleep their primary concern. The result is that very few get treated for their sleep problems. People need to become more aware of sleep and its disorders.

6. Treatment Options: Most practitioners are limited by the treatment options available for the treatment of the few diagnosed sleep disorders in the country. Apart from a few medications that are marketed for the treatment of other conditions but have been found effective in treating some sleep disorders, only melatonin is available in a few centers. More needs to be done in making drugs, and other modes of treatment available for patients in the country.

CONCLUSION

The prevalence of sleep disorders in the Nigerian population shows that a significant proportion of the population is affected, the occurrence of which may be associated with multiple factors. The practice of sleep medicine in the country, however, remains inadequate and challenging because the majority of Nigerians are quite unaware of the existence and importance of sleep disorders. The current practice of sleep medicine in Nigeria therefore is still rudimentary. The major barriers to the practice of sleep medicine in the country include the inadequate training of personnel, lack of diagnostic equipment and sleep laboratories, inadequate funding for health services, lack of a health insurance package with wide coverage, and the non-availability of drugs and devices for treatment such as CPAP. Also, there are threats to the practice of sleep medicine which include the national economic recession, a huge burden of communicable and non-communicable diseases competing for health resource allocation, and brain drain among others. Nevertheless, the practice of sleep medicine in Nigeria has a lot of opportunities. There is a growing interest of Nigerian researchers in Sleep medicine, especially in the last decade. Also, the large population of Nigerians, many of whom have risk factors for sleep disorders, suggest that they may be a significant contributor to the global burden of sleep disorders. Therefore, further efforts to identify the needs, barriers to practice, and challenges with the practice of sleep medicine in Nigeria are highly needed to improve the practice of sleep medicine in the country.

CONSENT FOR PUBLICATION

Not applicable.

CONFLICT OF INTEREST

The authors declare no conflict of interest, financial or otherwise.

ACKNOWLEDGEMENT

Declared none.

REFERENCES

[1]　Central Intelligence Agency (CIA). Country comparison: Area. The World Factbook 2020.

[2]　Akinyemi AI, Isiugo-Abanihe UC. Demographic dynamics and development in Nigeria. Afr Popul Stud 2014; 27(2): 239-48.
[http://dx.doi.org/10.11564/27-2-471]

[3]　Countries By Density 2020. World Population Review. World Population Review 2020.

[4]　Lysonski S, Durvasula S. Nigeria in transition: acculturation to global consumer culture. J Consum Mark 2013; 30(6): 493-508.
[http://dx.doi.org/10.1108/JCM-07-2013-0626]

[5]　Stranges S, Tigbe W, Gómez-Olivé FX, Thorogood M, Kandala NB. Sleep problems: an emerging global epidemic? Findings from the INDEPTH WHO-SAGE study among more than 40,000 older adults from 8 countries across Africa and Asia. Sleep 2012; 35(8): 1173-81.
[http://dx.doi.org/10.5665/sleep.2012]

[6]　Ramnathan Iyer S. Sleep and type 2 diabetes mellitus- clinical implications. J Assoc Physicians India 2012; 60: 42-7.

[7]　Z Assefa S, Diaz-Abad M, M Wickwire E, M Scharf S. The Functions of Sleep. AIMS Neurosci 2015; 2(3): 155-71.
[http://dx.doi.org/10.3934/Neuroscience.2015.3.155]

[8]　Krueger JM, Frank MG, Wisor JP, Roy S. Sleep function: Toward elucidating an enigma. Sleep Med Rev 2016; 28: 46-54.
[http://dx.doi.org/10.1016/j.smrv.2015.08.005]

[9]　Franken P, Kopp C, Landolt HP, Lüthi A. The functions of sleep. Eur J Neurosci 2009; 29(9): 1739-40.
[http://dx.doi.org/10.1111/j.1460-9568.2009.06746.x]

[10]　AlDabal L, Bahammam AS. Metabolic, endocrine, and immune consequences of sleep deprivation. Open Respir Med J 2011; 5(1): 31-43.
[http://dx.doi.org/10.2174/1874306401105010031]

[11]　Goel N, Rao H, Durmer J, Dinges D. Neurocognitive consequences of sleep deprivation. Semin Neurol 2009; 29(4): 320-39.
[http://dx.doi.org/10.1055/s-0029-1237117]

[12]　Aurora RN, Punjabi NM. Obstructive sleep apnoea and type 2 diabetes mellitus: a bidirectional

association. Lancet Respir Med 2013; 1(4): 329-38.
[http://dx.doi.org/10.1016/S2213-2600(13)70039-0]

[13]   Kasai T, Floras JS, Bradley TD. Sleep apnea and cardiovascular disease: a bidirectional relationship. Circulation 2012; 126(12): 1495-510.
[http://dx.doi.org/10.1161/CIRCULATIONAHA.111.070813]

[14]   Mume CO. Prevalence of sleepwalking in an adult population. Libyan J Med 2010; 5(1): 2143.
[http://dx.doi.org/10.3402/ljm.v5i0.2143]

[15]   Olorunmoteni OE, Fatusi AO, Komolafe MA, Omisore A. Sleep pattern, socioenvironmental factors, and use of electronic devices among Nigerian school-attending adolescents. Sleep Health 2018; 4(6): 551-7.
[http://dx.doi.org/10.1016/j.sleh.2018.09.002]

[16]   Oshinaike O, Akinbami A, Ojelabi O, Dada A, Dosunmu A, John Olabode S. Quality of Sleep in an HIV Population on Antiretroviral Therapy at an Urban Tertiary Centre in Lagos, Nigeria. Neurol Res Int 2014; 2014: 298703.
[http://dx.doi.org/10.1155/2014/298703]

[17]   Fawale MB, Ismaila IA, Mustapha AF, Komolafe MA, Ibigbami O. Correlates of sleep quality and sleep duration in a sample of urban-dwelling elderly Nigerian women. Sleep Health 2017; 3(4): 257-62.
[http://dx.doi.org/10.1016/j.sleh.2017.05.008]

[18]   Epstein LJ, Valentine PS. Starting a sleep center. Chest 2010; 137(5): 1217-24.
[http://dx.doi.org/10.1378/chest.09-2186]

[19]   Adewole O. Pattern of Sleep Disorders among Patients in a Nigerian Family Practice Population. Ann Med Health Sci Res 2017; 7.

[20]   Osaikhuwuomwan JA, Aina OI, Aziken ME. Sleep disorders in women attending antenatal care at a tertiary hospital in Nigeria. Niger Postgrad Med J 2014; 21(2): 155-9.

[21]   Sunmonu TA, Abubakar SA, Disu JO, *et al.* Sleep disturbances among patients with epilepsy in Nigeria. Ann Afr Med 2015; 14(2): 103-8.
[http://dx.doi.org/10.4103/1596-3519.149880]

[22]   Oluwole OSA. Lifetime prevalence and incidence of parasomnias in a population of young adult Nigerians. J Neurol 2010; 257(7): 1141-7.
[http://dx.doi.org/10.1007/s00415-010-5479-6]

[23]   Fawale MB, Ibigbami O, Ismail I, *et al.* Risk of obstructive sleep apnea, excessive daytime sleepiness and depressive symptoms in a Nigerian elderly population. Sleep Sci 2016; 9(2): 106-11.
[http://dx.doi.org/10.1016/j.slsci.2016.05.005]

[24]   Awopeju OF, Erhabor G, Awopeju O, Irabor I, Ashaolu O. Awopeju OF, Erhabor G, Awopeju O, Irabor I, Ashaolu O. Identifying The Risk Of Obstructive Sleep Apnoea And Its Determinants In A General Outpatient Clinic In Nigeria. Inb70. Sleep Disordered Breathing. Epidemiology And Outcomes: Bench To Bedside 2013 May A3450-0. American Thoracic Society.

[25]   Olufemi Adewole O, Hakeem A, Fola A, Anteyi E, Ajuwon Z, Erhabor G. Obstructive sleep apnea among adults in Nigeria. J Natl Med Assoc 2009; 101(7): 720-5.
[http://dx.doi.org/10.1016/S0027-9684(15)30983-4]

[26]   Desalu O, Onyedum C, Sanya E, *et al.* Prevalence, awareness and reporting of symptoms of obstructive sleep apnoea among hospitalized adult patients in Nigeria: A multicenter study. Ethiop J Health Sci 2016; 26(4): 321-30.
[http://dx.doi.org/10.4314/ejhs.v26i4.4]

[27]   Anyanwu OU, Ibekwe RC, Orji ML. Nocturnal enuresis among Nigerian children and its association with sleep, behavior and school performance. Indian Pediatr 2015; 52(7): 587-9.
[http://dx.doi.org/10.1007/s13312-015-0680-4]

[28]   Senbanjo IO, Salisu MA, Oshikoya KA, Adediji UO, Akinola AO. Nigerian sleep study found that children slept less and had more problems than children in other countries. Acta Paediatr 2018; 107(8): 1449-54.
[http://dx.doi.org/10.1111/apa.14313]

[29]   Seun-Fadipe CT, Mosaku KS. Sleep quality and psychological distress among undergraduate students of a Nigerian university. Sleep Health 2017; 3(3): 190-4.
[http://dx.doi.org/10.1016/j.sleh.2017.02.004]

[30]   Tobi Seun-Fadipe C, Samuel Mosaku K. Sleep quality and academic performance among Nigerian undergraduate students. J Syst Integr Neurosci 2017; 3(5): 1-6.
[http://dx.doi.org/10.15761/JSIN.1000179]

[31]   Balogun FM, Alohan AO, Orimadegun AE. Self-reported sleep pattern, quality, and problems among schooling adolescents in southwestern Nigeria. Sleep Med 2017; 30: 245-50.
[http://dx.doi.org/10.1016/j.sleep.2016.11.013]

[32]   Ayuk AC, Uwaezuoke SN, Kingsley Ndu I, *et al.* Sleep-disordered breathing and neurobehavioral symptoms in children in a Southeast Nigerian city. Indian J Child Health (Bhopal) 2019; 6(6): 259-64.
[http://dx.doi.org/10.32677/IJCH.2019.v06.i06.001]

[33]   Sogebi OA, Ogunwale A. Risk factors of obstructive sleep apnea among nigerian outpatients. Rev Bras Otorrinolaringol (Engl Ed) 2012; 78(6): 27-33.
[http://dx.doi.org/10.5935/1808-8694.20120029]

[34]   Igbokwe D, Ola BA, Odebunmi A, *et al.* Sleep disorders among adolescents in Nigeria: The development of an assessment instrument (Sleep Disorders in Nigeria Questionnaire [SDINQ]). Eur Psychiatry 2016; 33(S1): s267-7.
[http://dx.doi.org/10.1016/j.eurpsy.2016.01.700]

[35]   Komolafe MA, Sanusi AA, Idowu AO, *et al.* Sleep medicine in Africa: past, present, and future. J Clin Sleep Med 2021; 17(6): 1317-21.
[http://dx.doi.org/10.5664/jcsm.9218]

[36]   Alabi BS, Abdulkarim AA, Musa IO, *et al.* Prevalence of snoring and symptoms of sleep disordered breathing among primary school pupils in Ilorin, Nigeria. Int J Pediatr Otorhinolaryngol 2012; 76(5): 646-8.
[http://dx.doi.org/10.1016/j.ijporl.2012.01.029]

[37]   Kuti BP, Kuti DK. Is Childhood Obstructive Sleep Apnoea Properly Taught In Medical Schools? An Assessment Of The Knowledge And Perception Of Doctors On Obstructive Sleep Apnoea. InC105. Disorders Of Respiratory Physiology And Sleep In Children 2017; (May): A6887-7. [American Thoracic Society.].

[38]   Moturi S, Avis K. Assessment and treatment of common pediatric sleep disorders. Psychiatry (Edgmont) 2010; 7(6): 24.

[39]   Krishna J, Omlor GJ. Setting Up a Pediatric Sleep Lab. Journal of Child Science 2019; 9(1): e30-7.
[http://dx.doi.org/10.1055/s-0038-1675608]

[40]   Maduabuchi JC, Obu HA, Chukwu BF, Ebele A, Manyike PC, Chinawa AT. Sleep pattern and practice among adolescents school children in Nigerian secondary schools. Pan Afr Med J 2014; 19: 2-6.
[http://dx.doi.org/10.11604/pamj.2014.19.313.4603]

[41]   Ozoh OB, Iwuala SO, Desalu OO, Ojo OO, Okubadejo NU. An assessment of the knowledge and attitudes of graduating medical students in Lagos, Nigeria, regarding obstructive sleep apnea. Ann Am Thorac Soc 2015; 12(9): 1358-63.
[http://dx.doi.org/10.1513/AnnalsATS.201412-561OC]

[42]   Nwosu N, Ugoeze F, Ufoaroh CU, *et al.* Knowledge Attitude and Practice Regarding Obstructive Sleep Apnea among Medical Doctors in Southern Nigeria. West Afr J Med 2020; 37(7): 783-9.

[43]   Ohaeri JU, Adelekan MF, Odejide AO, Ikuesan BA. The pattern of isolated sleep paralysis among Nigerian nursing students. J Natl Med Assoc 1992; 84(1): 67.

[44]   Bower B. Slumber's unexplored landscape: People in traditional societies sleep in eye☐opening ways. Sci News 1999; 156(13): 205-7.
[http://dx.doi.org/10.2307/4011789]

[45]   Abad VC, Guilleminault C. Diagnosis and treatment of sleep disorders: a brief review for clinicians. Dialogues Clin Neurosci 2003; 5(4): 371-88.
[http://dx.doi.org/10.31887/DCNS.2003.5.4/vabad]

CHAPTER 18

Sleep Medicine and Surgery in Egypt: Evolution, Clinical Practice, Education and Research Services

Nevin Fayez Zaki[1,*] and **Nesreen Elsayed Morsy**[2]

[1] *ESRS Somnologist, Sleep Research Unit, Department of Psychiatry, Faculty of Medicine, Mansoura University, Mansoura, Egypt*

[2] *ESRS Somnologist, Pulmonary Medicine, Sleep Disordered Breathing Unit (SDB), Mansoura University Sleep Center (MUSC), Faculty of Medicine, Mansoura University, Mansoura, Egypt*

Abstract: All through Egyptian history, starting from the pharaohs, passing by the Coptic and Islamic eras up to modern Egypt, there have been different interests in healthy sleep and sleep hygiene. Myths about sleep medicine are common among cultures and in Egypt, lack of public awareness about sleep disorders makes most patients undiagnosed or ignorant about whom to consult about their symptoms. In this chapter, we aim to provide the reader with the current state of the art of sleep medicine in Egypt. We conducted a literature review, furthermore the opinion of sleep experts in Egypt was collected and stated in detail, and additionally Egyptian sleep centers were invited to answer a survey in order to collect information about the equipment and trained personnel presented in this chapter. There are three types of Egyptian medical education streams including, the public, private and Al-Azhar medical schools, in which undergraduate and postgraduate medical students can join and earn their degrees but there are no specialized degrees in sleep medicine yet, exact details about medical education in Egypt are provided below. Egypt has numerous health care system providers or sectors: public, private and financing agents' parastatal providers. Nevertheless, sleep studies remain expensive for the Egyptian public and most insurance companies do not fund it, which makes the expenses of polysomnography the duty of the patient to pay from his own pocket. Egyptian sleep laboratories are governmental and private labs, the governmental labs usually exist in university hospitals, financial and educational hassles make accreditation of these labs by AASM difficult. We provided statistics describing these labs and the type of equipment they use. We tried to discuss the clinical and research sleep status in Egypt, additionally, we tried to suggest solutions for these challenging issues.

Keywords: Egypt, Polysomnography, Sleep education, Sleep medicine.

* **Corresponding author Nevin Fayez Zaki:** Sleep Research Unit, Department of Psychiatry, Faculty of Medicine, Mansoura University, Mansoura, Egypt; Tel: +201283339789; E-mail: mernakero@mans.edu.eg

Hrayr P. Attarian, Marie-Louise M. Coussa-Koniski & Alain Michel Sabri (Eds.)

INTRODUCTION

Egypt is the land of civilization since the beginning of the history. In Egypt, you can find different cultural and religious variations throughout different historical eras. The oldest civilization in the history lived in Egypt (the ancient Egypt or pharaohs). Since the dawn of human civilization, Ancient Egyptians were great physicians and the best in the world, their medical knowledge and practice were the base of all medical practices and medical education in all other successive civilizations. They were concerned about sleep nature, sleep disorders and dreaming with its interpretations. Not only pharaonic Egypt but also Islamic Egypt had great concern about sleep. Sleep hygiene tips and sleep stages, *etc.* are part of Islamic religious practices. In the modern era, Egyptian doctors follow international guidelines and accompany the scientific development all over the world.

The data in this chapter was collected through three main methods:

The first: we did literature review using the relevant keywords by main search engines and database: Google, Google Scholar, Scopus, MEDLINE (PubMed), SAGE Research Methods, and ScienceDirect. We also scanned the official data available from governmental websites that issue official reporting *e.g.*: the Egyptian Central Agency for Public Mobilization and Statistics (CAPMS) and medical schools' records in different universities.

The second: was the opinion of two Egyptian sleep experts about the current situation of clinical practice, medical education and research of sleep medicine and surgery . We had to use this because we have a knowledge gap in the published work about this topic.

The third was conducted by communication with the known Egyptian sleep experts through WhatsApp application or direct phone calls for each known sleep laboratory head in different cities of Egypt as well as website visits, we asked them to fill up two semi-structured questionnaires, conducted through Google form. The first survey was about the type, the place, work force and available services of the sleep laboratory as well as the load of patients per year. The second survey was conducted to get the sleep physician expert (somnologist) and researchers' opinions about the sleep medicine service practice facilities, barriers and challenges as well the educational and clinical information sources, national societies or guidelines and lately the needs for the development of sleep medicine clinical and experimental studies. Results of the surveys will be discussed later in this chapter.

EGYPT IN WORDS

Geographical Position and Population

Egypt has a unique strategic geographical position, it lies in the eastern north part of the African continent, on its northern coasts lies the Mediterranean Sea and on its eastern coasts lies the Red Sea. The land area is around one million km^2. According to the central agency for public mobilization and statistics (CAPMAS), the number the of Egyptian population in January 2020 was around 100 million with approximately equal genders and around 74% are 35 years old or younger [1]. The official religion is Islam (Sunni). Muslims (predominantly Sunni) constitute 90% of the population, while Christians (majority Coptic Orthodox) 10% [2]. Ethnic Egyptians account for 91% of the total population [3]. The official language is Arabic (Modern Standard) and the Egyptian Dialect or accent is the most widely spoken among Egyptians. English is generally understood [4].

Medical Education System

Undergraduate Medical Education (UGME)

For doctors to attain a medical degree with a clinical practice license, Egypt has three types of medical schools: public (governmental, non-profit schools), Al-Azhar (the oldest continuously operating university in the world and the main Islamic religion teaching university in the world plus all non-religious scientific knowledge), and private (with profit aim). Before 2018, Egyptian medical schools followed the French model, which consists of a six-year program featured as a preclinical–clinical dichotomy and a 12 months internship program, English is the language of instruction. The program was a discipline-based curriculum, in which large-group lectures and apprenticeship approaches to clinical teaching were the main methods of instruction, except at Suez Canal medical faculty which applied an integrated curriculum that features project-based learning. An alternative model using student-centered teaching approaches, *e.g.* The PBL parallel track at Mansoura Faculty of Medicine began in 2006, the integrated curriculum at Alexandria Faculty of Medicine in 2009, the modular parallel track at Ain Shams University in 2014, and the Integrated Program of Kasr Al-Ainy (IPKA) in 2015. After the Egyptian Parliament issued a statement that the number of years required for a medicine bachelor's degree has been reduced to five years and will be calculated through credit hours and an integrative system combining basic science with clinical studies then it will be followed by a 2-year internship to follow the requirements of world's federation of medical education [5 - 8].

Postgraduate Medical Education (PGSM)

The aim of this type of medical education is the specialization of the medical school graduate. The graduate can choose either one of the two main pathways.

The first pathway is the academic pathway, leading to a scientific degree: Master (MSc.) or Doctorate (MD, PhD). This pathway is under the auspices of the universities. The students should have residency of three years for clinical training and attend at least 75% of their learning system requirements including practical skills activities and provide evidence of continuity and progress in their professional practice. They also should conduct a research thesis. Finally, all students must undertake a summative assessment, usually comprising written, practical, and clinical exams. Previously, the theoretical learning system was the conventional contact-hour system, which requires physical attendance at indicated activities at a university hospital, a minimum number of study years, passing examinations (mostly in two parts administered at different times), but nowadays, in credit hour system, in which the graduate undertakes and is examined in a group of courses. The academic supervisor is an integral component of the credit-hour system.

The second pathway is the Fellowship of the Egyptian Board (FEB) program, leading to membership of the national board of medical specializations of the high committee of medical specialties. It is coordinated by the Ministry of Health. The FEB training program duration ranges between three and seven years, depending on the specialty, and graduates are granted a professional degree. No research thesis is required. Clinical training in the FEB is conducted in accredited training centers by the FEB council. Training of fellows must be supervised by one or more consultants or professors in the same specialty. Theoretical Education is conducted as in-job training using different instructional methods, such as lectures, small-group discussions, and library activities [9 - 11].

Continuous Medical Education (CME)

It is the professional long-life process of acquiring new knowledge and skills. After 2017, Egypt developed a regulatory system for the provision, and accreditation of CME activities and centers as well as endorsement of obtained CME credits with a subsequent award of licenses to practice medicine. This is conducted by the Egyptian Authorities for Compulsory Training of Doctors [6].

Health Care System

Egypt has numerous health care system providers or sectors: public, private and financing agents' parastatal providers [12].

The government sector represents services of the Ministry of Health and Population (MOHP) which is funded by the Ministry of Finance (MOF). The parastatal sector is composed of semi-governmental institutions, syndicates and different organizations which are governed by their own set of rules and regulations, and have independent budgets but they are still under control of the ministry of higher education and MOHP, *e.g.* University' hospitals, Health Insurance Organization, Curative Care Organization, and the Teaching Hospitals and Institutes Organization [12].

The private sector includes profit and non-profit organizations. The profit organizations are under control of MOHP too, they include everything from traditional midwives, private pharmacies, private clinics, private polyclinics or centers, to private hospitals of all sizes. The non-profit organizations include: religiously affiliated clinics or hospitals and other charitable organizations i.e. red crescent hospitals *etc.*, all of which are registered with the Ministry of Social Affairs (MOSA) [12 - 14].

The Percentage of Public expenditure on Health is 4%. However, in the private sector, the health care costs are paid by patients themselves or insurance companies [1]. In 2011, the percentage of Private expenditure on health of the total health care expenditure is 60% due to the privatization policies of the country. The percentage of private primary health care clinics and centers of total primary health care units is 78%. The number of doctors, pharmacists, dentists and nurses who work at general office ministry, directorates of health affairs and bodies related to MOHP in 2018 was around 90.000, 50.000, 20.000 and 80.000, respectively [1, 13, 14].

Scientific Research System

Egypt's Science, Technology and Innovation system (STI system) comprises: 1- the National Council of Scientific Research and Education (NCSRE), 2- the Ministry of higher education and Scientific Research, 3- the Academy of Scientific Research and Technology (ASRT), 4- Science and Technology Development Fund (STDF), and 5- Research Institutions and Universities. Egypt's research community include around 127,000 theoretical and applied scientists in 26 state (governmental) universities and academies and 12 national research centers according to the ministry of higher education and scientific research in their last statistics of years 2014-2017. The research work divided into postgraduate studies (master and doctorate thesis), free researches or research projects. According to the Central Agency for Public Mobilization and Statistics (CAPMAS) 119,759 post graduate studies (diploma, master and doctorate) were awarded for Egyptian researchers in the year 2018 and in medicine, around 886

Egyptian researchers were awarded (master = 644, doctorate = 242). The number of internationally published researches by Egyptians was 18,876. The Egyptian research publications count for Egypt published between 1 June 2019 - 31 May 2020 which are tracked by Nature Index are as follows: The count is equal to 183 and the share is 13.3. Egypt currently ranks 37th in the world of scientific research published in 240 countries worldwide. Based on reports from scientific indicator SJR (SCImago journal and country rank) up to the year 2019. Egypt's international ranking is 30 in Medicine. On Publons, there are 250 Egyptian verified reviewers for international journals. The expenditure on scientific research is 17.56 billion pounds which equals 0.72% of GDP (Gross Domestic Product) according to the World Bank statistics and Egyptian Ministry of Finance. The ministry supported the establishment of 56 central labs with funding of LE 240 million for universities, institutes and research centers. Funding, Grants and Scholarships for scientific research and development of the Egyptian researchers' skills are divided into two main sectors, national or international opportunities. The national opportunities for example: Universities funding of research projects, Science and Technology Development Fund (STDF), cultural affairs and missions' sector and the Bibliotheca Alexandrina Research Grants Program. The international opportunities exclusive for Egyptians are for example: Fulbright Commission in Egypt, DAAD Egypt, European commission different funds, grants and Newton-Mosharafa Fund. Moreover, the Egyptian researchers also compete for other international funding opportunities offered for researchers from developing countries. For sure many pharmaceutical companies contract with Egyptian researchers in multicenter studies in different phases especially phase 3. The Egyptian Ministry of Higher Education and Scientific Research supports around 175 researchers per year in scientific missions to developed countries, with a total funding of 26.8 million pounds [15 - 31].

Egyptian Knowledge Bank(EKB), which was launched in 2015, is an online library archive that has an access to a huge number of databases or publishers' resources that provide an access to a huge number of scientific journals, books, *etc.* Every researcher has an online account for EKB to be able to retrieve the required data or literatures either at work or home [32]. Many other libraries show different services for researchers, for example: Egyptian Public Library (Maktabah Masr 'Ammah), Bibliotheca Alexandrina, Greater Cairo Library, Library of United States Embassy, each university library *e.g.* Cairo university, American university in Egypt. Any library in Egypt is recorded in the Egyptian libraries network website [33 - 35]. Egyptian scientific journals are usually released by Egyptian societies or universities and published through a well-known publisher for example: The Egyptian Journal of Chest Diseases and Tuberculosis which is the official journal of Egyptian Society of Chest Diseases and Tuberculosis and Arab Thoracic Association published by Medknow, part of

Wolters Kluwer Health, being one of the largest open access publishers worldwide [36]. Research Ethics Committees (RECs) in Egypt were introduced in some institutions in 1980s. In Egypt, ethical committees are well-distributed over the country. The Egyptian national ethical committee collaborates with the United Nations Educational, Scientific and Cultural Organization (UNESCO). The Ministry of Health and Population (MOHP) has its own ethical committee. The Egyptian Network of Research Ethics Committees (ENREC) was created in 2008. Now every university, or institution has a regulatory committee for approval of research conduction using international guidelines in this regard [37, 38].

EVOLUTION OF SLEEP MEDICINE IN EGYPT ACROSS THE AGES

Ancient Egypt Era

The ancient Egypt (pharaonic) medicine was known as one of the earliest records of medicine in human history. The Archaeologists discovered the engravings and paintings in the Egyptian tombs dating back to 2500 B.C.E. One of the famous premier examples of these records is the Edwin Smith Surgical Papyrus, which is part of the New York Academy of Medicine's collection. It dates back to 1600 B.C.E. and was a copy of a much earlier work. Another one, The Ebers Papyrus, (Figs. **1a** and **1b**) dating back to 1550 BCE, is among the oldest and most important medical papyri in ancient Egypt and it is currently maintained at the University of Leipzig Library in Germany. It includes information on different diseases, medical prescriptions, medicinal herbs, magic spells, and potions against evil spirits.

In a book released in conjunction with the exhibition (the art in ancient Egypt) held at the metropolitan museum of art, New York 2006, a catalogue section for exploring different potions, methods, tools and bowls used by ancient Egyptian doctors can be seen in Figs. (**2a,2b** and **2c**). Doctors have had the education and training in medicine as well as in other disciplines of life such as the arts, religion, architecture, administration and warfare in The Mystical School of Life. The physician called 'Hsi Ra', from the third dynasty (about 2700 BCE), is considered the oldest example of a physician in ancient Egypt. The greatest physician of Ancient Egypt is Imhotep the Royal Chamberlain of the third dynasty King Djoser and the architect of the step pyramid at Saqqara. In the Ptolemaic Period, the Greeks identified him as Asklepios, their god of medicine because of his unique pioneering medical skills, they built a shrine to Imhotep at the great temple of Hatshepsut in Deir el Bahari, which became a place of pilgrimage by the sick. Egyptian theories and practices influenced the Greeks, who provided many of the physicians in the Roman Empire, and through them Arab and European medical thinking for centuries to come [39 - 45]. The ancient Egyptians believed in the ability of the ba (soul) to travel beyond the physical body during sleep. Sleep was viewed to be similar, in some aspect, to death, in which the person is in a different state or a different world. They used to get the interpretation of their patients' dreams to diagnose the problem and to suggest treatment in their temples, these were known as Sleep temples or dream temple therapy which were hospitals for placing the patient into a hypnotic state, and analyzing their dreams in order to determine treatment. This therapy was dated from the time of Imhotep. The temple at Deir el-Bahri is an example of a place where one could go for healing [46, 47]. They used Poppy (Papaver somniferum) to relieve insomnia as well as Lavender, and Chamomile. They also drank a brew of lactucarium, a milky and psychoactive latex that oozes from wild lettuce stems. It contains a hint of lactucin, a sedative Thyme that was thought to be beneficial in reducing snoring [48].

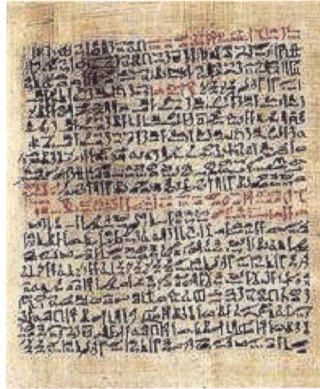

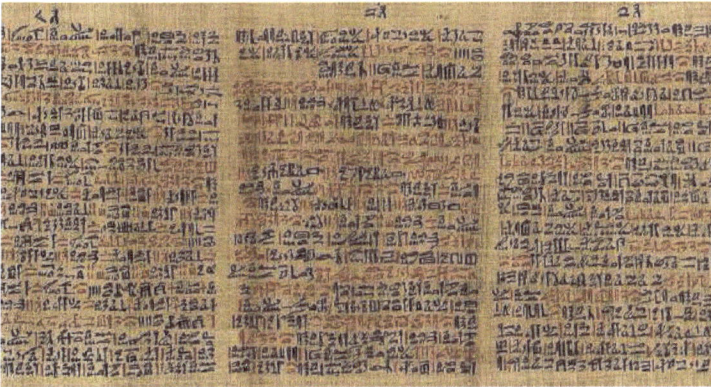

Fig. (1). (a, b): Fragments from the Ebers Papyrus, dating back to 1550 BC, it is among the oldest and most important medical papyri in ancient Egypt and it is currently maintained at the University of Leipzig Library in Germany.

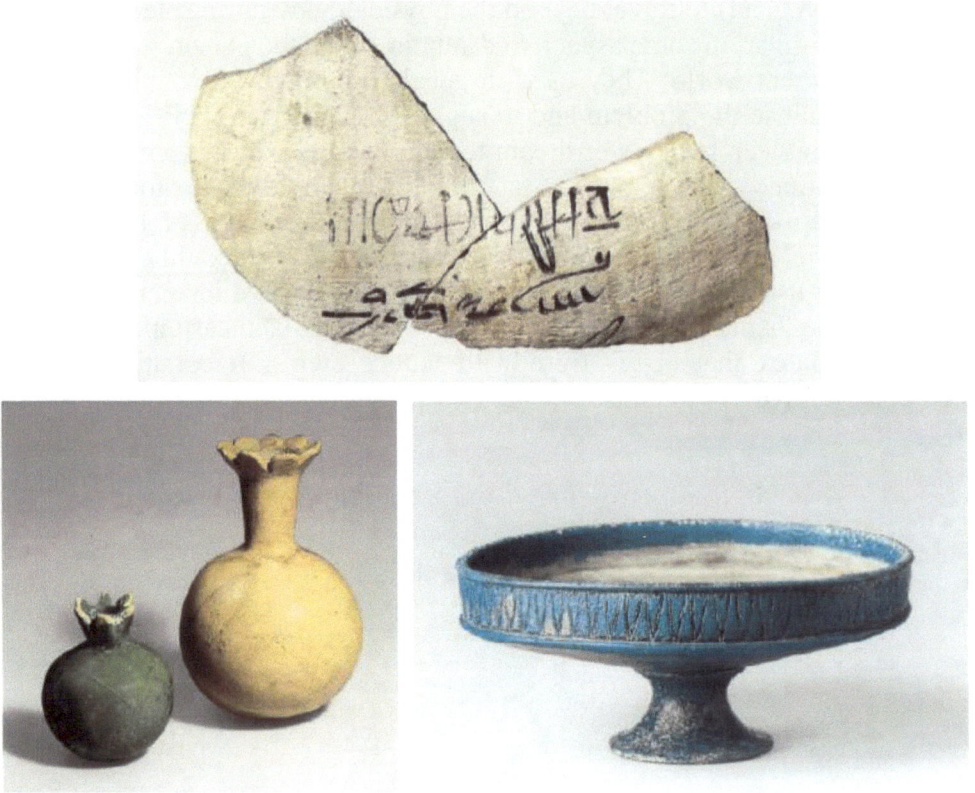

Figs. (2). (a, b & c) represent tools used by Ancient Egyptian doctors in preparing medicine for their patients.

Ancient Greek (Ptolemaic) and Romanian Era

During the Greek (Ptolemaic) occupation of Egypt, they imported much of their medical knowledge from the Egyptians because they were not as skilled as the Ancient Egyptians, whom even Homer recognized as the greatest healers in the world. Egyptian people and their medical knowledge are often mentioned in the Iliad and Odyssey of Homer. So Egyptian medicine is considered the base of Greek medicine. Many Greek doctors, such as Melampus, Asclepius as well as Hippocrates visited Egypt to study and understand medicine. Herodotus (484-420 BCE) in the second book of "The Histories" describes Egypt and the medical knowledge of its doctors. However, Hippocrates, was one of the most famous Greek physicians, and his famous oath is still used by doctors today in Egypt (Figs. (**3** and **4**) are two versions of the Hippocratic Oath). His most important contribution to medicine was the separation of medicine from the magic or spiritual side. In the following century, the work of Aristotle was regarded as the first great biologist. Following Aristotle's time, Alexander the Great, (Aristotle's pupil) built Alexandria and made it the intellectual capital of the world. The famous medical school of Alexandria was established in about 300 BCE by its two founders and the best medical teachers were Herophilus, who is known as the first anatomist in history, and Erasistratus, whom some regard as the founder of physiology. The Egyptian and Greek knowledge was passed down to the Romans, who preserved the medical skills and refined them. Galen, the famous Roman physician studied in Alexandria before practicing in Rome. His teachings and writings survived well into the sixteenth century and formed the basis of more modern medical practices during the Renaissance. These writings were conserved partly by Christian monks and partly by Arab and Jewish scholars of the middle-ages. The medical school of Alexandria was still active until late in the 3rd century CE [45, 49 - 51].

Fig. (3). The Hippocratic oath on papyrus.

In the Greco-Roman myth, Sleep god was Hypnos. Dionysius of Heracleia, an ancient Greek tyrant (360 BCE) had morbid obesity, difficulties breathing and significant daytime sleepiness such that his physicians are said to have prescribed him the insertion of long, fine needles into his flesh, in order to awaken him whenever he fell into a deep sleep. Dreams were thought to be internally reflective of body states. Physicians of that era inherit the same idea of ancient Egyptians that analyzing the content of a patient's dream makes the physician able to diagnose bodily disturbances and direct treatment accordingly. Disturbances in sleep are frequently noted in the Hippocratic corpus collections as a symptom. Galen described sleep as a cooling method of the brain to increase its moisture. He explained the cause of insomnia by excessively warm and dry brain. He distinguished natural sleep from that of commas and other forms of unconsciousness, as well as from sleep induced by hypnotics. Aristotle and Dioscorides in their work (De material medica) used the opium poppy, saffron, aloe mandragora, henbane, rush, wine, and darnel to induce sleep [52, 53].

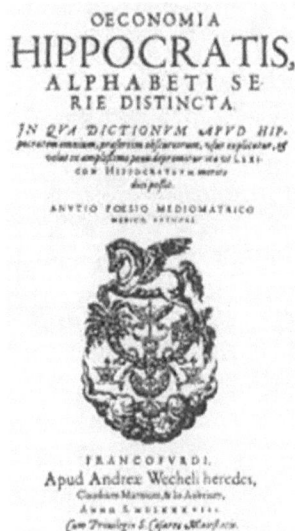

Fig. (4). Hippocratic corpus.

Christian (Coptic) Era

It was a short period around two and a half centuries only. The principal source of the information for this era is retrieved from a fine papyrus discovered in 1892 and now in the French archeological institute at Cairo. The Cairo papyrus is in good condition and contains 237 prescriptions and was written in the 9th century CE. Another two leaves of parchment in the Vatican library once formed part of a book contain 45 prescriptions. A third medical papyrus was discovered in 1887, at Deir-el-Abiad, and published by Bouziane; and has 11 prescriptions. The last is a series of tiny fragments present now in many places, *i.e.,* the British Museum, the John Rylands Library at Manchester, and the Berlin Museum [54].

Islamic Medieval Era

Islamic civilization covers a time-frame between the seventh and the eighteenth centuries spreading through the middle east up to China in the east and Spain in the west and Europe in the north, including Egypt. During the golden age of Islamic civilization, the other nations were in the dark ages and the Islamic civilization paved the way for the European Renaissance. However, the Muslim physicians inherited their knowledge from Greek, Roman, Persian Indian, Chinese and byzantine resources. In addition, they add their observations, experiments and clinical practice including different innovative methods of diagnosis and treatment and recognition of previously unknown diseases. They also found out many discoveries like the discovery of pulmonary circulation by Ibn El-Nafis. Most of them were skilled in medical writing and produced encyclopedic works which became standards for medical practice. The idea of hospitals previously called (Bimaristan) was adopted by the early Muslim caliphs for example: Al-Walid and Harun-ul-Rashid. In Egypt, one of the largest hospitals was ever built by Mamluk Sultan Qalawun. These hospitals were medical schools for students. Also, these hospitals were managed by great physicians like Al-Razi (864 – 935 CE), who wrote the al-Hawi book in 25 volumes long, the third oldest preserved medical book in the world. He discussed the bed-wetting problem in detail and described many therapeutic behaviors or remedies. He also provided a detailed description of sleep paralysis, although in this era this problem was thought to be caused by a demon's presence in bed. Al-Bokhari (983 CE) in his book Hidayat al-muta'allemin fi al-Tibb, designated a chapter for a discussion of nightmares and sleep paralysis, he analyzed the etiology scientifically and discussed the available therapeutic approaches to resolving it. Before them, Ibn al-Jazzar (895–979 CE) wrote an entire book about sleep disorders that was unfortunately lost. Also, Ibn al-Ash'ath (975 CE) realized the importance of sleep in maintaining good health in his book Quwa al-Adwiyyah, to be one of the principles of sickness and health.

The greatest physician in the Islamic era ever was Avicenna or Ibn Sina (980 – 1037 CE) who wrote the main medical textbook al-Qanun fi al-Tibb in five volumes. Fig. (**5**) represents an excerpt from this book, which was translated into Latin and used for centuries by physicians all over the world. He wrote a full chapter about sleep and vigilance. He explained the importance of sleep for body's health and as a therapeutic method. He also described many sleep disorders and behavioral and pharmacologic ways for treatment of people suffering from insomnia and circadian rhythm problems. He also suggested sleep hygiene rules and described the daytime sleepiness and its relation to illnesses. He described many drugs, potions, and remedies for sleep problems in another volume of the book [55 - 58].

The Muslims gained their knowledge mainly from the Holy Quran and the prophet Mohammed's sayings and traditions (Hadith or Sunna). We can find in the teachings of the Islamic religion. The sleep pattern of Muslims is influenced by prayer times. Going to bed early and waking-up early are strongly encouraged in Islam. The sleep stages have been recently discovered to be mentioned in the holy Quran, referring to sleep by different synonyms which uncovered a new audit to them by the Arabic linguists. The circadian rhythm idea was established by the holy Quran verse which says: "Do they not see that we made the night that they may rest there in and the day giving sight?". In Sunnah, Naps also recommended in the midday but for a short period and long nap is prohibited which is scientifically proved nowadays. Dream interpretation is an established science in Muslim literatures, and considered to be a kind of supernatural perception. The most famous dream interpreter in the Islamic history was Ibn Sirin (653–728 CE) [59 - 61].

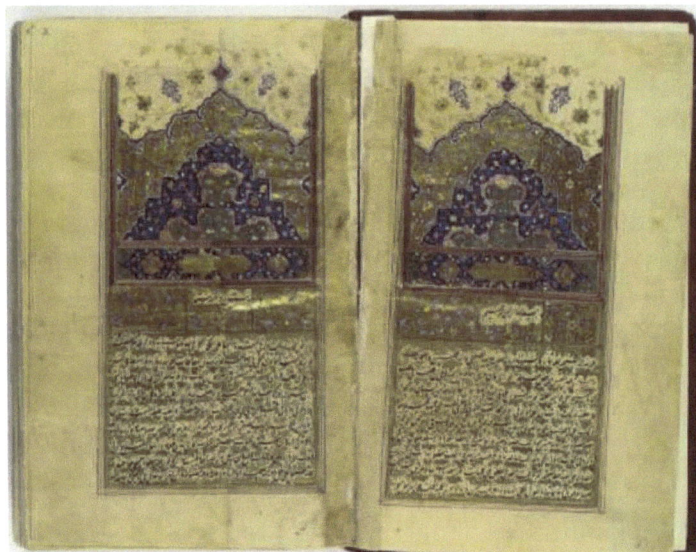

Fig. (5). Excerpt al-Qanun fi al-Tibb by Avicenna or Ibn Sina.

Modern Era

The modern western medical education and training in Egypt was founded over a 7-year period by Antoine-Barthelemy Clot Bey better known as Clot-Bey in 1837 and became part of the university programs in 1925. Clot Bey was a French physician and the son of a sergeant major in Napoleon Bonaparte's incursion army of Egypt in 1798 who was recruited to Egypt in 1825 as a Surgeon-in-Chief (later he was given the army rank of general then commander of the Legion of Honor and the title "Bey," the title of Mameluke chieftains) of the Egyptian Armies by Mohammed Ali, viceroy of Egypt in this period. He created a council of health and reorganized hospitals to make them consonant with the Western medicine of the day. Also, he found a medical school with a 6-year study program on the assembly of the Paris Medical School for 300 students at the 1500 bed in 1827, at Kasr Al-Ainy (cairo university medical school later) a military teaching hospital in Abu-Zaabal, to the northeast of Cairo [62 - 64]. In 1832, Clot Bye sent the distinguished 12 graduates wearing turbans and flowing robes to Paris to complete their studies and then returned back to be the first nucleus of the Egyptian medical academic staff. By the year 1837, the number of graduates reached 430 doctors. Then the school of medicine was moved from Abou Zaabal to Kasr El-Ainy for more expansion and it was the first medical school in Egypt, however during the next decades, the medical education was deteriorated again and the Egyptian physicians have been educated abroad, mostly in France [65]. In 1882, the school was rebuilt by Dr Sandwith and Dr Milton to accommodate 500 students. In 1885, the doors of the outpatient clinic were reopened to the public. In 1896, the Government decided to spend about £27 000 on reconstruction of the hospital. In 1925, the school of medicine was incorporated into the Egyptian university and was called the Faculty of Medicine. In 1927, it was decided that a new hospital with 1200 beds and a new modern medical school should be established. King Fouad laid the foundation of the new faculty and its hospital on December 16th 1928 [66, 67]. These advances in the twentieth century were executed by Sir Prof. Dr. Ali Pasha Ibrahim (1880 - 1946) (see Fig. **6**), the Iconic pioneer and the father of the modern medical renaissance in Egypt and the Middle East. He was the first Egyptian dean of Kasr El-Ainy faculty of medicine who reconstructed and organized medical education in Egypt, as well as established the Physicians' Syndicate. Also, he was involved in the issuance of the first law for medical practicing in Egypt. He became the minister of health, and the director of Cairo University (Kasr El-Ainy) and Red Crescent society. He allowed the girls to study medicine.

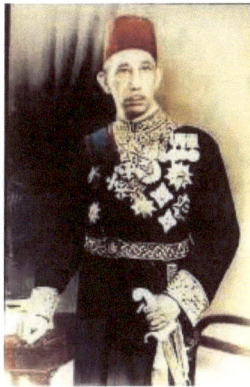

Fig. (6). Sir Prof. Dr. Ali Pasha Ibrahim.

He planned and successfully started a new full-scale medical school at Alexandria [68, 69]. Since then, different medical schools in all governorates of Egypt have evolved. Nowadays, these medical schools or faculties are well known in the whole world and a lot of the Egyptian universities got a high rank among the world's universities of medical sciences (401-500) [70]. During this era, sleep medicine was based on the new development and discoveries in sleep physiology and disorders.

SLEEP MYTH AND PUBLIC MISCONCEPTIONS IN EGYPT

The Egyptian false concepts or misconceptions about sleep are nearly the same as in other nations all over the world [71]. Egyptians consider sleep as an additional luxurious act and not a priority. It can be skipped especially if you have work or study and you can catch up on missed sleep over the weekend. Even Arabic phrases or quotes encourage you to not sleep because it is a waste of precious time and sleep will not lengthen your life span and staying up late will not decrease it as in the famous song of the most famous female singer Umm Kulthum (Rubaiyat (quadruplets) of al-Khayyám) which was abstracted of the Poetry of Omar Al-Khayyám [72, 73].The mental image of the intelligent person or the thinker is a man who drinks a lot of Turkish coffee and who does not sleep at night except for a few hours because it is a waste of time for such a great responsible man. Snoring is a normal trait in men and no need for medical consultation. Even among the educated, it is just due to adenoid enlargement and it is optional to treat it. However, females are usually embarrassed to admit snoring; they can even totally deny it due to the belief that it's a masculine criterion and will reduce their femininity. The morning person (early bird) is an active ambitious person and the evening person (night owl) is lazy reckless one. Daytime sleepiness or falling asleep at any time of the day or in any place is a criterion of laziness or means you did not get enough sleep with no other causes. The elders are usually sleepy all over the day and this is a normal trait in this age group. Falling asleep once you enter the bed or in any place any time means you are a good sleeper. Do not wake a sleepwalker it will harm him/her very much. Watching television or using smartphone applications is a method of relaxation before sleep. A very dangerous concept among commercial drivers is you can drive with no night sleep to reach your destination faster and there is no problem with using stimulants, opening the car windows, and listening to the radio while driving, *etc.* and the other you can fix your hand on the Steering wheel on the double highway roads to rest. Shift work jobs is very bad for your health. The sleep paralysis as in different cultures is believed to be caused by the devil (Jenn), who are malevolent spirit-like creature specifically attacking teenage girls and called (the loving jenny) [74, 75]. There is no link between major health problems like hypertension, diabetes mellitus, *etc.* or major psychiatric diseases like depression to sleep. Even among the physicians, the idea of sleep medicine is comic and a mocking material.

SLEEP MEDICINE EDUCATION IN EGYPT

Sleep medicine is a relatively recent medical specialty. The current situation of medical education can be divided into three parts:

Undergraduate Sleep Medicine Education

During the medical school, the student can be introduced to the sleep world through different courses or modules for example, the sleep stages are studied in physiology curriculum and the melatonin hormone is discussed in the biochemistry curriculum, *etc.* The famous sleep disorders are explained during other medical curricula for example obstructive sleep apnea is learned during pulmonology curriculum and the insomnia is taught in the psychiatry curriculum. At the end of the medical school, the graduate will be able to recognize the outlines of sleep medicine [76, 77]. Articles describing the status of sleep medicine education in undergraduate Egyptian students are scarce. We could only identify one article by Zaki *et al.*, [84] where sleep medicine knowledge was tested in seven Egyptian universities and it was found that there was no difference in the knowledge between final year students and house officers according to the geographic location and the study year of the students. The research team assumed that house-officers might show more knowledge regarding sleep medicine since they are more exposed to the clinical setting during their year of clinical rotations and the possibility of encountering a patient with sleep complaints is higher. Nevertheless, the results showed no significant differences between the two groups. Most recently during the production of this chapter, there has been an invention of the Egyptian Medical Licensing Examination, which is an exam that medical graduates have to pass before they are able to practice as GPs in Egypt. Further rules and eligibility criteria of the exam are being modified during the production of this chapter.

Postgraduate Sleep Medicine Education

To date, there is no accredited specialized postgraduate degree or certified degree in sleep medicine. Most Egyptian sleep experts were educated and trained in Europe or USA. Actual well-constructed education is gained through postgraduate studies. However, this knowledge is divided according to the different categories of groups of diseases; for example, sleep-related breathing disorders: obstructive and central sleep apnea as well as obesity hypoventilation syndrome comprise the main course in pulmonology masters or doctorate courses. In addition, the practical and clinical experience is developed through the participation of students in the daily work of sleep lab, such as overnight monitoring sessions or morning manual revision of the recorded studies and epochs or, the sleep clinic work in interviewing new patients, diagnosis of the disease after sleep study and management and follow-up of the patients [78, 79].

Continuous Medical Education of Sleep Medicine

Any specialist of pulmonology, psychiatry, or neurology who is interested in sleep medicine and wants to improve his skills in order to be a sleep expert only has one way to reach this goal, mainly by attending conferences, courses or workshops or even by getting an internal scholarship to be trained in a well-known sleep lab or center. During these sessions, the intern usually learns the missing skills being either theoretical, technical or clinical. Usually these conferences, courses and workshops are part of the continuous medical education programs certified by faculties of medicine, doctors, syndicates *etc.* The authors of this chapter are members of the World Association of Sleep Medicine (WASM) and both act as regional coordinators of the World Sleep Day. They were awarded the World Sleep Day (WSD) distinguished activity Award in 2017; for the activities and educative workshops, they organized targeting sleep medicine awareness both on the professional level and also public education (check this website http://worldsleepday.org/egypt-2017-dr-nevin-zaki.).

Sleep Technology Education

Fresh graduates of nursing faculty are usually invited to work in a sleep laboratory in order to be qualified sleep technicians with good medical background. Those new sleep technicians are trained through theoretical courses conducted in different sleep laboratories and by practice throughout participating in the daily activities of the laboratory. They are usually well-trained to deal with any emergency during their study and should be certified for different life saving courses and certificates.

Barriers and Solutions

The main challenges faced by sleep trainees is the non-availability of an individualized residency and diploma in sleep medicine. The importance of sleep medicine is not widely popular among physicians making them hold back and less interested in this branch of medicine. Also, the earned knowledge mainly depends on one's passion and usually it costs the more effort, time and money expenditure than his peers. Insufficient resources or available funds to hold sleep specified conferences, workshops and courses as usually the fund is targeted towards other specialties that are considered more popular or important. The low number of interested audience usually leads to lack of sponsorship. The international certificates for example The American board of sleep medicine require conditions that are difficult to be implemented in Egypt. Other international societies certificates like world sleep society also consider the existence of a local sleep society to accept your application which is not applicable in Egypt. Sleep technician education is not introduced in any targeted education programs. This problem leads to lack of experienced sleep technicians who are the main pillar for the attended sleep study.

The proposed solution requires the establishment of a separate university graduate degree for sleep medicine with a curriculum and training in specialized centers and Increasing the number of sleep experts by increasing awareness about the importance of sleep medicine among physicians and medical students. It will increase also the attendance to workshops and conferences and encourage funding of such scientific activities. Conduction of American sleep board examination for international physicians and the local facilitation to be taken into the account of the international certificate providers will help the Egyptian sleep physicians get certified by these international societies. The Sleep technician diploma will enhance the quality of Sleep centers and will open new job opportunities for youth.

SLEEP MEDICINE PRACTICE IN EGYPT

The practice of sleep medicine in Egypt began in the mid to late 1990s, and it has been rapidly expanding since then. However, it is still not significant (Tables **1** & **2**).

Sleep Medicine Services Structure

Types of Sleep Medicine Services Facilities and Accreditation

Usually the sleep labs or centers are either governmental or private. Most of the government centers are built in universities as part of pulmonology, neurology or psychiatry departments' services for the public. Up to our knowledge, no specified governmental or university sleep center for sleep medicine and surgery exists in Egypt except in Mansoura university. A sleep research unit and an additional Sleep Medicine center were both founded through two capacity building grants, funded by Mansoura University and established by the authors of this chapter and others. However, there are a few small private centers which may be either specialized only for sleep medicine or may be integrated within larger multispecialty medical centers. These centers (both governmental and private) are usually licensed by medical syndicate and university different councils (for university labs. and centers). However, there are no specific national accreditation sleep certificates to be granted for these centers. The international accreditation for example offered by the American academy of sleep medicine is difficult to be applied due to financial issues and lack of American board-certified physicians. Fig. (**7**) is a map showing the distribution of sleep centers in different Egyptian areas.

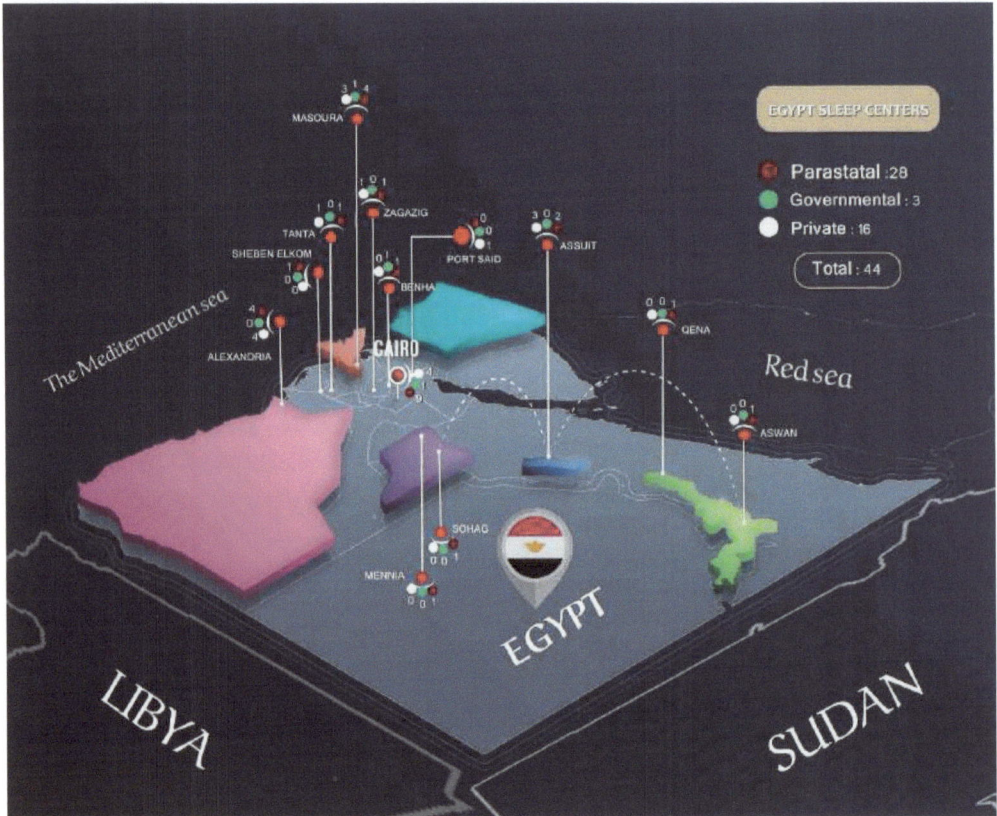

Fig. (7). Distribution of sleep labs in different Egyptian governorates.

Types of Sleep Medicine Practitioners

Sleep medicine practitioners are divided into physicians and sleep technicians. As previously mentioned, no specific certificates can prepare them for this practice. However, the interested personnel of pulmonology, neurology, and psychiatry departments are the main pillars of this practice. Usually, sleep experts are located in different universities and work as part time in private centers. So, the total number of sleep experts is generally much less than the requirement as there is no specialized sleep technician diploma.

Patients

The majority of sleep disorder patients lack awareness about these disorders for many reasons: they might have misbeliefs about sleep, and sleep complaints as previously mentioned in the sleep myth and public views section. They are unaware of this branch of medicine and if anyone gets a sleep complaint; they usually do not seek medical advice. Because even if a well-educated person is familiar with sleep medicine, he/she usually is unaware of the existing centers for diagnosing and treating such diseases. In addition, there is a lack of awareness of the medical community about sleep medicine. Patients usually consult several physicians before reaching the sleep specialist. According to the country's constitution, no discrimination is made upon religion, gender or ethnicity to reach full medical services. However, residents of remote places (whatever their group) can face difficulties to reach a good medical service which is usually located in a major city and not in a nearby towns. Many patients are sharing the same locality, we have another obstacle, which is the socioeconomic status. The rich patient can afford the cost of the diagnosis and the treatment (pharmacological or therapeutic devices, *etc.*) because the insurance companies are not covering this group of diseases. Second, the gender differences in complaining like females are less likely to confess about their snoring problem. The female patients usually take into consideration the social aspects especially if she is young.

Sleep Medicine Practice Guidelines

The sleep experts in Egypt have no national or local guidelines, however, they follow the international guidelines released by the main international sleep societies like the American academy of sleep medicine during their clinical work. The practice depends on the updated resources provided to sleep specialists by these societies. However, for the local problems especially financial problems, physicians use their initiatives to find an alternative method to help their patients even if it is not the ideal solution. For example oral appliances which are usually indicated in mild or moderate obstructive sleep apnea are used even in severe obstructive sleep apnea. These are financially more affordable than positive airway pressure devices.

Sleep Surgery in Egypt

Sleep surgery (synonymous snoring surgery) in Egypt is well practiced by otolaryngologists (ORL) especially that the surgery could be a good substitute for expensive positive pressure devices and that surgical operations are usually covered by medical insurance companies. Usually snoring patients attend the outpatient clinic (OPC) of otolaryngology specialty either by themselves or as referrals from a sleep medicine clinic. Sleep experts try to establish an efficient collaboration between the two sides of the coin sleep medicine and surgery experts for the aim of providing the best quality of management for the patient. Usually, the involved primary physicians meet in a collaborative seminar to discuss the decision of the treatment approach and the management plan especially the complicated cases. Another established collaboration is the Drug-Induced Sleep Endoscopy (DISE), which is conducted either in the operating theater of ORL or in the interventional pulmonology unit (fiberoptic bronchoscopy theater). Multiple integrated educational programs were conducted with sleep medicine and surgery experts to educate the juniors of different specialties. Numerous research inter-projects are being conducted between sleep medicine and surgery experts to reach optimal clinical services and research's results.

Other Specialties Collaboration

Sleep specialists evaluate the patients with a complete work up in order to diagnose comorbidities and refer the patient to the appropriate specialist providing a multidisciplinary comprehensive care.

Sleep Professional Societies and Regulatory Bodies

Egyptian Scientific Society for Sleep Medicine and Research (EGYPTSLEEP) was launched in March 14th, 2014. It was a nice trial for gathering sleep experts in Egypt. However, the society activities were not as expected although it started in a good way. Another small society was launched in 2012 Society of Sleep Disordered Breathing and Respiratory Failure chaired by sleep disordered breathing unit staff in The Pulmonary Department at Mansoura university [80]. But no active national society exists. Nowadays, the activities of the sleep medicine or sleep surgery education is conducted by the main pulmonary, neurology or psychiatry Egyptian societies. No national guidelines or regulatory bodies exist. However, the experts follow the international norms in their practice and education. Egyptian Laryngological & Sleep Surgery Society was launched in 2017 and it conducts two conferences with multiple cadaveric educational workshops on the sidelines of the conferences.

Barriers to Appropriate Care and its Solutions

The main problem in the proper management of sleep problems is the cost involved in the diagnosis and the treatment because sleep related diseases are not under the coverage of insurance companies. Increasing lobbying at the national authorities and insurances to increase the awareness about the cost of untreated sleep diseases will help allowance of coverage of the diagnosis and treatment of these diseases. The numbers of sleep specialists, trained sleep technicians and well equipped sleep laboratories should be increases along with their visibility to the public. Another obstacle is the awareness of the patients about the sleep medicine and the presence of sleep disorders and the possibility of the treatment with highlighting the complications of untreated diseases, for example, obstructive sleep apnea not only has negative effects on the patient's health but is also bad for society. Also, the lack of knowledge about sleep medicine facility among both patients and physicians will delay the diagnosis and increase the burden of medical services cost. Awareness must be provided by health educational campaigns in the crowded areas like clubs and shopping malls and with the use of the media channels to reach the patients to overcome this problem. Increasing the CME certified courses, workshops and conferences directed to non-specialized physicians will help to increase their awareness and widen the possibilities for differential diagnosis during the management of such patients. Launching an active society of sleep to gather all the sleep experts both from the field of medicine and surgery to shape the practice in Egypt and release local guidelines which will be more suitable for the actual practice with regard to the local barriers to especially help the juniors for proper management. These societies can also help in the release of official different educational publications or even Egyptian sleep journals.

SLEEP MEDICINE RESEARCH IN EGYPT: REAL SITUATION, BARRIERS IN THE SLEEP MEDICINE RESEARCH AND PROPOSED SOLUTIONS

Happily, the last decade has witnessed noticeable growth in sleep research in Egypt since the last survey in 2014 of the Egyptian-published sleep papers which were 12 only after Robert and his colleagues searched in EMBASE and Medline. Although we conducted a rapid search on only Medline database on 12 August 2020 by author affiliation (Egypt) and title (sleep) and we found 141 published sleep researches starting from 2005. Although, it is still relatively low, however, if we had used other search engines, the number would have been much higher [81, 82]. The research studies are variable in their design (observational, experimental or theoretical i.e. reviews and books or book chapters) and in nature (sleep physiology, medicine or surgery). However, there is still no available published work about sleep medicine services or research output in Egypt.

Moreover, as a branch of medicine, the sleep medicine research faces challenges and barriers experienced by researches of other specialties. There are also unique constraints related to the nature of sleep disorders themselves or the absence of facilitating equipment or equipped clinical and experimental laboratories. The challenges, barriers and gaps noticed during our experience in sleep research in Egypt are:

Funding

Although there are many sources for national funding, but the opportunities for sleep research are lower than other topics such as liver diseases and cancer due to the national concern for these common diseases plus low awareness about the importance of the sleep and sleep disorders. Concerning international grants, the high competition with other colleagues in developed countries usually is the main problem especially with their highly encouraging work environments and backgrounds. Moreover, the pharmaceutical companies or companies manufacturing therapeutic devices are not including Egyptian researchers in their multicenter studies. Increasing the national awareness among authorities and physicians can increase sleep researches opportunities. International grants should be divided into two classes for developed and developing countries to get more fairness. Finally, the attention of the pharmaceutical companies to include Egyptian researchers in their clinical trials projects is needed.

Lack of Well-equipped Clinical and Experimental Laboratories

As a consequence of the lack of resources, there are insufficient well-equipped sleep laboratories and lack of beds. Most established sleep laboratories have single beds and the availability of this bed is divided into two sections: the first for the diagnosis, follow-up or titration session of sleep clinic patients and the second for the research population which means a very long time to recruit a suitable number of participants for a research idea. Plus, lack of after sale technical maintenance of the polysomnography hardware is very difficult because of the unavailability of well-trained engineers or technical maintenance workers or spare parts in Egypt and the device needs to be maintained in the manufacturing country and this consumes much more time and cost. Moreover, there is no experimental sleep laboratory available for experimental animals, day and night studies, *etc.* The solutuion of such problems mainly depends on increasing the capacity building fund or grants to improve the infrastructure and increase the sleep laboratory bed capacity plus the establishment of specialized sleep experimental laboratory. The availability of spare parts or well-trained personnel will accelerate the after-sale services process of laboratories' devices.

Lack of Well-trained Somnologists, Sleep Technicians, Full-time Job Sleep Researcher, Researcher Assistant or Research Nurses

Moreover, the research assistant or research nurse positions are not available. There is lack of medical research skills and journals' high rejection rate. However, the interested researchers can personally develop their own experience by different CME workshops or by supplementary research skills introduced by masters and doctorate learning system in addition to increase their practice under experienced supervisors. Appropriate training for research in the university curriculum should be introduced.

Samples Collection

Patients' recruitment and informed consent are very difficult. This popular refusal is because of the popular heritage or scientific fiction movies that these researches will be harmful, and they will be like an experimental animal, especially the clinical trials which are more difficult to conduct and persuade than observational studies. The rejection could also be due to the absence of the expected benefits like a financial reward. Another problem is the compliance of the participants to consecutive sessions in the follow up studies. Also, the costly devices which are needed in treatment trials restrict the clinical trials especially that it is not covered by the medical insurance companies. The survey study needs free unoccupied researchers for this field study. The experimental studies are very difficult because of the funding issues and lack of valid experimental labs and materials. Multicenter studies are difficult to conduct because of lack of Egyptian sleep researcher's registries or networks and lack of cooperation in between different universities [83].

THE CURRENT SITUATION IN NUMBERS

We designed an online survey with structured questions. The survey was directed to sleep specialists in Egypt about how they see the current situation in sleep.

Results of the survey can be seen in (Tables **1a** and **1b**).

Table 1a. Charecteristics of sleep experts approached during the survey.

	Survey Question	N	%
	What is your original specialty	-	-
-	Pulmonology	14	70
-	Otolaryngeology	2	10
-	Neurology	2	10
-	Psychiatry	2	10
	What is the type of facility providing the sleep service	-	-
-	University hospital	16	80
-	Educational hospital	2	10
-	Ministry of health	2	10
-	Private	6	30
-	Governmental	14	70
	Do you have any practice guidelines? if yes please specify	-	-
-	Yes	15	75

Survey Question	N	%
- No	5	25
- International guidelines	15	75
- Local guidelines	5	25
Do you have any professional societies or regulatory bodies as regard sleep medicine	-	-
- Yes	6	30
- No	14	70
- International society	6	30
- Local society	6	30
In your opinion how can the patients reach the sleep medicine service?	-	-
- Referrals	7	35
- Media	3	15
- Health education	4	20
- OPC of other specialties	2	10
- Sleep clinics	4	20
In your opinion the patients are oriented about the sleep disorders and the possibility of the treatment	-	
- Yes	3	15
- No	11	55
- Maybe	6	30
In your opinion the patients are oriented about the presence of sleep medicine service	-	-
- Yes	3	15
- No	11	55
- Maybe	6	30

Table 1b. Sleep physicians expert opinion about sleep medicine in Egypt.

Survey Question	N	%
Why the patients are not really oriented about the sleep medicine and the sleep disorders? please specify your reasons		
Lack of education and health awareness	9	45
sleep problems is a new thing in the Egyptian culture and a new specialty	5	25
Sleep disorders are considered as a normal variant for some people in the Egyptian society	2	10
Lack of physician knowledge about sleep medicine	2	10
patient think that sleep is a symptom of another medical problem that needs treatment	2	10
Are the the diagnostic methods covered by the general health insurance		
Yes	3	15

(Table 1b) cont.....

Survey Question	N	%
No	15	75
Maybe	2	10
Are the treatment methods covered by the general health insurance		
Yes	3	15
No	15	75
May get it later	2	10
In your opinion what is the barriers of the appropriate clinical care?		
Knowledge and awareness	10	50
financial	10	50
Are other specialty physician familiar to sleep medicine and its disorders		
Yes	5	25
No	3	15
I am not sure	12	60
Is there any gender differences in searching and access for the service please explain why there is a difference		
Yes	5	25
No	15	75
Higher incidence in Male	3	15
Female refuse to admit complaints	2	10
Cultural reason	5	25
Is there any difference between high and low socioeconomic class in searching and access for the service please explain why		
No	1	5
Yes	19	95
The Cost of the Sleep service is the reason	19	95
In your opinion what is the unique needs to improve the sleep research situation in Egypt		
Funding	9	45
Establishing more clinical sleep labs	5	25
Establishing more experimental sleep labs	4	20
Lack of experienced sleep experts	1	5
Others	1	5
Do you prefer sleep medicine to be a separate specialty with separate residency, training, certificate and degree		
Yes	17	85
No	3	0

Table 2a. Summary of sleep lab logistics in Egypt.

Quantatitive data of Sleep centers	Min	Max	Mean (±SD)
Number of sleep specialist per center	1.00	10.00	3.4(2.58)
Number of sleep technicians per center	0.00	32.00	4.35(6.95)
Number of beds per center	1.00	5.00	1.5(0.94)
Number of patients attending the sleep clinic per year	0.00	1200.00	169.5(290)
Number of sleep. Studies per year	10.00	700.00	210.8(186.7)

Table 2b. Summary of PSG devices in Egyptian sleep labs.

Specification of PSG devices	N	%
Level 1 Sleep Lab	13	65
Level 2 Sleep Lab	4	20
Level 3 Sleep Lab	10	50
Level 4 Sleep Lab	4	20
Pediatric kit	11	55
Capnography	4	20
Erectile dysfunction	1	1
Autotitration	16	80
Manual titration	11	55

Furthermore, Tables (**2a** and **2b**) summarize the state of art of sleep: laboratories in Egypt.

In Fig. (**7**), we summarize the geographic distribution of sleep labs around the country.

CONCLUSION

Interest in sleep medicine and sleep disorders in Egypt dates back to the ancient Egyptian pharos and developed gradually through the eras of Egyptian history, where religious and cultural aspects influenced its progress. Additionally the occupation of the Egyptian land by different cultural backgrounds had its imprint on sleep practices. Nevertheless, sleep medicine in Egypt remains underdeveloped in comparison to European countries and North America.

The current status of sleep medicine regarding undergraduate and postgraduate education indicates the necessity to establishing a professional degree for sleep physicians and sleep technologists. Recognition of this degree by international sleep bodies is also a required task, in addition to establishing a proper licensing pathway for healthcare providers who are willing to work in the sleep field.

Professional sleep societies have been established but more attention toward their roles in public and the professional services they provide is needed. Sleep laboratories, facilities and equipment are in fair condition but far beyond the real needs of the country, and the preparation of requirement and eligibility criteria for accreditation of the facilities by AASM or ESRS is an urgent need. Polysomnography should be included in the health insurance plan of Egyptians, to solve the financial burden of patients who can't afford the fees of the sleep study services.

Research in the field of sleep has been discussed and the obstacles have been reviewed with our view of improvement. Research is needed in a wider scope because it will show the extent of the sleep problem in the country and the needed corrective actions to improve sleep medicine services in Egypt. We think that the critical appraisal provided in this chapter will act as a guide for politicians, ministers of health and decision makers in the country to give more attention to sleep medicine and improve healthcare services provided to Egyptian patients suffering from sleep disorders.

CONSENT FOR PUBLICATION

Not applicable.

CONFLICT OF INTEREST

The authors declare no conflict of interest, financial or otherwise.

ACKNOWLEDGEMENTS

We acknowledge the time and effort of sleep experts and sleep technologist who helped with answering the survey questions. Authors would also like to express their gratitude to Dr. John Zaki (Assistant Professor of Electronic Engineering, Mansoura University for his efforts designing the map of Egypt showing the goegraphical distribution of sleep centers in Egypt.

REFERENCES

[1]   "Capmas," 2020.. https://www.capmas.gov.eg/Pages/StaticPages.aspx?page_id=5035 (accessed Jul. 10, 2020).

[2]   Central Intelligence Agency, "Field Listing: Religions — The World Factbook," 2015.. https://www.cia.gov/library/publications/the-world-factbook/fields/401.html (accessed Sep. 20, 2020).

[3]   World poulation review, "Egypt Population 2020 (Demographics, Maps, Graphs)," 2020.. https://worldpopulationreview.com/countries/egypt-population (accessed Sep. 06, 2020).

[4]   WorldAtlas, "Languages Spoken In Egypt -," 2017.. https://www.worldatlas.com/articles/languages-spoken-in-egypt.html (accessed Sep. 20, 2020).

[5]   Abdalla ME, Suliman R. Ali, "Overview of medical schools in the Eastern Mediterranean Region of the World Health Organization," East. Mediterr. Heal. J., vol. 19, no. 12, 2013, Accessed: Aug. 03, 2020.   [Online].   Available:. http://www.emro.who.int/emhj-vol-19-2013/12/overview-of-medical-schools-in-the-eastern-mediterranean-region-of-the-world-health-organization.html

[6]   Abdelaziz A, Kassab SE, Abdelnasser A, Hosny S. Medical Education in Egypt: Historical Background, Current Status, and Challenges. Health Prof Educ 2018; 4(4): 236-44. [http://dx.doi.org/10.1016/j.hpe.2017.12.007]

[7]   Abd El-Galil T. Egypt Prescribes Changes for Doctors in Training - Al-Fanar Media 2018. https://www.al-fanarmedia.org/2018/09/egypt-prescribes-changes-for-doctors-in-training/

[8]   WFME, "World Federation for Medical Education | Enhancing Quality Worldwide,". Http://Wfme.Org/, 2018. http://wfme.org/ (accessed Aug. 03, 2020).

[9]   Lai Y, Ahmad A, Da Wan C. Higher education in the Middle East and North Africa: Exploring regional and country specific potentials 2016. [http://dx.doi.org/10.1007/978-981-10-1056-9]

[10]   Cupito E, Langsten R, Langsten R. Inclusiveness in higher education in Egypt. Springer 2011; 62: pp. 183-97. [http://dx.doi.org/10.1007/s10734-010-9381-z]

[11]   Richards A. Higher education in Egypt 1992.

[12]   E. G. Gericke C.A.. Health System in Egypt Health Care Systems and Policies, B R van Ginneken E, Ed New York, NY:. New York: Springer 2018.

[13]   World Health Organization. Assessing the regulation of the private health sector in the Eastern Mediterranean Region Egypt 2014.

[14]   World Health Organization. Analysis of the private health sector in countries of the Eastern Mediterranean: Exploring unfamiliar territory 2014.

[15]   D.- Egypt, "Find Funding," 2020.. https://www.daad.eg/en/find-funding/ (accessed Aug. 09, 2020).

[16]   "Egypt | Country outputs | Nature Index," 2020 https://www.natureindex.com/country-outputs/Egypt (accessed Aug. 07, 2020).

[17]   M of higher education and S Research, "Scientific Research in Numbers," 2018 http://portal.mohesr.gov.eg/en-us/Pages/Scientific-research-in-numbers.aspx (accessed Aug. 09, 2020).

[18]   Ranking S-IS. "counteries ranks," 2020 https://www.scimagojr.com/countryrank.php (accessed Aug. 09, 2020).

[19]   Publons, "Researchers- Egypt," 2020. https://publons.com/researcher/?country=197&is_core_collection=1&is_last_twelve_months=1&order_by=num_reviews (accessed Aug. 09, 2020).

[20]   Finance MO. "The state General Budget," 2020. http://www.mof.gov.eg/english/pages/home.aspx (accessed Aug. 09, 2020).

[21]   World bank, "Research and development expenditure (% of GDP) | Data," 2020. https://data.worldbank.org/indicator/GB.XPD.RSDV.GD.ZS (accessed Aug. 09, 2020).

[22]   CAPMAS. Annual Bulletin of the Graduates of Higher Education and Higher Degrees 2019.https://www.capmas.gov.eg/Pages/Publications.aspx?page_id=5104&YearID=23413

[23]   European Commission. Egypt | International Cooperation - Research and Innovation 2020. https://ec.europa.eu/research/iscp/index.cfm?amp;pg=egypt#projects (accessed Aug. 13, 2020).

[24]   http://portal.mohesr.gov.eg/en-us/Pages/governmental-universities.aspx (accessed Aug. 07, 2020).

[25]   Council of research centers and Institutes. research centers and institutes 2020. http://www.crci.sci.eg/?page_id=815 (accessed Aug. 07, 2020).

[26]   S. and T. D. F. (STDF). Science, Technology and Innovation (STI) System in 2020. http://stdf.org.eg/page/?p=60 (accessed Aug. 09, 2020).

[27]   Alexandrina B. Research Grants Program - Bibliotheca Alexandrina 2020. https://www.bibalex.org/en/Project/Details?documentid=181 (accessed Aug. 09, 2020).

[28]   S. and T. D. F. (STDF). STDF - Open Grants 2020. http://stdf.eg:8080/web/grants/open (accessed Aug. 09, 2020).

[29]   F. C. in Egypt. Fulbright Commission in Egypt 2020. https://fulbright-egypt.org/ (accessed Aug. 09, 2020).

[30]   https://cdm.edu.eg/cdm/category/granting/ (accessed Aug. 09, 2020).

[31]   Council B. Newton-Mosharafa Fund 2020. https://www.britishcouncil.org.eg/en/programmes/education /newton-mosharafa-fund (accessed Aug. 09, 2020).

[32]   Bank EK. Egyptian Knowledge Bank | Publons 2015. https://publons.com/publisher/12110/egyptian-knowledge-bank?page=8& (accessed Sep. 26, 2020).

[33]   https://library.aucegypt.edu/home (accessed Sep. 26, 2020).

[34]   Bibliotheca Alexandrina. Home - Bibliotheca Alexandrina 2020. https://www.bibalex.org/en/default (accessed Sep. 26, 2020).

[35]   Egyptian Libraries Network. Egyptian Libraries Network 2020. http://www.egyptlib.net.eg /Site/Home. aspx (accessed Sep. 26, 2020).

[36]   The Egyptian Journal of Chest Diseases and Tuberculosis, "The Egyptian Journal of Chest Diseases and Tuberculosis: About us," 2020.. http://www.ejcdt.eg.net/aboutus.asp (accessed Sep. 26, 2020).

[37]   Marzouk D, *et al.* Overview on health research ethics in Egypt and North Africa European Journal of Public Health. (1)87-91.Oxford University Press 2014; 24: pp.
[http://dx.doi.org/10.1093/eurpub/cku110]

[38]   Abdel-Aal W, Ghaffar EA, El Shabrawy O. "Review of the medical research ethics committee (MREC), national research center of Egypt, 2003-2011," *Current Medical Research and Opinion*, vol. 29, no. 10. Curr Med Res Opin 2013; 29(10): 1411-7.
[http://dx.doi.org/10.1185/03007995.2013.815158] [PMID: 23777313]

[39]   Kirkpatrick BA. History of the development of medical information 1985. https://www.ncbi.nlm.nih.gov/pmc/articles/pmc1911841/

[40]   Allen J. The art of medicine in ancient Egypt. New York, NY: Yale university press 2005; 75.(1953)

[41]   Amin OM. Ancient Egyptian Medicine. Explore (NY) 2003; 12(5): 1-9.

[42]   Scott N, Leake CD. The Old Egyptian Medical Papyri. (2)Lawrence. Kansas: Lawrence. Kansas: University of Kansas Press 1953; 57.

[43]   Hasan NAEGA. Medicine in ancient Egypt. Egypt J Intern Med 2017; 29(1): 33-4.
[http://dx.doi.org/10.4103/ejim.ejim_23_17]

[44]   Saunders J. The transitions from ancient Egyptian to Greek medicine 1963.

[45]   https://brill.com/content/books/b9789004232549s002

[46]   Reeves D. Hypnosis in Ancient Civilizations - Ecstatic Trance: Ritual Body Postures https://www.cuyamungueinstitute.com/articles-and-news/hypnosis-in-ancient-civilizations/

[47]   Scott E. The natural way to sound sleep 1996; 182.

[48]   Aboelsoud N H. Herbal medicine in ancient Egypt J Med Plants Res 2010; 4(2): 082-6.

[49]   Serageldin I. Ancient Alexandria and the dawn of medical science. Glob. Cardiol. Sci. Pract 2013; Vol. 47: pp. 395-404. [Online] https://www.ncbi.nlm.nih.gov/pmc/articles/PMC3991212/

[50]   Rossi M. "Homer and Herodotus to Egyptian medicine," Vesalius, vol. Suppl 2010; pp. 3-5. [Online] https://europepmc.org/article/med/21657099

[51]   W. A. SCOTT. THE PRACTICE OF MEDICINE IN ANCIENT ROME. Can Anaesth Soc J 1955; 3(2): 281-90.

[52]   Barbera J. The Greco-Roman Period in Sleep Medicine 47-53.2015; [http://dx.doi.org/10.1007/978-1-4939-2089-1_8]

[53]   Barbera J. Sleep and dreaming in Greek and Roman philosophy. Sleep Med 2008; 9(8): 906-10. [http://dx.doi.org/10.1016/j.sleep.2007.10.010] [PMID: 19014776]

[54]   Dawson WR. Egyptian Medicine under the Copts in the early Centuries of the Christian Era 1924; 17: 51-7. [http://dx.doi.org/10.1177/003591572401701704]

[55]   Majeed A. How Islam changed medicine. BMJ 2005; 331(7531): 1486-7. [http://dx.doi.org/10.1136/bmj.331.7531.1486] [PMID: 16373721]

[56]   N. Husain F.. Islamic medicine history and current practice 2003; 19-30.

[57]   Loza S. Sleep Medicine in the Arab Islamic Civilization. Sleep Med 2015; pp. 21-4. [http://dx.doi.org/10.1007/978-1-4939-2089-1_3]

[58]   BaHammam A, Almeneessier A, Pandi-Perumal S. Medieval Islamic scholarship and writings on sleep and dreams. Ann Thorac Med 2018; 13(2): 72-5. [http://dx.doi.org/10.4103/atm.ATM_162_17] [PMID: 29675056]

[59]   BaHammam A, Gozal D. Qur'anic insights into sleep. Nat Sci Sleep 2012; 4: 81-7. [http://dx.doi.org/10.2147/NSS.S34630] [PMID: 23620681]

[60]   BaHammam A. Sleep from an islamic perspective. Ann Thorac Med 2011; 6(4): 187-92. [http://dx.doi.org/10.4103/1817-1737.84771] [PMID: 21977062]

[61]   Heidari MR, Norouzadeh R, Abbasi M. Sleep in the Quran and Health Sciences 2014. https://doaj.org/article/b828c644f18e45fab0b3e4e4793597d8

[62]   Burrow GN. Clot-Bey: Founder of Western Medical Practice in Egypt 1975. https://www.ncbi.nlm.nih.gov/pmc/articles/PMC2595236/

[63]   Barnard H. B. H. [Medical education in Egypt]. Ned Tijdschr Geneeskd 2002; 146(24): 1147-9. [PMID: 12092309]

[64]   Aboul-Enein BH, Puddy W. Contributions of *Antoine Barthélémy Clot (1793–1868)* : A historiographical reflection of public health in Ottoman Egypt. J Med Biogr 2016; 24(3): 427-32. [http://dx.doi.org/10.1177/0967772015584708] [PMID: 26025850]

[65]   Necessary C. Medical Education in Egypt. 1749-37.Br. Med. J. 1894; 2: pp.

[66]   El Dib N. Kasr Al Ainy, the story of a palace that became a medical school. Kasr Al Ainy Medical Journal 2015; 21(1): 1. [http://dx.doi.org/10.4103/2356-8097.155653]

[67]   Sandwith FM. Records of the Egyptian Government, Faculty of Medicine 1927.

[68]   R. C. of S. of England Ibrahim, Sir Ali (1880 - 1946) 2013. https://livesonline.rcseng.ac.uk/client/en_GB/lives/search/detailnonmodal/ent:$002f$002fSD_ASSET $002f0$002fSD_ASSET:376426/one?qu=%22rcs%3A+E004243%22&rt=false%7C%7C%7CIDENTI FIER%7C%7C%7CResource+Identifier

[69]   I. S.. Sir Ali Ibrahim Pasha, KBE 1947; 159(4042): 531-1.
        [http://dx.doi.org/10.1038/159531a0]

[70]   https://www.timeshighereducation.com/student/best-universities/best-universities-world

[71]   Sleep   Foundation.   Myths   and   Facts   about   Sleep   2020.
        https://www.sleepfoundation.org/articles/myths-and-facts-about-sleep

[72]   https://www.britannica.com/biography/Omar-Khayyam-Persian-poet-and-astronomer

[73]   Wikipedia. Umm Kulthum 2020. https://en.wikipedia.org/wiki/Umm_Kulthum

[74]   de Sá JFR, Mota-Rolim SA. Sleep paralysis in Brazilian folklore and other cultures: A Brief Review.
        Front Psychol 2016; 7(SEP): 1294.
        [http://dx.doi.org/10.3389/fpsyg.2016.01294] [PMID: 27656151]

[75]   Jalal B, Hinton DE. Rates and characteristics of sleep paralysis in the general population of Denmark
        and Egypt. Cult Med Psychiatry 2013; 37(3): 534-48.
        [http://dx.doi.org/10.1007/s11013-013-9327-x] [PMID: 23884906]

[76]   http://www1.mans.edu.eg/facmed/dept/anatomy/under.htm

[77]   Mansoura   PD-U.   Physiology   undergraduate   courses   specification
        http://www1.mans.edu.eg/facmed/dept/physiology/under.htm

[78]   http://www1.mans.edu.eg/facmed/dept/thoracic-new/md.html

[79]   http://www1.mans.edu.eg/facmed/dept/neurology-new/post.html

[80]   http://www2.mans.edu.eg/hospitals/muh/depts/sdbu/

[81]   https://pubmed.ncbi.nlm.nih.gov/?term=(egypt%5BAffiliation%5D)

[82]   Robert C, Wilson CS, Gaudy JF, Arreto CD. The evolution of the sleep science literature over 30
        years: A bibliometric analysis. Scientometrics 2007; 73(2): 231-56.
        [http://dx.doi.org/10.1007/s11192-007-1780-2]

[83]   European Sleep Research Society. European Sleep Research Laboratories 2020.
        https://esrs.eu/european-sleep-research-laboratories/

[84]   Zaki NWF, Marzouk R, Osman I, *et al.* Sleep Medicine Knowledge among Medical Students in Seven
        Egyptian Medical Faculties. J Sleep Disord Ther 2016; 5: 239.

CHAPTER 19

Practice of Sleep Medicine in Zambia

Kondwelani John Mateyo[1,*]

[1] *Department of Internal Medicine, University Teaching Hospital, Nationalist Road, Lusaka, Zambia*

Abstract: Zambia, a southern African country with a resource-strained healthcare system that for the past three decades has been tailored to fight the HIV pandemic, is grappling with an increasing non-communicable disease burden. The practice of sleep medicine in Zambia, with sleep disorders being a cause of some of the cardiovascular and motor-vehicle-related morbidity and mortality, has long lagged behind the significant HIV-related disease burden. Sleep disorders in Zambia have therefore remained under-researched, and unquantified and thus are not considered a significant clinical problem.

Against a background of scarce specialized sleep practitioners, the absence of a specific regulatory framework for the practice of sleep medicine, and the absolute lack of equipped sleep centers, the diagnosis of sleep disorders is based on the use of validated clinical risk questionnaires. The availability of treatment devices in the country is also scarce. Further, population-wide and practitioner knowledge-gaps have exacerbated the stagnation of the practice of sleep medicine and research. These deficiencies however present an opportunity to finally harness the practice of sleep medicine and the conduct of sleep-related research, and make them a priority.

Keywords: Sleep disorders, Sleep medicine, Sleep research, Zambia.

INTRODUCTION

Sleep disorders have been on the rise globally, accounting for significant morbidity and mortality [1]. A seventh of the world's population is estimated to have obstructive sleep apnoea, which is the commonest form of sleep disorder [2]. Obstructive sleep apnoea (OSA) has had profound footprint on the global rise in non-communicable disease morbidity and mortality. Sleep disordered breathing and obstructive sleep apnea have been found to be independent risk factors for systemic hypertension [3, 4], heart failure and stroke [5, 6], while obstructive sleep apnea is associated with a significantly increased risk of motor vehicle accidents [7].

---

[*] **Corresponding author Kondwelani John Mateyo:** Department of Internal Medicine, University Teaching Hospital, Nationalist Road, Lusaka, Zambia; Tel: +260966611097; Email: kondwelanimateyo@yahoo.co.uk

Hrayr P. Attarian, Marie-Louise M. Coussa-Koniski & Alain Michel Sabri (Eds.)

Africa is unlikely to be an exception to the rising global burden of sleep disorders and obstructive sleep apnoea, given the high prevalence of obesity in sub-Saharan Africa [8], and the rise in obesity and its associated co-morbidities [9]. Further, Africa is the leading continent in both cardiovascular disease and motor vehicle accident-related morbidity and mortality [10]. That some of this morbidity and mortality is attributable to sleep disorders, is beyond question, given the weight of global evidence to this effect [10, 11]. However, in the face of a greater burden of infectious diseases on the continent, sleep disorders have long been under-researched, and unquantified. They thus have remained under-recognized as a distinct clinical entity on the continent [12]. This has further worsened sleep-disorder-attributable morbidity and mortality.

Zambia is a land-locked country in southern Africa with a population of 17.86 million), spread across its $752,000m^2$ land mass. This population is mostly concentrated in the urban cities that have the attraction of job opportunities for the country's predominantly youthful population [13]. It is a lower middle-income country, with an economy heavily dependent on copper mining and a gross national income (GNI) per capita of US$1,300 (/country/zambia?view=chart).

The public healthcare system in the country is decentralized, comprising three levels; hospitals, health centers and health posts. The hospitals are separated into primary (sub-district or district), secondary (provincial or general) and tertiary (central or specialist or university). The three levels are linked by a referral system with the latter at the top [14].

Zambia is implementing a universal healthcare package for its citizens, to mitigate the burden of paying for life-saving treatments by individuals. The government-run health facilities therefore offer a basic healthcare package. Services included in the basic healthcare package are provided free-of-charge or on a cost-sharing basis, depending on the location of the healthcare facility (rural or urban) and the level of the system (primary, secondary or tertiary). In rural districts, these services are free. However, this is challenged by the chronic under-funding from the national budget which results in inadequate services. Recently, a national health insurance scheme was launched to supplement government funding, but its benefits are yet to come to full fruition. Alongside the public healthcare system exists private healthcare facilities that are mainly concentrated in the urban areas. Specialized medical care is offered mainly in the tertiary level healthcare facilities in the public sector, and to a lesser extent in the private healthcare facilities.

This chapter aims to give a synopsis of the practice of sleep medicine in Zambia. It is divided into three parts; the current practice of sleep medicine in the country, the challenges to practice of sleep medicine, and finally highlighting the possible interventions to filling existing research and clinical gaps.

CURRENT PRACTICE OF SLEEP MEDICINE

The practice of Sleep Medicine in Zambia is nearly exclusively done at the University Teaching Hospital (UTH) in Lusaka, a 1700-bed facility national referral tertiary-level hospital. It is the only hospital in the public sector with specialist Neurology and Respiratory clinics, respectively, which are the points of referral for patients with sleep disorders.

The UTH, and by default the whole country, has five Neurologists and one Pulmonologist. The Neurology team has two foreign and four local Neurologists. Three of the Zambian Neurologists are products of a local Neurology Residency program which was launched in 2018, as a collaboration by the UTH, several academic medical centers in the USA and the US National Institute of Neurological Disorders and Stroke [15]. The program is ongoing and has residents in training. The Pulmonologist at the UTH was trained in The Netherlands, and runs (with Internal Medicine Residents in rotation) the Pulmonology clinic that sees the majority of patients with sleep disorders, predominantly obstructive sleep apnoea. There are future plans to develop a Pulmonology training program, in partnership with academic centers in the West.

In view of the fact that both the Neurology and Pulmonology services are in their infancy, the practice of sleep medicine is yet to fully develop, following years of long neglect. In priority, sleep medicine fell far behind both other non-communicable, and infectious diseases, particularly the HIV-related ones. HIV, given its high burden in morbidity and mortality in the past 30 years, has been of greater priority for the healthcare system. However, since the provision of free antiretroviral treatment in the country beginning in 2004, HIV-related morbidity and mortality have declined and life-expectancy has increased [16, 17]. As people live longer, they have more opportunity to be in gainful economic livelihoods, which have brought with them lifestyle-related non-communicable diseases (NCDs) such as obesity and cardiovascular conditions [17]. The rising NCD epidemic has borne a tremendous and increasing burden on the thin specialized human resource available to manage these diseases in this setting, not to mention the absence of equipment.

Zambia has no dedicated sleep laboratory or other diagnostic equipment, either in the public or private healthcare sector. Polysomnography or home sleep study facilities or gadgets are absent. Therefore, diagnostic workup comprises mainly the use of sleep questionnaires for OSA. This is wrought in poor specificity.

Further, these tools are uninformative and inadequate in the diagnosis of sleep disorders besides OSA.

Practice guidelines are adopted from professional societies elsewhere and adapted to this setting. This adaptation has been guided by local consensus. There are no sleep medicine-specific regulatory bodies. The practice of medicine and practitioners in Zambia is regulated by the Health Professionals Council of Zambia. The Council accredits both health facilities and practitioners. Given the absence of specialized sleep medicine practitioners, the practice is regulated under the ambit of the more established specialties of Internal medicine, Pulmonology or neurology. Sleep technicians would be also regulated under the 'medical technologist' category.

There is the absence of a sleep professional society, in view of a lack of specialized practitioners. However, the importance of establishing such a society cannot be overstated as it would serve as a catalyst to the development of this specialty, notwithstanding the lack of highly specialized practitioners.

Challenges to Practice of Sleep Medicine

The practice of sleep medicine in a developing country such as Zambia is hampered by several factors which hinder patient access to appropriate care. These factors are patient or practitioner-driven, but are all largely perpetuated by an overwhelmed healthcare system.

Patient Factors

Patients with sleep disorders often do not regard their illness as a medical problem worth presenting to healthcare facilities for. This is against a background of poor general health-seeking behavior generally in the population [18]. Further, snoring (with or without breath cessation), a paramount feature of OSA, is also not commonly perceived as a medical problem. There exists generally in Africa misconceptions and myths about sleep disorders. Most of these are deep-rooted in spiritual beliefs [19]. Therefore, patients are more likely to seek care for these from religious or spiritual mediums than healthcare facilities. Given the fact that patients have to meet part of the cost of medical care, the majority of the poor but afflicted generally tend to prioritize which problems to present to healthcare facilities for attention. Sleep disorders are likely to fall down the ladder of priority.

Practitioner Factors

The primary health care level is likely to be the first point of call for patients with sleep disorders in Zambia. The primary health care facilities are managed by community health workers, nurses, clinical officers or unspecialized junior doctors, depending on whether they are a health post, health center, sub-district/district hospital, and also whether they are located in a rural or urban area. Inevitably, the level of knowledge and experience in these healthcare cadres is often inadequate to diagnose and let alone manage sleep disorders. A multicenter survey carried out by Chan *et al.* among primary care physicians in South Africa, Nigeria, and Kenya revealed that while they considered obstructive sleep apnoea to be important, they had modest knowledge about it, and a low perceived confidence in its management [20]. This is likely to be the case in Zambia. Further, healthcare facilities are often inadequate to manage non-communicable diseases (NCDs), as was revealed by a cross-sectional survey by Mutale *et al.* assessing primary healthcare capacity to manage NCDs in three districts in Zambia. Only six out of 46 facilities were deemed adequate to manage NCDs, with most failing to reach the minimum threshold [21].

Healthcare System Barriers

The absence of equipped sleep centers is a profoundly significant barrier to care in Zambia. It leaves confirmation of diagnosis elusive. CPAP machines for treatment are not routinely available in the country, let alone in the public health sector, save for occasional donations by foreign partners. When available, they are used on patients diagnosed based on risk assessment *via* questionnaires, without sleep study confirmation. Neither are oral devices available. As a result, only patients with international health insurance or those able to afford care in specialized centers outside the country have access to sleep diagnostics and devices for care. However, the effect of COVID-19 on travel has hampered this access, and a slowly increasing number of these patients have had to resort to follow-up of care at the UTH.

Clinical and Research Knowledge Gap

In view of the gross inadequacies in diagnostics and treatment in-country, gaps in care are inevitable. However, these are only part of the problem, as they are further impacted by patient and practitioner misperceptions and knowledge insufficiency of sleep disorders. An area that has subsequently lagged behind is the assessment for sleep disorders in commercial motor vehicle drivers. It is not done by the Road Traffic and Safety Agency (RTSA), which is the national road safety regulator in the country. Sleep disorders therefore remain a possible cause of a large number of road traffic accidents. The 2020 Zambian annual Road

Transport and Safety Report attributed human error to 86.55% of road traffic crashes [22]. Of these, 91.71% were due to driver errors. That only 0.42% of driver errors were attributed to the driver falling asleep while driving may be down to the fact that these require the presence of a witness to report the sleepiness. However, the numbers could be more and sleeping could have weighed in on the other cited causes of driver error in the report such as failure to keep to the near side, misjudging clearance distance, failure to obey traffic signals, turning without due care and other errors of judgment.

Research in sleep disorders has paralleled the inadequacies in clinical care. However, a yet to be unpublished study by Simpamba and Mateyo was recently done to assess daytime somnolence in commercial motor vehicle drivers and the likelihood of obstructive sleep apnoea in this group. The authors found that 22.8% of 136 commercial motor vehicle drivers had high risk for OSA on the STOP-BANG questionnaire. Further, they found that 67.7% of the respondents with a high risk of OSA had a statistically significant association with a past history of being involved in a road traffic accident. These findings are significant for the fact that sleep disorders are perhaps more prevalent than suspected, and therefore call for the need for more baseline studies to be conducted. Current research gaps include quantification and delineation of the problem of sleep disorders, associated risk factors, assessment of simple, cheap diagnostic tools in this resource-constrained setting, and future interventional studies across the spectrum of sleep disorders.

CONCLUSION

The practice of sleep medicine in Zambia is wrought with patient and practitioner knowledge gaps on sleep disorders, diagnostic and management gaps, and the failure of the health system to recognize, quantify and thus invest in sleep disorder management and research in the country. However, these gaps present an opportunity research to answer the many questions that exist and subsequently improve the care of patients with sleep disorders in the country. for harnessing and developing this area and answering the many research questions that arise subsequent to these gaps.

CONSENT FOR PUBLICATION

Not applicable.

CONFLICT OF INTEREST

The authors declare no conflict of interest, financial or otherwise.

ACKNOWLEDGEMENT

Declared none.

REFERENCES

[1]   Hossain JL, Shapiro CM. The prevalence, cost implications, and management of sleep disorders: an overview. Sleep Breath 2002; 6(2): 085-102.
[http://dx.doi.org/10.1055/s-2002-32322] [PMID: 12075483]

[2]   Lyons MM, Bhatt NY, Pack AI, Magalang UJ. Global burden of sleep☐disordered breathing and its implications. Respirology 2020; 25(7): 690-702.
[http://dx.doi.org/10.1111/resp.13838] [PMID: 32436658]

[3]   Peppard PE, Young T, Palta M, Skatrud J. Prospective study of the association between sleep-disordered breathing and hypertension. N Engl J Med 2000; 342(19): 1378-84.
[http://dx.doi.org/10.1056/NEJM200005113421901] [PMID: 10805822]

[4]   Nieto FJ, Young TB, Lind BK, *et al.* Association of sleep-disordered breathing, sleep apnea, and hypertension in a large community-based study. Sleep Heart Health Study. JAMA 2000; 283(14): 1829-36.
[http://dx.doi.org/10.1001/jama.283.14.1829] [PMID: 10770144]

[5]   Shahar E, Whitney CW, Redline S, *et al.* Sleep-disordered breathing and cardiovascular disease: cross-sectional results of the Sleep Heart Health Study. Am J Respir Crit Care Med 2001; 163(1): 19-25.
[http://dx.doi.org/10.1164/ajrccm.163.1.2001008] [PMID: 11208620]

[6]   Yaggi HK, Concato J, Kernan WN, Lichtman JH, Brass LM, Mohsenin V. Obstructive sleep apnea as a risk factor for stroke and death. N Engl J Med 2005; 353(19): 2034-41.
[http://dx.doi.org/10.1056/NEJMoa043104] [PMID: 16282178]

[7]   Karimi M, Hedner J, Häbel H, Nerman O, Grote L. Sleep apnea-related risk of motor vehicle accidents is reduced by continuous positive airway pressure: Swedish Traffic Accident Registry data. Sleep 2015; 38(3): 341-9.
[http://dx.doi.org/10.5665/sleep.4486] [PMID: 25325460]

[8]   Ajayi IO, Adebamowo C, Adami HO, *et al.* Urban–rural and geographic differences in overweight and obesity in four sub-Saharan African adult populations: a multi-country cross-sectional study. BMC Public Health 2016; 16(1): 1126.
[http://dx.doi.org/10.1186/s12889-016-3789-z] [PMID: 27793143]

[9]   Adeboye B, Bermano G, Rolland C. Obesity and its health impact in Africa : a systematic review : review article. Cardiovasc J Afr 2012; 23(9): 512-21.
[http://dx.doi.org/10.5830/CVJA-2012-040] [PMID: 23108519]

[10]   Lagarde E. Road traffic injury is an escalating burden in Africa and deserves proportionate research efforts. PLoS Med 2007; 4(6): 170.
[http://dx.doi.org/10.1371/journal.pmed.0040170] [PMID: 17593893]

[11]   World report on road traffic injury prevention.pdf. 2007.

[12]   Aragón-Arreola JF, Moreno-Villegas CA, Armienta-Rojas DA, De la Herrán-Arita AK. An insight of sleep disorders in Africa. eNeurologicalSci 2016; 3: 37-40.
[http://dx.doi.org/10.1016/j.ensci.2016.02.006] [PMID: 29430534]

[13]   Crankshaw O, Borel-Saladin J. Causes of urbanisation and counter-urbanisation in Zambia: Natural population increase or migration? Urban Stud 2019; 56(10): 2005-20.
[http://dx.doi.org/10.1177/0042098018787964]

[14]   Health-Sector-Profile.pdf.

[15] DiBiase RM, Salas RME, Gamaldo CE, *et al.* Training in Neurology: Implementation and Evaluation of an Objective Structured Clinical-Examination Tool for Neurology Postgraduate Trainees in Lusaka, Zambia. Neurology 2021; 97(7): e750-4.
[http://dx.doi.org/10.1212/WNL.0000000000012134] [PMID: 33931541]

[16] Bendavid E, Seligman B, Kubo J. Comparative analysis of old-age mortality estimations in Africa. PLoS One 2011; 6(10): e26607.
[http://dx.doi.org/10.1371/journal.pone.0026607] [PMID: 22028921]

[17] Venkat Narayan KM, Miotti PG, Anand NP, *et al.* HIV and noncommunicable disease comorbidities in the era of antiretroviral therapy: a vital agenda for research in low- and middle-income country settings. J Acquir Immune Defic Syndr 2014; 67 (Suppl. 1): S2-7.
[http://dx.doi.org/10.1097/QAI.0000000000000267] [PMID: 25117958]

[18] Household_Health_Seeking_Behavior_in_Zambia.pdf.

[19] Komolafe MA, Sanusi AA, Idowu AO, *et al.* Sleep medicine in Africa: past, present, and future. J Clin Sleep Med 2021; 17(6): 1317-21.
[http://dx.doi.org/10.5664/jcsm.9218] [PMID: 33687322]

[20] Chang JWR, Akemokwe FM, Marangu DM, *et al.* Obstructive Sleep Apnea Awareness among Primary Care Physicians in Africa. Ann Am Thorac Soc 2020; 17(1): 98-106.
[http://dx.doi.org/10.1513/AnnalsATS.201903-218OC] [PMID: 31580702]

[21] Mutale W, Bosomprah S, Shankalala P, *et al.* Assessing capacity and readiness to manage NCDs in primary care setting: Gaps and opportunities based on adapted WHO PEN tool in Zambia. PLoS One 2018; 13(8): e0200994.
[http://dx.doi.org/10.1371/journal.pone.0200994] [PMID: 30138318]

[22] RTSA-2020-Annual-Road-Transport-and-Safety-Status-Report-v3-23.03.2021-Printed-1.pdf. 2021.

CHAPTER 20

Sleep Medicine in Brazil

Helena Hachul[1,*], Daniel Ninello Polesel[1], Karen Tieme Nozoe[1], Dalva Poyares[1], Monica Levy Andersen[1] and Sergio Tufik[1]

[1] Department of Psychobiology, Universidade Federal de Sao Paulo, Sao Paulo, SP, Brazil

Abstract: Sleep Medicine has only recently become a medical specialty in Brazil. There are few qualified professionals in this field, and they are mainly concentrated in metropolitan areas. Access to the diagnosis and treatment of sleep disorders is not yet homogeneous for the entire population. In Brazil, there is a public health system called the *Sistema Único de Saúde (SUS)* that offers free and universal health access to all. Although it can be difficult and time-consuming to access a sleep assessment, *SUS* offers free diagnosis and treatment for sleep disorders. However, private clinics and hospitals provide more treatment options and faster access compared to the public sector, but at a high cost. Sleep Medicine is not yet a mandatory discipline in medical training, and most specialized courses and professional development in sleep are not free. With respect to the sleep research being carried out in Brazil, most basic research is concentrated on the effects of sleep deprivation, and clinical research into the health consequences of sleep disorders and possible interventions. Modern society is increasingly subject to sleep restriction and the consequences of sleep disturbances. As a result, sleep has attracted more attention and interest from the media and the general population. Sleep Medicine in Brazil has experienced a significant expansion in knowledge over the last 20 years, and the prospects are positive in relation to future research and the training of specialized professionals.

Keywords: Brazil, Bruxism, Diagnosis, Insomnia, Latin America, Polysomnography, Professional associations, Public health system, Questionnaires, Restless legs syndrome, Sleep, Treatment.

TEXT

Geopolitical Data

Brazil is the largest country in Latin America and the fifth largest in the world in terms of size, with an area of 8.5 million square kilometers. It is divided into five regions (north, northeast, midwest, southeast and south) and 27 federative units. According to the Brazilian Institute of Geography and Statistics (Instituto

---

* **Corresponding author Helena Hachul:** Department of Psychobiology, Universidade Federal de Sao Paulo, Sao Paulo, SP, Brazil; Tel: +55 (11) 2149-0155, Fax: +55 (11) 5572-5092; E-mail: helenahachul@gmail.com

Hrayr P. Attarian, Marie-Louise M. Coussa-Koniski & Alain Michel Sabri (Eds.)

Brasileiro de Geografia e Estatística), Brazil has a population of 211.8 million distributed among 5,570 municipalities. In the latest United Nations report, Brazil was considered the sixth most populous country in the world, has a human development index of 0.699 and currently occupies the 73rd place in the world ranking. Among the municipalities, the metropolitan area of Sao Paulo stands out, with approximately 21.5 million inhabitants (about 10% of the Brazilian population), and is among the 10 most populous metropolitan areas in the world. The official language of the country is Portuguese and the annual per capita income is USD 8,920.76 according to the World Bank.

Fig. (**1**) shows the distribution of the Brazilian population by sex and age. It is noteworthy that in Brazil the demographic census is carried out every 10 years, the last one being carried out in 2010, and a census was scheduled to be carried out in 2020, but has been postponed due to the SARS-COV 2 pandemic. Thus, we present the projection for 2020 created by the Department of Informatics of the Ministry of Health.

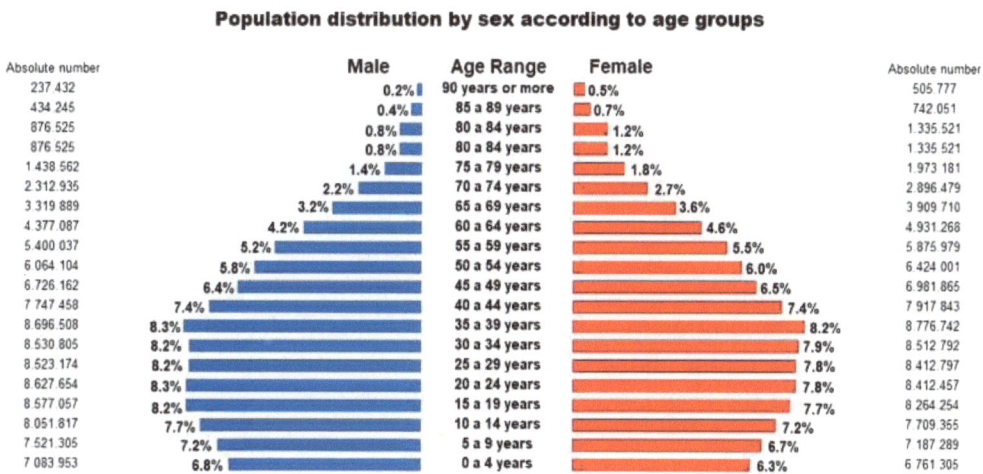

Population distribution by sex according to age groups

Absolute number	Male	Age Range	Female	Absolute number
237.432	0.2%	90 years or more	0.5%	505.777
434.245	0.4%	85 a 89 years	0.7%	742.051
876.525	0.8%	80 a 84 years	1.2%	1.335.521
876.525	0.8%	80 a 84 years	1.2%	1.335.521
1.438.562	1.4%	75 a 79 years	1.8%	1.973.181
2.312.935	2.2%	70 a 74 years	2.7%	2.896.479
3.319.889	3.2%	65 a 69 years	3.6%	3.909.710
4.377.087	4.2%	60 a 64 years	4.6%	4.931.268
5.400.037	5.2%	55 a 59 years	5.5%	5.875.979
6.064.104	5.8%	50 a 54 years	6.0%	6.424.001
6.726.162	6.4%	45 a 49 years	6.5%	6.981.865
7.747.458	7.4%	40 a 44 years	7.4%	7.917.843
8.696.508	8.3%	35 a 39 years	8.2%	8.776.742
8.530.805	8.2%	30 a 34 years	7.9%	8.512.792
8.523.174	8.2%	25 a 29 years	7.8%	8.412.797
8.627.654	8.3%	20 a 24 years	7.8%	8.412.457
8.577.057	8.2%	15 a 19 years	7.7%	8.264.254
8.051.817	7.7%	10 a 14 years	7.2%	7.709.355
7.521.305	7.2%	5 a 9 years	6.7%	7.187.289
7.083.953	6.8%	0 a 4 years	6.3%	6.761.305

Fig. (1). Population distribution by sex and age groups according to the DATASUS projection for 2020. Source: DATASUS, 2021.

Brazilian Public Health System

The 1988 Brazilian constitution established a public health system called the Unified Health System (in Portuguese the *Sistema Único de Saúde - SUS*), which provides free universal health care. Any citizen can access the service, as can foreigners in Brazil who need health assistance. The Brazilian Health System is one of the largest public health systems in the world. *SUS* serves more than 190 million people, 80% of whom depend exclusively on this system for their health care, and is financed through taxes, public resources and other supplementary sources of finance.

SUS is organized into three main parts:

1) Primary care, provided by the Basic Health Unit (*Unidade Básica de Saúde – UBS*), which is responsible for routine care, vaccination, prenatal care and prevention actions, including actions in the community and home visits;

2) Secondary care, provided by the Emergency Care Unit (*Unidade de Pronto Atendimento*), which is responsible for the care of intermediate complexity in outpatient clinics and hospitals;

3) Tertiary care, provided by large hospitals, which are responsible for complex care, including high-cost procedures and those using state-of-the-art technology such as transplantation and cancer treatment.

SUS also provides a range of other services that include pharmacy services, immunization, hemotherapy, organ transplantation and a human milk bank. In *SUS*, especially at the level of the *UBS*, health service delivery is focused on the Family Health Strategy program (*Estratégia da Saúde da Família*). The data contained in *SUS* databases guides the actions of public policy.

The standard procedure used by *SUS* in relation to diagnosis and treatment initially consists of the patient being seen at a *UBS* and, if necessary, referred to a specialized health service for treatment; one of the areas of specialized health is sleep assessment and the treatment of sleep disorders. However, few Brazilian cities offer polysomnography (PSG), the gold-standard sleep assessment, funded by *SUS*, and those that do have high demand with wait times in months, making access difficult for the population.

Sleep Education and Knowledge Diffusion in Brazil

Although Sleep Medicine is recognized as a medical specialty, it is not an essential component of medical school or health sciences curriculum. Few Brazilian universities teach sleep medicine in their health-related courses. The *Universidade Federal de Sao Paulo* was a pioneer in integrating sleep medicine into its undergraduate curriculum. However, there are only about 20 sleep medicine training sites in the whole country, with the majority being concentrated in the southeast region. There is a relatively low demand among newly graduated doctors to study this specialty, which is possibly related to their low exposure to Sleep Medicine during their medical training [1].

Since 2014, the Brazilian Association of Sleep (*Associação Brasileira do Sono - ABS*) has promoted Sleep Week, a week of activities aimed at spreading knowledge about sleep. This represents an extension of the World Sleep Day, an initiative of the World Sleep Society. This annual event is held in March and aims to disseminate scientific information about sleep to the entire Brazilian population. Currently, it has the support of a number of Brazilian celebrities, which helps to ensure that information reaches the widest possible audience.

Recently, there has been a great deal of media interest in various topics related to sleep health and sleep disorders, and several experts and researchers have had the opportunity to spread information on these subjects through interviews. A number of support groups have been created through pioneering initiatives by patients and their families/friends with the aim of exchanging experiences in relation to various sleep problems, such as narcolepsy, idiopathic hypersomnia, and sleep apnea, among others.

The Brazilian Sleep Congress is a national, biannual event aimed at health professionals, researchers and students, and includes contributions from renowned national and international sleep experts. It is currently in its 18th annual edition, and provides space for the presentation of scientific research in the area of sleep, the discussion of clinical cases, sleep pathologies, diagnoses and the latest treatments. In even years, the Sao Paulo Congress of Sleep Medicine is another major scientific event in the area of sleep. These two congresses are attended by an estimated 2,000 participants.

The *ABS* promotes continuing education with a multidisciplinary introduction to sleep course, and courses for professionals in the fields of medicine, speech therapy, psychology, physiotherapy and dentistry. It has also published the *Revista Sono* since 2015, which is a magazine-type periodical that aims to disseminate knowledge about sleep to professionals and the population in general. In 2008, the *ABS* and the Latin American Federation of Sleep Societies (*Federación Latinoamericana de Sociedades de Sueño*) created Sleep Science, an interdisciplinary, international open-access journal dedicated to the investigation of sleep, chronobiology, and related topics.

Several centers specializing in the diagnosis and treatment of sleep disorders have been created. One of the earliest of these was the *Instituto do Sono* (the Sleep Institute), which is located in Sao Paulo. The *Instituto do Sono* was a pioneer in the training of doctors and other health professionals in Sleep Medicine, with the first training course being held in 1996, and is now the largest sleep center in Brazil with 77 beds available for PSG exams. It offers more than 20 training courses in sleep related subjects, including both theoretical and practical classes.

In addition, it provides professionals the opportunity to follow specific teaching clinics. This diagnostic and research center has carried out more than 350,000 PSG exams since its foundation and trained more than 4,000 professionals.

Another specialized center is the *Núcleo Interdisciplinar da Ciência do Sono,* located in the city of Sao Paulo. It has a multidisciplinary team of sleep specialists, such as cardiologists, otolaryngologists, dentists, speech therapists and psychologists, all focused on the diagnosis and treatment of sleep disorders. They promote courses focused on Sleep Medicine, such as theoretical/practical courses for the treatment of snoring, sleep apnea and bruxism.

With respect to the public sector, there has not been a political commitment to promote courses and qualifications for health professionals working in the area of Sleep Medicine. There remains, therefore, much work to do in the public health system to improve and develop training in this area.

Courses promoted by the *ABS* and other private institutions are not free, and this can be a limiting factor in the mass qualification of professionals.

Professional Sleep Associations and Societies

Sleep Medicine in Brazil is represented by the following professional associations and societies:

● The *Associação Brasileira do Sono* (ABS) – ABS, the Brazilian Sleep Society, has a central unit in Sao Paulo and 22 regional units across the country, and its membership encompasses all health professionals working in the sleep field. It has different departments for psychologists, physical therapists, and speech therapists, but lacks a special division for researchers.

● The *Associação Brasileira de Medicina do Sono* (ABMS) – ABMS is a medical society and all its members are physicians. It deals with medical issues and policies in Sleep Medicine.

● The *Associação Brasileira de Odontologia do Sono* (ABROS) – which represents dental professionals involved in the treatment and research of sleep-disordered.

Epidemiological Data on Sleep Disorders

Sleep is essential for health and quality of life; scientific research from around the world has demonstrated its importance and the consequences of sleep deprivation or sleep disorders for health. Currently, there are more than 80 sleep disorders recognized by the International Classification of Sleep Disorders (ICSD), which are classified into seven classes: insomnia, respiratory sleep disorders, central hypersomnia disorders, sleep-wake circadian rhythm disorders, parasomnias, sleep-related disorders movement and other sleep disorders [2]. Surveys show that approximately 69% of Brazilians believe that sleep has an important impact on health and well-being. In addition, 50% of respondents believe that night rest is the most important factor for well-being (being ahead of items, such as good nutrition and physical exercise). Despite these findings, studies show that 36% of the population complains of recurrent insomnia. According to data collected by the *ABS*, the Brazilian population is sleeping less; decreasing from 6.6 hours/day in 2018 to 6.4 hours/day in 2019.

With respect to sleep data, the Epidemiological Study of Sleep (*EPISONO*) is considered the largest Brazilian epidemiological study aimed at investigating sleep disorders through objective (polysomnographic) and subjective (questionnaire) measures. The first edition was carried out in in 1987 and then repeated in 1995 and 2007, making it possible to perform comparative evaluations of a range of sleep parameters. The findings indicated a growing tendency towards increased insomnia (a higher prevalence of difficulty starting and maintaining sleep, combined with early awakening), sleep disorders related to movement, snoring and bruxism [3]. The Brazilian population is very diverse, comprising different races and ethnicities as a result of its historical formation. The survey, therefore, was designed to produce a representative sample of the population of the city of Sao Paulo in relation to ethnicity, as well as age, gender and socioeconomic class. Prior to the *EPISONO* study, worldwide estimates indicated that the prevalence of obstructive sleep apnea (OSA) in the population ranged from 2-4%. A sample size of volunteers was calculated that would allow prevalence estimates with a 3% precision. Studies in the literature related to sleep disorders indicate that specific populations may have different characteristics according to gender, age and socioeconomic criteria. Thus, it was necessary that the sample was representative of the selected population. These considerations resulted in a sample that comprised 1,042 participants aged between 20 and 80 years old, all of whom were evaluated by laboratory PSG.

The main results of this study demonstrated that excessive daytime sleepiness affects about 39.2% of the inhabitants of the city of Sao Paulo and is the main symptom of sleep disorders, directly affecting work productivity, the quality of life and increasing the risk of accidents [4]. There was a high prevalence of OSA that was associated with non-restorative sleep, tiredness on waking and sleep fragmentation, affecting almost 1 in 3 individuals (32.9%) [5]. *EPISONO* showed moderate to severe OSA frequencies of about 28% in men and 10% in women. Another study based on the 2012 AASM criteria for severe OSA (an apnea-hypop nea index higher than 15 events/hour) projected a prevalence of severe OSA in excess of 25 million people in Brazil [6].

Compared to men, women have proportionately less severe OSA and report nonspecific symptoms more frequently, which may lead to clinicians not recognizing the sleep disorder. Women with OSA report 2 to 3 times less of the classic symptoms of the disease, such as snoring, suffocation and apnea, when the results have been adjusted for the level of severity of OSA. However, they are more prone to complications and have a higher demand for health services compared to men. In the female population after menopause, there is an increase in sleep disorders, mainly insomnia and/or OSA [7].

Among the main causes that contribute to the increase in the prevalence of sleep-disordered breathing are: overweight/obesity, age, sedentary lifestyle, comorbidities due to chronic non-communicable diseases and ethnic/genetic factors, such as craniofacial factors and soft tissue abnormalities. Of these factors, obesity, especially abdominal obesity, is considered the main risk factor. However, this is a potentially modifiable parameter, especially in young patients. Obese individuals with sleep apnea who can reduce their waist circumference to within the desirable limits are likely to have a milder form of the disease.

Regarding insomnia, based on the *EPISONO* sample and according to the last criterion established by the Diagnostic and Statistical Manual of Mental Disorders, Fifth Edition, on insomnia, 48.6% of women had symptoms of persistent insomnia, and 18.1% were classified as having insomnia that resulted in significant impairment in daily functions. In men, these percentages were 47.2% and 10.7%, respectively [8].

Restless Legs Syndrome (RLS) is one of the most prevalent sleep disorders in Brazil. This syndrome is classified in the class of sleep disorders related to movement (ICSD-3). RLS is a chronic disease characterized by exclusively subjective symptoms, with sensations of discomfort and paresthesia in the limbs, especially the lower limbs, which are present at rest and relieved with movement. In Brazil, a study showed a prevalence of 6.4%, with greater prevalence in women than in men [9]. This difference possibly reflects the higher perception and reporting of the condition by women, hormonal differences between genders and a higher probability of iron deficiency in women.

Bruxism is another syndrome that is prevalent in Brazil, and is classified as a sleep disorder related to movement (ICSD-3). This syndrome is defined as the repetitive activity of the masticatory muscles characterized by the clenching or grinding of teeth and/or jaw movements. In Brazil, a study indicated a prevalence of about 12.5% of this disorder through the use of a questionnaire. However, when these results were associated with the results of a PSG test, this prevalence decreased to 5.5% [10]. In this same study, no statistically significant difference was found between genders.

In addition to the *EPISONO* study previously described, another important study in epidemiological terms is *ELSA-Brasil*. This is a longitudinal study of adult health and includes an assessment of the sleep of its participants. This was approved in 2008 and will be conducted over 20 years, evaluating about 15,000 public employees between 35 and 74 years of age who work in the six Brazilian universities/research centers that are part of this consortium, namely: the Oswaldo Cruz Foundation, the *Universidade Federal da Bahia*, the *Universidade Federal do Espírito Santo*, the *Universidade Federal de Minas Gerais*, the *Universidade Federal do Rio Grande do Sul* and the *Universidade de São Paulo*. It is currently the largest epidemiological study in Latin America on chronic non-communicable diseases. With respect to sleep, volunteers are being evaluated for one night by portable home polygraphy (airflow monitoring through a nasal cannula, abdominal thoracic breathing effort by inductance straps, pulse oximetry, pulse/heart rate and body position). They will also complete the Berlin questionnaire, the Lausanne NoSAS (neck circumference, obesity, snoring, age, sex) test and the Epworth Sleepiness Scale (ESS) for sleep assessment, in particular the risk for OSA. This large study was approved and financed by the Brazilian Ministry of Science and Technology and the investment exceeds USD 4 million. This study is important because chronic non-communicable diseases account for the largest part of the expenditures of *SUS* [11, 12].

Finally, the third important epidemiological study is the observational and longitudinal Baependi Heart Study. The Baependi Heart Study was set up in 2005 to develop a longitudinal family-based cohort study. The study aims to evaluate genetic and environmental influences on cardiovascular disease risk factor traits. Participants were recruited in Baependi, a small town in the state of Minas Gerais, Brazil. The first follow-up wave took place in 2010, and the second in 2016. At baseline, the study evaluated 1,691 individuals across 95 families. It included an objective assessment of sleep using a portable polygraphy exam with the following parameters: pulse oximetry, chest piezoelectric strap (for detection of respiratory effort), airflow through a nasal cannula, body position sensor, and heart rate. For subjective sleep evaluation, questionnaires were used, including the ESS, the Berlin Questionnaire and the Pittsburgh Sleep Quality Index (PSQI) [13, 14].

Professionals in the Field of Sleep Medicine

In Brazil, despite the scientific evidence showing the importance of sleep in relation to health, Sleep Medicine has not been recognized as an area of medical practice by the National Council of Medicine (*Conselho Federal de Medicina - CFM*) until 2011. To be a sleep specialist, it is necessary to have 1-year training and fulfill the prerequisites for medical residency in one of the following areas: internal medicine, neurology, otorhinolaryngology, pediatrics, pulmonology or psychiatry. The title of a sleep specialist is awarded by the respective medical society in conjunction with the Brazilian Medical Association (*Associação Médica Brasileira - AMB*). PSG technicians are certified by the *ABS* to work in sleep laboratories. Other health professionals can act as sleep specialists, such as:

• Dentists, who receive certification from the Brazilian Sleep Dentistry Association;

• Speech Therapists, who are certified by the ABS in partnership with the Brazilian Speech Therapy Society, the Brazilian Association of Orofacial Motricity and the National Speech Therapy Council;

• Physiotherapists, who are certified by the *ABS* in partnership with the Brazilian Association of Cardiorespiratory Physiotherapy and Physiotherapy in Intensive Care;

• Psychologists, who are certified by the ABS and the Brazilian Psychological Society.

According to the *CFM,* there are 555,213 doctors authorized to work in Brazil. Of these, only 396 doctors are accredited by the *ABS* to work in sleep medicine, 189 of whom are from otorhinolaryngology, 83 from pulmonology, 73 from neurology, 19 from psychiatry, 17 from pediatrics and 15 from clinical medicine. Although we estimate that there are over 500 private sleep laboratories in Brazil, only 37 are accredited by the *ABS* to perform diagnostic sleep tests, and only 4 to perform home PSG.

Although the number of clinics offering type 3 and type 4 PSG has substantially increased, it is not possible to determine the exact number as certification of sleep laboratories by the *ABS* is not mandatory.

Diagnosis of Sleep Disorders

Insomnia, OSA, bruxism and RLS are among the main sleep disorders in the country. In general, doctors across the country rely on clinical evaluation and the use of questionnaires to diagnose sleep disorders. Questionnaires are quick, inexpensive tools with good screening capacity. The most commonly used questionnaires are: the Sleep Apnea Clinical Score (SACS), the PSQI, the Berlin Questionnaire, and the Stop-Bang Questionnaire, which are all screening tools for OSA; the Insomnia Severity Index (ISI); and the ESS, which assesses excessive daytime sleepiness. The results of the questionnaires should be used together with anamnesis and symptoms to diagnose sleep disorders.

Consensus and guidelines for the diagnosis and treatment of insomnia in Brazil were developed by the *ABS* in conjunction with sleep specialists. However, the Brazilian Medical Association is officially responsible for the main treatment guidelines in the country.

There are 3 types of insomnia: chronic insomnia disorder, short-term insomnia disorder and other insomnia disorders. With respect to the diagnosis of insomnia, a clinical evaluation is recommended to assess sleep. The diagnosis of insomnia occurs when there is a complaint of dissatisfaction with sleep; difficulty falling asleep, staying asleep, waking up early or non-restorative sleep; the impairment of social or professional activities the following day; and the insomnia must happen at least 3 times a week, for at least 3 months and not be attributed to another cause or disease. A sleep diary, the insomnia severity index (ISI), actigraphy or PSG can be used to evaluate insomnia.

The ISI is a subjective assessment in the form of a validated questionnaire comprising a brief, simple self-administered scale that measures the patient's perception of their insomnia and the degree of concern and stress it causes due to difficulties with sleep. However, it is not used routinely, being useful only in some cases. Likewise, PSG can also be indicated for some cases of insomnia disorder, being recommended only when other sleep disorders are suspected, when treatment is refractory or when there is a discrepancy between subjective and objective sleep data. A sleep diary is considered the "gold standard" for the subjective assessment of a patient's sleep pattern and consists of daily monitoring of the habits and times of the sleep-wake cycle. It is recommended that the patient fills in the diary retrospectively, for example in the morning he/she writes about the previous night. Actigraphy has some advantages due to the size of the actigraph and its portability. It is used to register muscle activity correlated with sleep and circadian rhythm. The following parameters related to sleep are evaluated by the actigraph: total sleep time, sleep efficiency, latency to sleep onset and awake time after sleep onset. Its use on the non-dominant arm is recommended for at least 2 weeks. The use of actigraphy in insomnia is more for differential diagnosis between insomnia disorder and circadian rhythm disorders, identification of patients with poor perception of their sleep and for assessment of response to treatment.

With respect to RLS, the diagnosis is based on the following criteria: An intense urge to move the legs, usually due to a feeling of discomfort. These symptoms are observed to start or worsen during periods of inactivity, are relieved with movement and occur predominantly or exclusively in the evening or at night; Symptoms due to other medical conditions, such as leg cramps, myalgia or leg swelling need to be excluded; RLS symptoms can have a significant impact on an individual's life, causing worry, sleep disturbance or even mental, physical, social, educational or behavioral impairment. Complementary tests, such as serum ferritin dosage can aid in the diagnosis, since values below 50 mg/L are associated with an increased risk of RLS.

Polysomnographic findings related to RLS with a periodic limb movement index greater than 15 events/hour in adults or greater than 5 events/hour in children suggest the disorder. The diagnosis of RLS is predominantly clinical, and subjective symptoms are the factor that guides the treatment.

Sleep bruxism is diagnosed based on the following criteria: the presence of grinding sounds or teeth clenching during sleep; the presence of abnormal tooth wear, muscle pain or fatigue of the jaw; and headache or jaw block on waking, consistent with reports of grinding or clenching teeth (ICSD-3). Bruxism is classified according to its origin as primary or secondary. The primary type has an idiopathic origin and is not associated with any evident medical or psychiatric condition. The secondary type is associated with other clinical conditions, such as depression, Parkinson's disease, sleep apnea and drug use.

Finally, with respect to the diagnosis of sleep-disordered breathing, the criteria established by the 2014 ICSD-3 are used in Brazil. A diagnosis of OSA, the main sleep breathing disorder, uses the presence of criteria A1 and A2, or B, as described below:

A1. The Presence of at least one of the following parameters:

● A complaint of drowsiness, non-restful sleep, fatigue or insomnia symptoms;

● Waking up with shortness of breath;

● A report of habitual snoring, apneas or both during sleep;

● Hypertension, mood disorders, cognitive dysfunction, coronary heart disease, stroke, congestive heart failure, atrial fibrillation or type 2 diabetes mellitus.

A2. PSG examination or examination with a portable monitor, showing:

• Five or more respiratory events with a predominance of obstruction (obstructive and mixed apneas, hypopneas or arousals related to respiratory effort) per hour of sleep;

B. PSG examination or examination with a portable monitor, showing:

• Fifteen or more respiratory events with a predominance of obstruction (obstructive and mixed apneas, hypopneas or arousals related to respiratory effort) per hour of sleep;

PSG is the gold standard method to diagnose sleep disorders and is subdivided into 4 types:

• Type I: PSG performed in a sleep laboratory under the supervision of a technician. This type monitors 7 channels or more using an electroencephalogram (EEG), electrooculogram (EOG), chin and leg electromyogram (EMG), electrocardiogram (ECG) or heart rate (HR), an airflow channel, peripheral oxygen saturation (SpO_2), respiratory effort and additional position sensors;

• Type II: PSG performed at the patient's residence without supervision by a technician. This type also monitors 7 channels or more (EEG, EOG, chin and leg EMG, ECG or HR, airflow channel, SpO_2, respiratory effort and additional position sensors);

• Type III: PSG performed in the patient's home without supervision by a technician. This type monitors 4 channels or more (2 breathing effort channels or 1 breathing effort + 1 airflow channel, ECG and SpO_2);

• Type IV: PSG performed at the patient's residence without supervision by a technician. This type monitors 1 or 2 channels (airflow channel and/or SpO_2).

Full-night PSG is performed in only a few sleep laboratories, as it needs to be supervised by qualified professionals and requires an appropriate structure for carrying out and validating the results. Each type of PSG has advantages and disadvantages, as shown below:

Type II PSG has the following advantages: the possibility of recording a longer total sleep time, greater sleep efficiency, excellent correlation of the respiratory disorder index and access to hospitalized patients. Among the disadvantages of the methodology: the possibility of signal loss during the exam and high cost.

Both type III and type IV PSG demonstrate the following advantages: reduced cost, speed and less technical training for interpretation. The disadvantages are a higher rate of false negative results, higher risk of signal loss, and their unsuitability for patients with a low probability of OSA and other disorders.

Other methods also commonly used are:

Actigraphy: A non-invasive sleep assessment method used to monitor rest-activity cycles, in which long periods of rest have a good correlation with periods of sleep. The individual is instructed to use the device on the non-dominant arm for a few consecutive days to check their wake-sleep cycle pattern. Data are then collected and information is read in epochs of 1 minute [15]. In addition, a sleep diary is kept and its findings are analyzed together with the actigraphy data.

Peripheral Arterial Tonometry (PAT): the results are based on a sensor that continuously measures changes in arterial volume on the finger, thus reflecting sympathetic activity due to awakenings.

Watch-PAT: A technology that uses PAT, oximetry and actigraphy to assess an individual's sleep by measuring up to seven channels (PAT signal, heart rate, oximetry, actigraphy, body position, snoring, and chest motion) *via* three points of contact.

In Brazil, there is still no consensus in the public health system regarding the criteria for requesting a PSG exam, with each municipality having its own rules. For example, in the city of Campinas/SP (located in the southeast of the country), PSG can be requested only by specialists in pulmonology, neurology and otorhinolaryngology. Additionally, the PSG request must meet the following criteria: 1) Apnea with comorbidities, 2) Occupation (high risk), or 3) A high Berlin questionnaire score. On the other hand, in the city of Goiânia/GO (located in the midwest of the country), the medical specialties authorized to request the exam are: pneumology, neurology, neuropediatrics, otorhinolaryngology, nutrology, and bariatric surgeon. The referral of the patient must contain the medical report with clinical data, videonasolaryngoscopy, comorbidities, pulmonary function parameters and arterial blood gas analysis.

In general, in the public health system, the waiting time for PSG is very long due to the high cost of the exam and the limited number of beds that are available. Access to PSG in private clinics is expensive and beyond the reach of most Brazilians. The typical cost of PSG is around USD 180, which represents approximately 85% of the minimum wage. Thus, sleep disorders in the country are still underdiagnosed in the population.

Practice Guidelines - Treatment of Major Sleep Disorders in the Country

The patient's evaluation and diagnosis will depend on the type of sleep disorder, symptoms, severity and the comorbidities associated with each individual. Adequate treatment will also depend on the possibility of access to appropriate resources. The use of available medicines depends on the approval of the Brazilian National Health Surveillance Agency (*Agência Nacional de Vigilância Sanitária*), the regulatory agency linked to the Ministry of Health. This agency has the function of inspecting medicines, pesticides and cosmetics, aiming to eliminate or reduce risks to the population's health and to decide which drugs can be prescribed for which medical conditions.

The standard treatment for insomnia is cognitive behavioral therapy (CBT). When necessary, pharmacological treatment is indicated, but not all the sedative-hypnotics that are available in other countries, such as the USA, are available in Brazil [16]. If there is a mental disorder or clinical morbidity, these must be treated first.

Regarding the treatment of RLS, there are good results from drug use associated with physical activity. Dopamine agonists are the most commonly used drugs in the treatment of RLS, and these agonists can be divided into two groups: non-ergot and ergot derivatives. In Brazil, the non-ergot agents used are pramipexole and piribedil, and the ergots are pergolide, lisuride and bromocriptine [17].

Sleep bruxism is treated with: behavioral therapy with psychological support, such as sleep hygiene, relaxing therapies and others; the use of a stabilizer plate on the teeth or a mandibular advancement device when associated with OSA; or, less often, drug therapy is used with the use of relaxants, or benzodiazepines.

The treatment of OSA depends on its severity; Behavioral measures such as weight loss, regular physical activity, sleep hygiene and alcohol abstinence can directly influence the apnea-hypopnea index [18]. The initial approach, therefore, focuses on increased physical activity and weight loss. In mild to moderate cases, the use of intraoral devices may be indicated. Orthodontic professionals have shown good results with the use of a mandibular advancement device in patients with upper airway resistance syndrome, with primary snoring and mild or moderate OSA. The device keeps the jaw protruded during the night, enlarges the size of the pharynx, improves snoring and reduces upper airway obstruction [19]. More recent approaches with speech therapy have shown promising results, while the use of medications and electrostimulation are still under study. In general, OSA is treated with non-invasive ventilation during sleep. This equipment can be purchased for around USD 500 or borrowed through *SUS* only for patients with severe apnea. However, due to a number of bureaucratic procedures, this can take several months from the moment that the doctor indicates treatment with non-invasive ventilation until its effective use.

Use of Internet Technologies

The internet is already part of the daily lives of most individuals worldwide. According to Brazilian estimates for 2019, 79.1% of Brazilian households already have access to the internet and this percentage grows every year. This technology represents a paradox, as although it has brought many benefits, its overuse can cause impaired sleep quality and shortened sleep duration. Every year, the relationship between sleep and the use of technology grows stronger. One example is the use of smartwatches, which have been developed with several functions, among them, being the self-assessment of sleep, producing reports with information about total sleep time and awakenings, similar to actigraphy. A range of Internet-connected equipment has been developed for use by professionals that can monitor or even diagnose patients or be used to ensure adherence to treatment.

Telemedicine, whose use has recently been approved by regulatory agencies in Brazil, can allow patients in one part of the country to have consultations with specialists from another location. This promotes greater accessibility to the entire population in the country, and may be especially important in Sleep Medicine due to the small number of specialists and their concentration in specific geographical areas.

A recent initiative concerns CBT performed online for the treatment of chronic insomnia. Individuals with insomnia often develop negative thoughts and behaviors about sleep and CBT is the first line treatment. Some applications to treat insomnia are in the final stages of development and may be offered free of charge to the population.

Main Areas of Basic and Clinical Sleep Research

Brazil has several research groups on sleep, evaluating mechanisms associated with normal sleep and with lack of sleep in humans and experimental animals, as well as seeking innovative methods of diagnosing and treating sleep disorders. The main studies are directed to the biochemical and behavioral effects of sleep deprivation, as well as the consequences regarding molecular and cellular parameters. Brazilian clinical studies in the area of sleep involve mainly the relationship between sleep disorders, and health and quality of life in different groups of specific individuals, as well as therapeutic measures for sleeping disorders. Most research addresses OSA and insomnia, due to the high prevalence of these disorders. The number of basic research and clinical studies in the area of sleep has been rapidly increasing. A search of the PubMed database shows that 95 studies were published with the word "sleep" and "Brazil" between 1990 and 1999, increasing to 782 between 2000 and 2010, and 3,023 between 2010 and 2019.

Fig. (2) shows the top nine universities with the highest scientific production in the area, according to a search for articles in the Web of Science database, considering the keyword "sleep" in the period from 1990 to 2020. In the same period, Fig. (3) depicts the top 10 researchers in the sleep field in terms of scientific production. The main research areas are the prevalence of sleep disorders and interventions that can provide better quality sleep for the population.

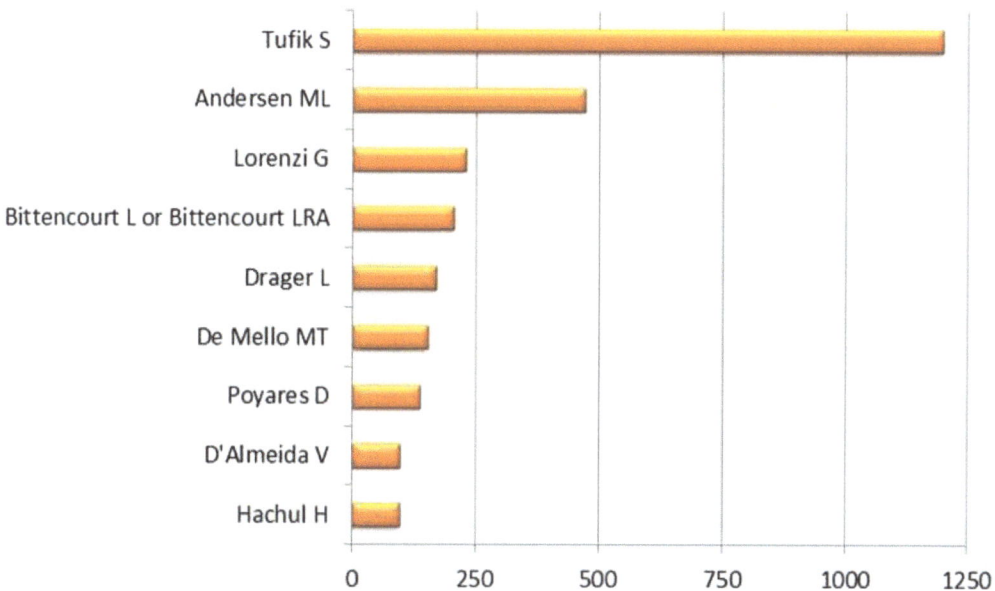

Fig. (2). Top 9 universities with greater scientific production in sleep research, based on the period from 1990 to 2020. Source: Web of Science, 2021.

Regulation of Driving Licenses

Based on the findings of sleep studies into the association between accidents and sleep disorders, the National Traffic Council issued resolution 267 in February 2008 which required the inclusion of a sleep disorder examination in the qualification process for professional drivers of large and/or heavy vehicles such as trucks, buses and trailers. Driving with sleep or signs of fatigue substantially increases the risk of accidents, and is as dangerous as driving under the influence of alcohol or other drugs. The objective of including this assessment was to reduce the number of road accidents caused by drivers who fall asleep while driving, particularly truck and bus drivers. A sleep assessment using a questionnaire was included with the other physical and mental fitness exams required to obtain a license to drive these vehicles. Depending on the severity of the sleep problem, drivers are referred to a more specific medical evaluation and a PSG exam. The resolution 267 of 2008 represented the first political act to consider the relevance of sleep disorders as possible cause of traffic accidents [20].

According to the Brazilian Highway Police, in the period 2017-2019, traffic accidents due to tiredness/lack of attention by the driver or by the driver falling asleep while driving represented approximately 41% of the total road accidents. About 4% of traffic accidents every year are related to the driver falling asleep while driving, which represents in absolute numbers more than 3,000 accidents due to this cause alone per year.

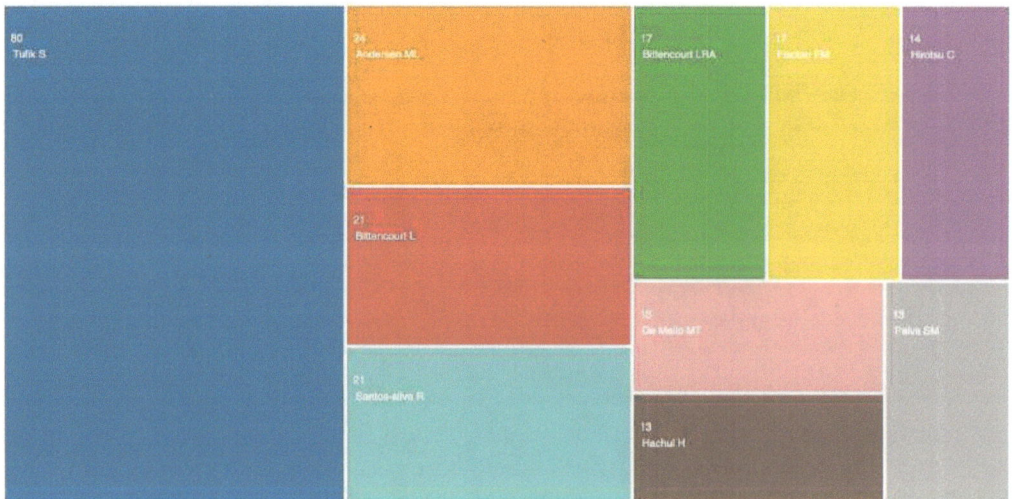

Fig. (3). Top 10 researchers with greater scientific production in sleep research, based on the period from 1990 to 2020. Source: Web of Science, 2021.

Authors' Ambulatory Experience

The authors of this chapter have had great success in the treatment of sleep disorders in the middle-aged female population, and belong to a group, which has established an outpatient clinic to treat women with sleep disorders. The group is formed by a multidisciplinary team, including physicians, biomedical scientists, pharmacists, physiotherapists, nutritionists and psychologists, all under the supervision of the physician responsible for the outpatient clinic; It comprises professionals who have graduated in their specific health field and are considering their specialization in postgraduate studies, as well as those who are interested in attending to learn more about this area and conduct their own clinical research projects. The Women's Sleep Disorders Integrative Treatment Outpatient Clinic uses an integrative interdisciplinary methodology for individual treatment [21]. All patients who seek medical attention for sleep complaints are given information on the importance of sleep hygiene practices. Practical experience at the outpatient clinic suggests that the poor quality of life of the patients is often associated with anxiety, moderate depression and complaints of symptoms resulting from menopause.

CBT is currently considered the main non-pharmacological treatment for insomnia. Other integrative approaches are performed as part of routine outpatient care according to the patient's need and acceptance, such as acupuncture, mindfulness, physiotherapy (urogynecology, global posture reeducation, myofascial release, kinesiotherapy, manual therapy, and chiropraxy) and psychotherapy. This approach is used in association with conventional treatments such as medications or hormonal therapy when indicated. This broad analysis allows differentiated and individualized treatment for each patient, promoting good outcomes.

When necessary, pharmacological treatment possibilities include, for example, antidepressants, non-benzodiazepine hypnotics, benzodiazepine hypnotics, melatonin agonists and hormone therapy.

Integrative is a term which refers to increasing the harmony and coherence of the whole being, and integrative care is focused on the person, not on the disease or a therapy. The intention with integrative care is to promote and enhance wellbeing, resilience, and the realization of an individual's potential capacities for self-care, self-regulation, and self-healing. The integrative care model includes the concept of integrated care, which brings together inputs, delivery, management and the organization of services related to diagnosis, treatment, care, rehabilitation and health promotion.

CHALLENGES

Brazil is a very large country, which makes the dissemination of information, accessibility to treatment and the diagnosis of sleep disorders very difficult for the whole population. Although there is a widespread lack of knowledge about sleep and its disorders, the level of this knowledge is gradually growing, mainly because of the significant increase in the coverage of the subject by the media in recent years. Although sleep disorders can cause sleep fragmentation, impair daily activities and reduce the quality of life, many people still do not realize how important sleep is to their lives. There is a great deal of ignorance regarding the signs and symptoms of sleep disorders in many individuals, for example, snoring and teeth grinding during sleep are still seen as normal sleep events. Increasingly, researchers, with the help of the media, are able to publicize the importance of having quality sleep, with good efficiency and minimal disturbing events that cause sleep fragmentation.

The main challenges that the country faces in respect of the treatment of sleep disorders can, therefore, be summarized as:

● A lack of professionals specialized in Sleep Medicine, thus decreasing rates of diagnosis and treatment;

● The limited number of sleep specialists that do exist in metropolitan centers, making it difficult for people from other regions to access treatment;

● The high cost and lengthy bureaucratic procedures often associated with the acquisition of specialist equipment from SUS, such as that used in Continuous Positive Airway Pressure (CPAP) therapy, and a lack of adherence to treatments by patients;

● The fact that Sleep Medicine is not yet a mandatory part of the medical school curriculum;

● The general absence of health awareness policies focused on the importance of sleep that also provides information on the consequences of sleep disorders. This is an important area as even basic advice on sleep hygiene measures may be sufficient to cure a significant portion of sleep complaints.

● Some drugs and equipment used to treat some sleep disorders are not easily available in Brazil.

CONCLUSION

Sleep Medicine is a growing area of interest in the medical literature due to the association between sleep and a wide range of pathologies, including diabetes, hypertension and cardiovascular diseases.

Studies show that people have been spending less and less time sleeping, either of choice or necessity. It is estimated that over the past 50 years, there has been a decrease of about 2 hours of sleep per day. Currently, sleep debt and various sleep disorders are very prevalent in our modern society. Humanity suffers from the consequences of these problems, such as the increase in cardiovascular comorbidities and metabolic syndrome, among others. The consequences impact the social and professional environment, and even increase the risk of accidents. It is essential that doctors responsible for primary and secondary care assist in the screening and treatment of sleep disorders.

In Brazil, there is an increasing need to train more sleep experts and pay more attention to the role of sleep, given the growing evidence indicating its multiple impacts on health. Moreover, some evaluation methods and treatments, such as those aimed at improving sleep hygiene, might be relatively simple and cost-effective to put in place, yet have significant outcomes.

LIST OF ABBREVIATIONS

ABMS	*Associação Brasileira de Medicina do Sono*
ABROS	*Associação Brasileira de Odontologia do Sono*
ABS	*Associação Brasileira do Sono*
CBT	cognitive behavioral therapy
CPAP	Continuous Positive Airway Pressure
ECG	electrocardiogram
EEG	electroencephalogram
EMG	chin and leg electromyogram
EOG	electrooculogram
EPISONO	the Epidemiological Study of Sleep
ESS	Epworth Sleepiness Scale
HR	heart rate
ICSD	International Classification of Sleep Disorders
OSA	obstructive sleep apnea
PAT	Peripheral Arterial Tonometry
PSG	polysomnography
PSQI	the Pittsburgh Sleep Quality Index
RLS	Restless Legs Syndrome
SpO$_2$	peripheral oxygen saturation
SUS	*Sistema Único de Saúde*
UBS	*Unidade Básica de Saúde*

CONSENT FOR PUBLICATION

Not applicable.

CONFLICT OF INTEREST

The authors declare no conflict of interest, financial or otherwise.

ACKNOWLEDGEMENT

Declared none.

REFERENCES

[1]　Revista ABS. 2020. http://www.absono.com.br/assets/revista_sono_edicao_23_onlline.pdf

[2]　American Academy of Sleep Medicine. International classification of sleep disorders 3a ediç~ao ed Darien. American Academy of Sleep Medicine. IL: American Academy of Sleep Medicine 2015.

[3]　Santos-Silva R, Bittencourt LRA, Pires MLN, *et al*. Increasing trends of sleep complaints in the city of Sao Paulo, Brazil. Sleep Med 2010; 11(6): 520-4.
[http://dx.doi.org/10.1016/j.sleep.2009.12.011] [PMID: 20494615]

[4]　Kim LJ, Coelho FM, Hirotsu C, *et al*. Frequencies and associations of narcolepsy-related symptoms: a cross-sectional study. J Clin sleep Med 2015; 11(12): 1377-84.
[http://dx.doi.org/10.5664/jcsm.5268] [PMID: 26235160]

[5]　Tufik S, Santos-Silva R, Taddei JA, Bittencourt LRA. Obstructive sleep apnea syndrome in the Sao Paulo Epidemiologic Sleep Study. Sleep Med 2010; 11(5): 441-6.
[http://dx.doi.org/10.1016/j.sleep.2009.10.005] [PMID: 20362502]

[6]　Benjafield AV, Ayas NT, Eastwood PR, *et al*. Estimation of the global prevalence and burden of obstructive sleep apnoea: a literature-based analysis. Lancet Respir Med 2019; 7(8): 687-98.
[http://dx.doi.org/10.1016/S2213-2600(19)30198-5] [PMID: 31300334]

[7]　Vigeta SMG, Hachul H, Tufik S, de Oliveira EM. Sleep in postmenopausal women. Qual Health Res 2012; 22(4): 466-75.
[http://dx.doi.org/10.1177/1049732311422050] [PMID: 21917564]

[8]　Lucena L, Polesel DN, Poyares D, *et al*. The association of insomnia and quality of life: Sao Paulo epidemiologic sleep study (EPISONO). Sleep Health 2020; 6(5): 629-35.
[http://dx.doi.org/10.1016/j.sleh.2020.03.002] [PMID: 32335038]

[9]　Eckeli AL, Gitaí LLG, Dach F, *et al*. Prevalence of restless legs syndrome in the rural town of Cassia dos Coqueiros in Brazil. Sleep Med 2011; 12(8): 762-7.
[http://dx.doi.org/10.1016/j.sleep.2011.01.018] [PMID: 21824818]

[10]　Maluly M, Andersen ML, Dal-Fabbro C, *et al*. Polysomnographic study of the prevalence of sleep bruxism in a population sample. J Dent Res 2013; 92(7_suppl) (Suppl.): S97-S103.
[http://dx.doi.org/10.1177/0022034513484328] [PMID: 23690359]

[11]　Brasil ELSA. maior estudo epidemiológico da América Latina. Rev Saude Publica 2009; 43: 1.

[12]　Aquino EML, Barreto SM, Bensenor IM, *et al*. Brazilian longitudinal study of adult health (ELSA-Brasil): objectives and design. Am J Epidemiol 2012; 175(4): 315-24.
[http://dx.doi.org/10.1093/aje/kwr294] [PMID: 22234482]

[13]　Egan KJ, von Schantz M, Negrão AB, *et al*. Cohort profile: the Baependi Heart Study—a family-based, highly admixed cohort study in a rural Brazilian town. BMJ Open 2016; 6(10): e011598.
[http://dx.doi.org/10.1136/bmjopen-2016-011598] [PMID: 27797990]

[14]　Alvim Rafael de Oliveira. Prevalência de Doença Arterial Periférica e Fatores de Risco Associados em uma População Rural Brasileira: Estudo Corações de Baependi. Int J Cardiovasc Sci 2018; 31(4): 405-13.

[15]   de Souza L, Benedito-Silva AA, Pires MLN, Poyares D, Tufik S, Calil HM. Further validation of actigraphy for sleep studies. Sleep 2003; 26(1): 81-5.
[http://dx.doi.org/10.1093/sleep/26.1.81] [PMID: 12627737]

[16]   Pinto LR Jr, Alves RC, Caixeta E, *et al.* New guidelines for diagnosis and treatment of insomnia. Arq Neuropsiquiatr 2010; 68(4): 666-75.
[http://dx.doi.org/10.1590/S0004-282X2010000400038] [PMID: 20730332]

[17]   Fröhlich AC, Eckeli AL, Bacelar A, *et al.* Brazilian consensus on guidelines for diagnosis and treatment for restless legs syndrome. Arq Neuropsiquiatr 2015; 73(3): 260-80.
[http://dx.doi.org/10.1590/0004-282X20140239] [PMID: 25807136]

[18]   Bittencourt LRA. Diagnóstico e tratamento da síndrome da apnéia obstrutiva do sono: guia prático. São Paulo: Livraria Médica Paulista; 2008.

[19]   de Godoy LBM, Sousa KMM, Palombini LO, *et al.* Long term oral appliance therapy decreases stress symptoms in patients with upper airway resistance syndrome. J Clin Sleep Med 2020; 16(11): 1857-62.

[20]   de Mello MT, Bittencourt LR, Cunha Rde C, *et al.* Sleep and transit in Brazil: new legislation. J Clin Sleep Med 2009; 5(2): 164-1666.

[21]   Frange C, Banzoli CV, Colombo AE, *et al.* Women's Sleep Disorders: Integrative Care. Sleep Sci 2017; 10(4): 174-80.
[http://dx.doi.org/10.5935/1984-0063.20170030] [PMID: 29410750]

CHAPTER 21

Sleep Medicine in Argentina

Arturo Garay[1,*], **Carlos Franceschini**[2], **Stella Valiensi**[3] and **Vivian Leske**[4]

[1] *Sleep Medicine-Neurology, Centro de Estudios Médicos e Investigaciones Clínicas "Norberto Quirno" (CEMIC), Ciudad de Buenos Aires (CABA), Argentina*

[2] *Sleep Medicine-Mechanical Ventilation, Hospital Cosme Argerich, Ciudad de Buenos Aires (CABA), Argentina*

[3] *Sleep Medicine-Neurology, Hospital Italiano, Ciudad de Buenos Aires (CABA), Argentina*

[4] *Sleep Unit-Pediatric Pulmonology, Hospital de Pediatría S.A.M.I.C. "Prof. Dr. J.P. Garrahan", Ciudad de Buenos Aires (CABA), Argentina*

Abstract: In this chapter we describe the history, research, education, and practice of sleep medicine in Argentina, pointing out the importance of the role of public policies in the development of sleep medicine grounds. With the drawbacks of a developing or "emerging" country, sleep medicine in Argentina has been growing up in the past decades. This fact allows us to be optimistic despite the unfavorable scenarios that our country usually goes through. Sleep medicine in Argentina is still rather young in the field of medicine and needs much more effort to consolidate as a specialty.

Keywords: Argentina, Accreditation, Demographics and practice, Health system, Research, Sleep medicine.

INTRODUCTION

Eighteen years ago, the first survey carried out by a group of Argentine researchers, explored the presence of sleep disturbances and the attitudes towards the problem that people who suffered in urban areas of Latin America (LA) (Mexico City, Buenos Aires, São Paulo). At present times, we can affirm that: in our country, around 20% of the general population sleeps little or badly, and this percentage goes up to 50% or more in groups considered at risk, in which the consequences of sleep deprivation will surely be manifested on the physical, mental and social health [1, 2]. At this point, in the twenty-first century, we must ask ourselves, which are the debts we have regarding sleep medicine in our country, and what are we doing to solve them? Among others, the occurrence of

* **Corresponding author Arturo Garay:** Sleep Medicine-Neurology, Centro de Estudios Médicos e Investigaciones Clínicas "Norberto Quirno" (CEMIC), Ciudad de Buenos Aires (CABA), Argentina, Tel: +54115290100; E-mail: adcgaray@gmail.com

Hrayr P. Attarian, Marie-Louise M. Coussa-Koniski & Alain Michel Sabri (Eds.)

sleep alterations related to working conditions in the adult population, and the approach of sleep alterations in vulnerable populations stand out. In this chapter we describe the history, research, education, and practice of sleep medicine in Argentina, pointing out the importance of the role of public policies in the development of sleep medicine grounds.

A BRIEF STORY OF THE SLEEP MEDICINE

Although previously some researchers began to explore different aspects of sleep and its disorders, we could say that sleep medicine as we know worldwide emerged in Argentina in 1982, when the first laboratories began to work with professionals trained in sleep laboratories of the USA and European countries according, mostly, with standards of the Association of Sleep Disorders Centers (ASDC) and the Diagnostic Classification of Sleep and Arousal Disorders in 1979 [3].

More recently, in 1995, the Argentinean Sleep Society (AAS) was born, gathered by the interest of joint work for the knowledge of sleep and wake and its disorders. This was a product of the association of basic researchers in the field of sleep and chronobiology, neurologists, pneumologists, and pediatricians who worked at that moment in our country. The primary purposes of AAS included, among others, the following: 1) To gather all professionals whose activity is linked to the area of sleep and the sleep and wake cycle, normal or pathological, as well as to the diagnosis and treatment of related disorders, either at an experimental or healthcare level; 2) To encourage the exchange of scientific experience in this specialty, among their members as well as with other professionals, through congresses, periodic scientific meetings, dissemination, and edition of specialized scientific publications and; 3) To promote education and training in the field of sleep, being able to grant training certificates for the practice of the specialty; 4) To promote and enable the development of teaching centers, and different activities related to the field of research, diagnosis and treatment of normal and pathological sleep and those related to professional practice (Statutes of the Argentinean Sleep Society Civil Association, 1995).

In 1999, and contemporaneously, to the evolution of the American Sleep Association (ASDA) to the current American Academy of Sleep Medicine (AASM), the AAS was renamed the Argentine Association of Sleep Medicine (AAMS) in consonance with the emergency, -worldwide and in our country-, of sleep medicine as specialty/subspecialty.

ACCREDITATION SYSTEM OF PHYSICIANS ON SLEEP MEDICINE

In Latin América, the growth of sleep medicine has been important in recent decades. Good evidence for this is the growing number of member societies of the Latin American Federation of Sleep Societies (FLASS) [4]. Currently, there are members of the FLASS: The Mexican Society for Sleep Medicine and Research, the Uruguayan Sleep Association, the Chilean Sleep Medicine Society, the Peruvian Sleep Medicine Association, the Venezuelan Academy of Sleep Medicine, Sleep Medicine, Sleep of Panamá, the Brazilian Association of Sleep, the Ecuatorian Association of Sleep Medicine, the Argentine Association of Sleep Medicine, Sleep Medicine of Costa Rica and the Colombian Association of Sleep Medicine. FLASS is currently initiating a common certification system for Latin America. In 2018, according to FLASS rules, the AASM, initiated the process of accreditation taking into account three different instances: 1) A process of homologation of worthy sleep personalities in our country, 2) Regular Accreditation Process in Sleep Medicine and 3) an Extraordinary Accreditation Process in Sleep Medicine as a common path for the uniformity of our work at the national and regional level. Currently, instances number 2 and 3 are the formal procedures with which physicians are accredited in sleep medicine by the AAMS with the recognition of FLASS. Soon, we hope to be able to follow a similar procedure with members of different health areas related to sleep medicine, *i.e.* psychologists, dentists/orthodontics, and kinesiologists, with which, at least, with some of them, we have reciprocity agreements among societies that will facilitate joint work favoring to develop sleep medicine in all the areas involved.

EDUCATION

Analysis of LA training programs reveals that Brazil offers a sleep medicine residency and Mexico includes sleep training in the neurophysiology specialty and both countries offer sleep medicine certification. Sleep societies of Colombia and Argentina have developed their certification processes according to the FLASS guidelines [4]. Indeed, there are remarkable differences in sleep society consolidations, training programs, available certifications, terminology, regulatory entities, and requirements in LA. This is the main reason for considering great importance to standardize the training and accreditation system. We consider that the vehicle for achieving the purpose of having a common way of integration and application of sleep medicine in our continent is the FLASS and in the future, the World Sleep Society. Having said that, let us review the present situation of training in sleep medicine in our country. Currently, in Argentina, physicians interested in training in sleep medicine carry out their training in first-level centers, generally on a part-time schedule. They can take recognized courses of one year in sleep medicine and/or international postgraduate diplomas or master's degrees in sleep medicine. According to AAMS/FLASS criteria, to be accredited in sleep medicine, a candidate must accredit at least two years in a recognized center in sleep medicine, attained by the accomplishment of a fellowship of one year or at least two years of part-time (2000 hours) activity. The candidate must also take a leveling course in sleep medicine accomplished by AAMS and accredit the background that makes him meritorious to pass an exam (written-multiple choice) in sleep medicine. The candidate must renew this accreditation every five years.

RESEARCH

Bernardo Houssay, Argentine scientist, Nobel Prize in medicine in 1944, an icon of the development of science and technology in Argentina, left great reflections on the subject. One of them is "Rich countries are rich because they dedicate money to scientific-technological development; poor countries continue to be so because they don't. Science is not expensive, expensive is ignorance". Even though Argentina is considered an emerging country or being realistic, a developing country, science and the academic level of science and medicine in Argentina have a great tradition: Argentina has three Nobel Awards in science (Dr. Houssay in Medicine, Dr. Leloir in Chemistry and Dr. Milstein in Medicine) and is the second country, behind Cuba, in the number of medical residents per 100,000 population. Despite the endless cyclical economic crises, the country has tried to maintain this legacy, with increasing difficulty to do so. A search for publications in indexed journals (PubMed search) shows a progressive increase in publications on sleep, probably due to the increase in interest in sleep on clinical grounds and the presentation of different classifications of sleep disorders (Fig. 1). This increase parallels the growth in other countries of LA, Canada, and the USA, with the USA being in the first positions flowed by Canada, Brazil, Mexico, Argentina, and Chile. A great disparity in the number of papers separates the first three from the other three countries, probably reflecting differences between developed and underdeveloped countries, differences or rather deficiencies in public policies in spreading knowledge to the population, and low participation in public health policies for developing sleep medicine in countries of LA.

The Argentinean Health System

Argentina is considered a developing country with 44.2% of the total people living below the poverty line [5]. The Argentinean healthcare system is excessively fragmented, mainly into three major subsectors: the public subsector, the social security subsector, and the private subsector. Such fragmentation is evidenced by the many sources of funding, different coverage services, coinsurance, and copayments applied to different systems (Fig. 2).

**Trend of annual number of indexed articles
on sleep and sleep medicine**
(PubMed search, 547 articles from 1976 to 2020)

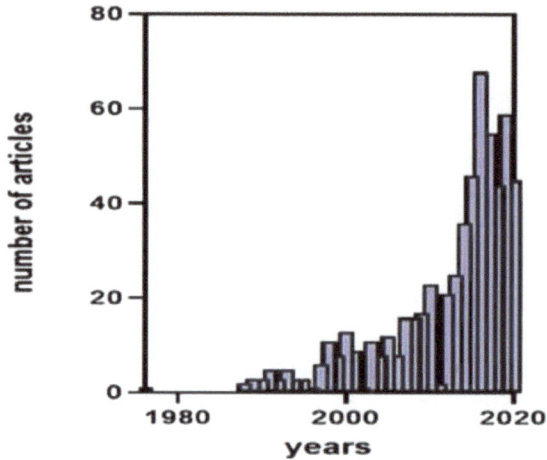

Fig. (1). The annual number of indexed articles on sleep and sleep medicine in Argentina from 1976 to 2020.

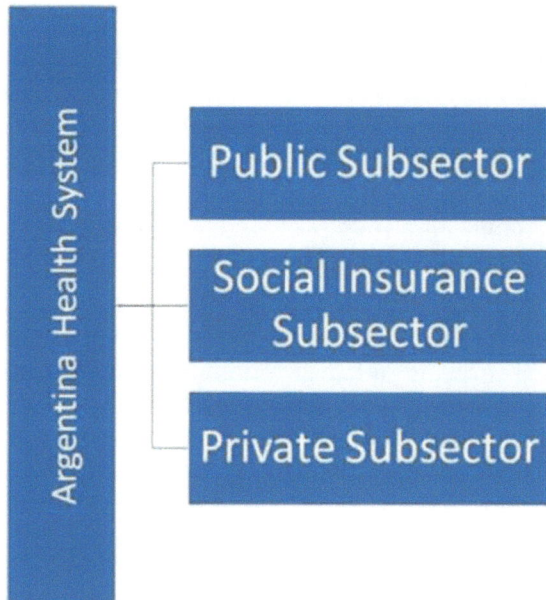

Fig. (2). Major Subsectors of the Argentinean Health System.

Fragmentation goes deeper inside each subsector: *the public subsector*, which is further fragmented at the country, province, and municipality levels, is subjected to the particular rules and regulations of the different jurisdictions. It is worth stating that half of the total population of the country lacks any social coverage, and therefore, they depend solely on the public subsector; *the social security subsector* involves four erent scenarios: 1) 285 nationwide health insurance providers covering eleven million people, including in particular, Argentinean's National Institute of Social Services for Retirees and Pensioners (a.k.a *PAMI*, an acronym in Spanish which stands for *"Plan de Atención Médica Integral"*, meaning "Comprehensive Healthcare Plan"), covering about three million inhabitants, 2) Provincial health insurance providers (one per province and one for the district of the Autonomous City of Buenos Aires), covering about five million people, 3) health insurance providers of the Security and Armed Forces, covering about eight hundred thousand people and 4) health insurance providers depending on national universities, on the judiciary and on the legislative branch of government, covering about three hundred and twenty thousand beneficiaries; *the private subsector* [6] consists of several entities providing voluntary insurance services (prepaid medical care providers), which cover about two million eight hundred thousand people. Healthcare providers depending on trade unions, the *PAMI*, and provincial healthcare providers jointly cover about 22 million people, as per the statistics made available by the Argentinean's Superintendence of Health Services.

Based on the 2010 Census (latest data available), 36% of Argentinean people lack any kind of healthcare coverage or social security service (*PAMI* and healthcare providers depending on trade unions), and they are not able to pay for any private healthcare services. They receive medical attention at public healthcare centers and hospitals.

The percentage of people receiving medical attention at public healthcare centers and hospitals throughout the country masks enormous inequalities, because there are huge disparities among provinces [7]. While less than 30% of the people in Chubut, Tierra del Fuego, and the Autonomous City of Buenos Aires lack any health insurance coverage, in the provinces of Chaco, Formosa, and Santiago del Estero, more than 50% of the people lack any health insurance coverage.

Sleep Medicine Services in Hospitals

Patients suffering from sleep disorders usually resort to different hospital services, such as neurology, pulmonology, pediatrics, otorhinolaryngology, internal medicine, and psychology (in order of frequency). Higher-complexity medical visits, diagnostic tests, manual titration of positive airway pressure, and treatment adherence and follow-up are performed at the sleep units which are only located in some hospitals. Patients are directly referred by other specialists within the same hospital, or they are referred by other hospitals or public healthcare centers.

Some pulmonology and cardiology services assess patients using validated sleep questionnaires, respiratory polygraphy tests, and auto-adjusting CPAP titration at baseline. However, if there are either any doubts about any patient's diagnostics or adherence to treatment or difficulty to conduct treatment follow-up, the patient in question is referred to sleep medicine units. The professionals working at sleep disorder units have received at least basic training on sleep medicine to be able to conduct assessments employing validated questionnaires, perform respiratory polygraphy tests and draft the resulting reports, and conduct auto-adjusting CPAP titration to initiate the relevant treatment.

Sleep medicine units are staffed with physicians specialized in sleep medicine, neurologists and/or pulmonologists who apply their expertise to the care of children and adults, EEG technicians with experience in performing Polysomnography tests (PSG) and titration with positive airway pressure devices, nursing staff, and bioengineering staff for telemedicine information technology and technical support. Sleep medicine specialist units have a patient care program that includes referrals to neurology, pulmonology, cardiology, nutrition, otorhinolaryngology, psychology, psychiatry, pediatrics, adolescence, endocrinology, and bariatric surgery. The studies conducted at sleep medicine units in hospitals are pulse oximetry, respiratory polygraphy, 6-channel EEG polysomnography for respiratory tests, and 20-channel EEG to assess the brain electrical activity in neurological pathologies, multiple sleep latency tests, split-night PSG tests, manual and auto-adjusting titration of positive airway pressure systems, end-tidal CO_2 capnography, and transcutaneous pressure of CO_2.

Adherence and follow-up of the use of positive airway pressure devices are supervised in person or *via* telemonitoring through wireless connectivity. Non-invasive mechanical ventilation (NIMV) and CPAP training are also performed. Patients who need to use ventilation devices, such as CPAP or NIMV, undergo pressure titration and proper interface testing. The required devices are requested from the health funders, if available; otherwise, the devices are requested from the relevant health authorities through the hospital's social services department, and after the devices have been granted, patients start to be trained on CPAP or NIMV with their own devices. Any treatment, studies, and devices related to sleep disorders are provided by health funders, and if a patient lacks any health coverage, the local health authorities will at all times be responsible for such treatment.

Patient treatment and follow-up are usually performed at sleep medicine units to ensure treatment adherence, provided that patients are at the training stage on NIMV devices or that their sleep pathologies require a specialist permanently, because of the difficulties in dealing with such pathologies. Any other patients showing good response to therapy and adapted to treatment are referred for follow-up to their primary care doctors, who will resort back to the sleep unit if there is any doubt.

Therefore, waiting lists for follow-up and personal appointments may be avoided because any questions may be answered by their primary care doctors, thus enabling access for first-time patients. Patients may currently make video calls with their doctors, thus avoiding waiting times in person-to-person appointments, loss of earnings, and board and lodging allowances in long-distance trips. These are some of the benefits of telemedicine with regard to sleep pathologies which are here to stay.

The sleep medicine units will be responsible for monitoring treatment compliance, maintaining the devices, restocking any disposable supplies, and replacing any necessary spare parts and interfaces of positive pressure devices. Such sleep medicine units will further any required proceedings before the health funders of patients or before the local health authority through the hospital's social services department.

Any patients who may need home mechanical ventilation will be assessed and adapted to ventilation upon startup, supervision of treatment adherence, and in-person follow-up by the sleep medicine unit in the event of hospitalization and *via* telemonitoring of home wireless connectivity. At some high-complexity hospitals with great demand for appointments, there are sleep medicine units for adults that also provide initial treatment of sleep disorders to pediatric patients, through physicians who have basic training on sleep disorders in children to provide outpatient care, report sleep studies, and initiate ventilation with positive pressure devices. However, if necessary, children may be referred to pediatric sleep units for a second opinion or to reassess the treatment effect. The care and monitoring of sleep disorder in adolescence and the transition to the adult hospital are particularly important and it needs to be properly instrumented.

Demography. The Argentinean Sleep Medicine Census of 2020

Last year we conducted with over 170 professionals the first census of professional or health workers in relation to the sleep health system in Argentina Members (82%) or nonmembers (18%) of the AAMS participated in this survey. We found that the dedication to different aspects of the sleep medicine activity was based on the following percentages from over 170 responses: clinicians 13.6%, cardiologists 0.6%, pulmonologists 34.3%, neurologists 37.9%, psychiatrists 3.6%, psychologists 1.2%, dentists 4.1%, respiratory physical therapist and sleep technicians 4.7%. 8.3% of the total reported worked with pediatrics, 60.1% with adults, and 31.5% with both pediatrics and adult patients.

The census reflects a growing field with multispecialty participation in sleep medicine. Regarding complexity for carried out studies, Level 1 in Institutions with three technicians by night involves 8% of the professionals, while Level 2 studies were performed by 33.8% and Level 3 and 4 conducted by 64.3% and 52.4%, respectively. Another question we asked was the number of rooms they have to carry out level 1 studies. The results of this question were that less than half (48.5%) reported carrying out studies in 3 or more rooms (up to 5 rooms), 46% reported a study capacity of 1 to 2 beds, and 6.5% reported having more than 5 study beds per night.

Regarding the question about the amount of CPAP equipment they have in their laboratory, 38.4% have 1 or 2 CPAP equipment, 49.4% reported having auto CPAP equipment for titling in their laboratory; 28.7% with 3 to 5 CPAP equipment, 42.6% did not have BPAP equipment, 84% did not have servo-ventilation equipment at the time of the survey.

Regarding the follow-up of patients with sleep breathing disorders requiring the use of CPAP, 39.2% used telemedicine for the follow-up of these patients.

Sleep medicine in Argentina has reached enough complexity, a fact that was demonstrated during the COVID-19 pandemic by conducting teleconsultations, studies, and treatments with protocols prepared ad-hoc.

CONCLUSION

Although the field of sleep medicine in Argentina was rapidly progressing in the past decades, it is still rather young in the field of medicine and needs much more effort to consolidate as a specialty. All this development has had little support concerning public policies partly due to ignorance and partly related to the continuous, cyclical, economic crisis in our country. The society of sleep medicine in Argentina has the responsibility to discuss and take action for these issues. As William Dement [8] states: "There is an enormous amount of good yet to be done. Let's do it!".

CONSENT FOR PUBLICATION

Not applicable.

CONFLICT OF INTEREST

The authors declare no conflict of interest, financial or otherwise.

ACKNOWLEDGEMENT

Declared none.

REFERENCES

[1] Blanco M, Kriber N, Cardinali DP. Encuesta sobre dificultades del sueño en una población urbana latinoamericana. Rev Neurol 2004; 39(2): 115-9.
[http://dx.doi.org/10.33588/rn.3902.2003649] [PMID: 15264159]

[2] Vigo DE, Cardinali DP. A diez años de la primera encuesta sobre prevalencia de alteraciones del sueño en poblaciones urbanas de América Latina: ¿Cómo dormimos los argentinos? Prensa Med Argent 2015; 101: 5.

[3] *Diagnostic Classification of Sleep and Arousal Disorders.* Prepared by the Sleep Disorders Classification Committee, Roffwarg HP. Sleep 1979; 2: 1-137.
[http://dx.doi.org/10.1093/sleep/2.1.1]

[4] Vizcarra-Escobar D, Fabián-Quillama RJ, Fernández-Gonzáles YS. Sleep societies and sleep training programs in Latin America. J Clin Sleep Med 2020; 16(6): 983-8.
[http://dx.doi.org/10.5664/jcsm.8422] [PMID: 32118575]

[5] Lavagna M, Lines PI, Viazzi MS, Costanzo M. Informes técnicos. (Technical Reports) Vol. 4, No. 181 ISSN 2545-6636 Condiciones de vida (Life Conditions). Vol. 4, No. 13 Incidencia de la pobreza y la indigencia en 31 aglomerados urbanos. Primer semestre de 2020 ISSN 2545-6660 (Incidence of poverty and indigence in 31 urban agglomerations. First Semester of 2020 ISSN 2545-6660) - National Institute of Statistics and Censuses (INDEC).

[6] Galli A, Pagés M, Swieszkowski S. Galli A, Pagés M, Swieszkowski S. El sistema de salud en Argentina. (The Argentine Health System). www.sadamweb.com.ar 2018.

[7] Arce HE. *Organización y financiamiento del sistema de salud en la Argentina MEDICINA (Buenos Aires) 2012; 72: 414-418* (The Argentine Health System: Organization and financial features. MEDICINE (Buenos Aires) 2012; 72: 414-8.

[8] Dement WC. The study of human sleep: a historical perspective. Thorax 1998; 53 (Suppl. 3): S2-7.
[PMID: 10193352]

CHAPTER 22

Sleep Medicine in Portugal

Miguel Meira e Cruz[1,2,*], **Cláudio D' Elia**[1] and **Amélia Feliciano**[1,3]

[1] *Portuguese Association of Chronobiology and Sleep Medicine, Portugal*

[2] *Sleep Unit, Centro Cardiovascular da Universidade de Lisboa, Lisbon School of Medicine, Lisbon, Portugal*

[3] *Católica Medical School, Lisbon, Portugal*

Abstract: Sleep science and sleep medicine have seen massive growth in the last century in the world, and Portugal is not an exception. In the last 20 years, we have assisted an exponential increase in sleep disorders due to the increase in obesity, lifestyle (24/7 society), massive media utilization, and individual, family, and social commitments. Simultaneously, the scientific community, population, and media have focused on sleep and sleep disorders leading to a progressive need to invest in Sleep Medicine, at the clinical, research, and educational levels.

Despite the increase in diagnostic and treatment capacity of sleep disorders, the National Health Service, and private groups still do not fulfill the real needs. Still, in Portugal, sleep and its disorders are not fully taught in pre-graduated education. Additionally, sleep medicine is not an individual medical specialty and is shared by several medical specialties, such as Pneumology, Pediatrics, Psychiatry, Neurology, Otorhinolaryngology, Maxillofacial surgeons, and Dentistry, among others. Training programs of the different clinical specialties do not offer sleep medicine even as an option being mandatory only in the pulmonology curriculum.

Considering the importance of sleep for physical, mental, and social health, the growth of sleep disorders and their individual, familiar, social, and economic impact, sleep medicine should be one of the focuses of health development and investment in this century.

This chapter focuses on the historical insights and current development of Portuguese Sleep Science and Sleep Medicine fields.

Keywords: Insomnia, Multiple Sleep Latency Test, Polysomnography, Public health system, Sleep therapies, Sleep medicine, Sleep apnea.

---

* **Corresponding author Miguel Meira e Cruz:** Portuguese Association of Chronobiology and Sleep Medicine, Portugal; Tel/Fax: +351217781714; Email: mcruz@medicina.ulisboa.pt

Hrayr P. Attarian, Marie-Louise M. Coussa-Koniski & Alain Michel Sabri (Eds.)

DEMOGRAPHIC AND GEOPOLITICAL DATA

Portugal is a country located on the Iberian Peninsula, in southwestern Europe. It has the twelfth biggest population (10.145 million inhabitants) and the thirteenth largest territory (92 211.9 km^2) in the European Union [1].

Portugal has been a member of the European Union since 1986. In 1999, it was one of the founding members of the euro area. The economy of Portugal was ranked 34th in the World Economic Forum's Global Competitiveness Report in 2019 [1].

The official language is Portuguese. The Portuguese language is widely diffused across the world. The community of Portuguese Language Countries has nine member states on four continents, including Brazil (with around 210 million inhabitants) and Angola (around 25 million inhabitants) [1].

The local authorities in mainland Portugal are 3092 parishes, within 308 municipalities, within 5 administrative regions. The constitution enshrines the principle of administrative decentralization and the financial autonomy of local authorities. The tasks of municipalities and parishes are associated with the fulfillment of the needs of local communities, for example regarding socio-economic development, spatial planning, utilities, sewage collection, culture, the environment, *etc* [1].

Portugal has two autonomous regions, namely the Azores and Madeira. By the reason of their geographical, economic, social, and cultural characteristics and the island populations' historic aspirations, they are granted a specific form of autonomous organization. They enjoy extensive legislative powers and define their own policies [1].

PORTUGUESE PUBLIC HEALTH SYSTEM

The Portuguese National Health Service (NHS) is the set of institutions and services, which are dependent on the Ministry of Health, warranting access to health care for all citizens, within the limits of human, technical and financial resources available [2].

It is a service whose core features are to be:

A. Universal and provide comprehensive global care or guarantee its provision.

B. Tendentially free, considering the economic conditions of the citizens.

C. Fairness, mitigating the effects of economic, geographic and any other inequalities in access to care, aiming to ensure the implementation of the state's responsibility in providing health care to individuals, family and to the community [2].

The traditional dichotomy between primary and differentiated health care proved to be not only incorrect, from a medical point of view, but also a source of dysfunctions, from an organizational point of view. Hence, the creation of integrated healthcare units which enable the essential articulation between personalized groups of primary care health centers and hospitals [2].

The growing demands of populations in terms of quality and readiness to respond to their health concerns and needs suggested that the management of resources should be made as close as possible to their recipients. Hence the creation of Health Regions, operated by administrations with decentralized competencies and attributions.

In Portugal, there are 5 health regions:

1. North, headquartered in Oporto

2. Center, in Coimbra

3. Lisbon and Tagus Valley, in Lisbon

4. Alentejo, in Évora

5. Algarve, in Faro

Regional Health Administration (RHA) is responsible for planning, distributing resources, guiding, and coordinating activities, managing human resources, technical and administrative support, as well as evaluating the functioning of institutions and services providing health care [2].

A Local Health System (LHS) is a set of health resources, articulated and organized according to a geographic-population criterion, implemented both in urban and rural areas, responsible for the care to be provided to individuals, families, and social groups, with the ability to coordinate available resources.

An LHS is made up of the set of:

1. Health Centers

2. Hospitals

3. Other services and public or private institutions, whether for profit or not, with direct or indirect intervention in the health domain.

The articulation aims to facilitate access, ensure the referral of clinical information, promote the professionals' qualification and the evaluation of provided services. As a result, the reduction of bureaucracy, the elimination of unnecessary or duplicated acts or the negative replacement of care (hospital centrism) is achieved [2].

The statistical data on health in Portugal in 2016 [3], obtained in the context of the National Statistical System is a large and very detailed dataset allowing for the following conclusions:

• There were 225 hospitals in Portugal, most hospitals were private (114 private hospitals, 107 public hospitals, and 2 hospitals in public-private partnership);

• However, the majority of beds available for hospitalization were in public hospitals (of a total of 35.3 thousand beds, 22.4 thousand were available in public hospitals, 11.3 thousand in private hospitals and 1.7 thousand in public-private partnership hospitals);

• By the end of 2016, the number of persons employed in hospitals accounted for 24.003 doctors, 39.670 nurses, 8.800 diagnosis and therapeutic technicians and 5.626 high technical professionals;

• The majority (68.6%) of doctors working in hospitals were specialist doctors, and the majority (85.8%) of nurses working in hospitals were generalist nurses;

• In the year under review, there were 50.239 doctors certified by the Portuguese Medical Association. The number of doctors per thousand inhabitants was 4.9. There were 9.177 dentists certified by the Medical Dentist Association, and the number of dentists per thousand inhabitants was 0.9.

The diseases of the circulatory system and the malignant neoplasms remained the two mains underlying causes of death in Portugal in 2016 [3].

SLEEP EDUCATION AND KNOWLEDGE DIFFUSION IN PORTUGAL

In Portugal, Sleep Medicine is recognized as a medical competency by the Portuguese Medical Association rather than a specialty. Sleep Medicine is however not included in general medical curricula and there are few fully pedagogic programs with a focus on sleep science and sleep health in postgraduate education. Medical School of Lisbon (University of Lisbon) was a pioneer in developing the first European Postgraduate Course on sleep medicine, designated as a Master in sleep science. The Post Graduated Program on chronobiology and sleep medicine is currently the leadership model in extensive sleep medicine education in Portugal. This post graduate program started in 2016 and is co-organized by CESPU, the European Sleep Center and Portuguese Association of Chronobiology and Sleep Medicine (APCMS). In 2020, the Portuguese Catholic University started a post-graduation in sleep psychology developed by the psychology department of this university. Another advancing postgraduate course is the Sleep Training Course: Medical and Technical aspects of Sleep Medicine organized by Instituto de Ciências da Saúde (Universidade Católica Portuguesa) that received the scientific sponsor of the European Research Sleep Society, European Society of Sleep Technologists, and several Portuguese Sleep Societies (Associação Portuguesa do Sono, Associação Portuguesa de Cronobiologia e Medicina do Sono, Associação Portuguesa de Técnicos de Neurofisiologia, Associação Portuguesa de Cardiopnneumologistas). Several other clinical and university-based institutions with a scope of practice in the sleep medicine field often offer some short courses with a distinct focus but mainly on sleep-disordered breathing.

The Portuguese Sleep Association (APS) has made several efforts to promote short courses to increase the objective of giving to the clinicians a capacity of detecting, diagnosing, and effectively treating sleep disorders in primary care and specialized centers. The Portuguese Sleep Societies, mainly APCMS and APS, the leading institutions representing sleep medicine practitioners and researchers are committed to spread the awareness and standardization of knowledge on the field together with university centers in Lisbon, Porto, and Coimbra. From the strict medical sleep medicine practice to the oral sleep medicine field as well as education strategies for technicians, psychologists and other professions with interest in sleep, since 2018 APCMS promotes an annual event providing a theoretical agenda and clinical workshops directed to different topics with interest and including renowned international speakers attended by an estimated number of 400 participants.

Additionally in Portugal, healthcare professionals working in the sleep field, such as physicians, technicians, and sleep scientists, have been looking for European certification in this area. This certification is possible by the European Sleep Research Society, through an examination for Sleep Experts – Somnologist and Somnologist-Technologist, and that has been occurring since 2012 for physicians and since 2014 for technicians. There are few qualified professionals in this field. Until now, 708 European physicians and 191 European technicians obtained this certification, and many of them are Portuguese professionals.

EPIDEMIOLOGICAL DATA ON SLEEP DISORDERS

There is a lack of robust epidemiological studies in Portugal.

SPECIALIZATION IN THE FIELD OF SLEEP MEDICINE

In Portugal, a medical degree takes 6 years, including a master's degree, ever since the Bologna Agreement of 2009. After this, and according to the Portuguese Medical Association (Ordem dos Médicos), one must complete 1 year of fully supervised clinical practice to be able to practice medicine. During this period, junior doctors rotate through several different medical and chirurgical specialties, after which and according to their grade on a national examination, they chose a specialty and location.

The Professional Area of Specialization is the field of technical-scientific differentiation that requires between 4 and 6 years (depending on the specialties) for the progressive acquisition of skills and a gradual increase in autonomy and responsibilities. The training follows a program prepared by the Specialty College, usually divided into a set of mandatory and optional internships subject to evaluation. To be recognized as a specialist, the intern doctor is submitted to a final exam, which involves a curricular test, a practical test and a theoretical test.

Sleep Medicine was recognized as competence by the Portuguese College of Physicians about 8 years ago. The main objectives were the elaboration of normative documents to allow the certification of Sleep Study Laboratories and Sleep Medicine Centers based on European guidelines.

There is still no specific Specialization Program in Sleep Medicine in Portugal, although criteria have been established for obtaining an expertise title that recognizes technical-professionals' qualifications common to some specialties and that can be obtained by any doctor. It is awarded after a curriculum assessment or examination whose contents were approved in 2018.

Physicians and dentists often begin their specialization path in postgraduate master's or doctoral programs in our country or abroad. The first sleep laboratory in Portugal in accordance with international recommendations, in 1987, and the first worldwide Master's in Sleep Sciences, in 2005, were coordinated by Professor Teresa Paiva. There is one extensive (1 year) postgraduate training in chronobiology and sleep medicine, coordinated by Dr. Miguel Meira e Cruz, in a joint organization between CESPU and European Sleep Center and supported by the Portuguese Association of Chronobiology and Sleep Medicine aiming to provide knowledge and practical skills in areas of chronobiology, physiology and sleep medicine, allowing students to be prepared for research purposes and, depending on their basic training, to integrate validated approaches and therapeutic models into their clinical activity and in accordance with the acquired skills.

The Portuguese Respiratory Training curriculum was updated in 2016, considering the impact of sleep medicine in clinical practice. Hence, a 3-month period exclusively dedicated to the diagnosis and treatment of sleep breathing disorders, with a dedication to obstructive sleep apnea, was included.

REQUIREMENTS FOR ACKNOWLEDGMENT OF COMPETENCE IN SLEEP MEDICINE

Without prejudice to the recognition of specialist titles and corresponding training, obtained by citizens of the Member States of the European Union and of the signatory States of the Agreement on the European Economic Area, under the terms of the applicable legislation, for the purposes of obtaining the title of competence in Sleep Medicine, a curriculum and exam assessments are required since there is no approved postgraduate specialization program.

The curriculum evaluation is carried out by the Board of the College of Competence in Sleep Medicine according to the criteria:

1 – The candidate must be registered with the Portuguese College of Physicians.

2 – The candidate must have a minimum period equivalent to 12 months in a full-time work regime in an accredited Sleep Medicine Center or equivalent, with full responsibilities. In cases where the specialty offers training in sleep medicine, depending on the degree of exposure, this period can be reduced to a time of not less than 6 months.

3 - Written statement, prepared by the Director of the Sleep Medicine Center (SMC) or equivalent where the training took place indicating the full and autonomous performance of the following functions:

a) Performing complete polysomnography (PSG) in 30 patients;

b) Staging, interpretation and reporting of 100 PSGs, including a spectrum of neurological, cardiorespiratory and psychiatric diseases in adults and children;

c) Complete Multiple Sleep Latency Test (MSLT) / Maintenance of Wakefulness Test (TMV) in 10 patients;

d) When applicable, 50 outpatient type 3 cardiorespiratory polygraphies;

e) Interpretation of relevant questionnaires and sleep diaries;

f) Familiarization with all techniques performed by technicians;

g) Experience in the follow-up of 100 patients with sleep/wake disorders, including cases of each of the following pathologies: sleep-disordered breathing, their treatment with continuous positive pressure, other intrinsic sleep disorders and sleep disorders secondary to physical and mental illnesses;

The knowledge assessment exam will consist of a test of 100 questions with 5 alternatives and a single correct answer, with 2 hours duration, which will focus on:

PHYSIOLOGICAL BASES OF SLEEP

- Physiology of sleep and wakefulness as a function of age;

- Age-dependent sleep regulation;

- Models of sleep ontogeny and biological function;

- Electroencephalographic activity during wakefulness and sleep and sleep staging;

- Usefulness and limitations of different sleep staging methodologies;

- Regulation of functional systems during sleep:

• Brain activity

• Motor control of skeletal muscles

• Sensation

• Autonomic nervous system activity

• Cardiac and circulatory function

• Respiratory function

• Metabolic activity

• Hormonal secretion

• Thermoregulation

• Effects of acute and chronic sleep deprivation

• Neuronal processes during REM (rapid eye movement) and non-REM sleep in sleep onset and on waking up: *e.g.* reflex activity, classic dreams, vivid dreams, nightmares, hypnagogic and hypnopompic hallucinations.

CHRONOBIOLOGICAL ASPECTS OF SLEEP

- Circadian rhythm, biological clock, and its influence on circadian rhythms such as temperature and various physiological functions;

- Chronobiological models of sleep regulation;

- Circadian variation of cognitive performance;

- Variation of tiredness and sleepiness during the day;

- Methods of recording variations, depending on time, drowsiness and alertness;

- Circadian rhythm disorders - diagnosis and treatment.

DIAGNOSIS AND ASSESSMENT PROCEDURES FOR SLEEP DISORDERS

- Ability to perform clinical history and psychological assessment (interview and examination);

- Adequate knowledge of the diagnostic approach to the diseases listed in ICSD-3

- Mastery of diagnostic procedures, including:

• PSG

• Cardiorespiratory polygraphy

• MSLT and MWT

• Sleep/Wake Questionnaires

• Basic knowledge about other diagnostic tests, such as neuropsychological tests

TREATMENT OF SLEEP DISORDERS

- Sleep hygiene;

- Influence of medication on sleep;

- Drug treatment for sleep disorders;

- Cognitive-behavioral therapy and other psychotherapy procedures;

- Nasal CPAP and other non-invasive ventilation modes;

- Surgical procedures;

- Mandibular advancement prosthesis;

- Phototherapy.

MANAGING A SMC

- The candidate must master the principles of managing a SMC and be familiar with the requirements relating to personnel and logistics.

DIAGNOSIS OF SLEEP DISORDERS

There is a lack of epidemiological studies in Portugal. Clinical practice shows that insomnia, obstructive sleep apnea, sleep deprivation and sleep-related movement disorders are the main sleep disorders in Portugal.

The approach of sleep patients starts with structured anamnesis and clinical evaluation, complemented by questionnaires and several objective diagnostic methods. Sleep diary consists of daily self-reported sleep habits and sleep-wake schedule, being important in assessing sleep patterns.

In terms of questionnaires, the Epworth Sleepiness Scale [4] and Stanford Sleepiness Scale [5] are the ones most used to assess excessive daytime sleepiness. The Berlin Questionnaire [6] and the Stop and the Stop-Bang Questionnaires [7], are used as quick and inexpensive screening tools for OSA. The Insomnia Severity Index [8, 9] and the Pittsburgh Sleep Quality Index [10] are the ones mostly used for Insomnia. In circadian rhythm disorders, the Morningness-Eveningness Questionnaire [11] is used and in restless legs syndrome RLS Screening Questionnaire [12] is used and the International Restless Legs Syndrome Study Group rating scale is used for RLS [13]. Some questionnaires are used to evaluate psychological states such as mood (anxiety and depression scales), such as Beck Depression Inventory [14] and General Anxiety Disorder 7-item [15]. Other questionnaires can also be used in specific settings or for research purposes.

In terms of objective evaluation, sleep services can offer polysomnography (type I and II), sleep polygraphy, actigraphy [16], MSLT and MWT [17]. Additionally, laboratory tests such as blood and urine analysis, and hormone determinations (such as melatonin) [18] can be prescribed. Globally the indications to prescribe these exams are those established by the American Academy of Sleep Medicine and European Sleep Research Society [19]. With respect to the diagnostic criteria of sleep disorders, Portugal used the criteria established by the 2014 ICSD-3. In

terms of scoring sleep and events those established in The AASM Manual for the Scoring of Sleep and Associated Events version 2.6 are used [20].

PRACTICE GUIDELINES - TREATMENT OF MAJOR SLEEP DISORDERS IN THE COUNTRY

The standard treatment (pharmacological and non-pharmacological) for sleep disorders follows the international indications published in Sleep Medicine Textbook, 2nd Edition, ESRS [21].

USE OF INTERNET TECHNOLOGIES

In occidental European countries most people cannot think of living without the internet. Everyone uses the internet as a multifunction tool for several contexts of daily lives.

The growth of the use of consumer sleep technologies included into cell phones or similar wearables give coarse information concerning sleep-wake cycles. Although, this information has alerted the community for the importance of sleep and can be used as an educational tool to warn the importance of healthy sleep habits.

In the last 5 years, especially since COVID-19 pandemic, we have assisted the growth of Telemedicine in Portugal applied to sleep medicine. In Portugal, urgently to reduce the underdiagnosis of sleep disorders, public and private health services have organized to offer on-line consultations specially in the first sleep evaluation and in stable patients under chronic treatment. Also, patients under nocturnal ventilation, have been followed in some centers with the help of new technologies, which allow downloading ventilation data helping monitor treatment.

It is important to regulate and define the clinical areas to perform Telemedicine in the sleep field. As said before, Portugal is a heterogeneous country in terms of sleep facilities and Telemedicine, if proper regulated and applied, is a quick and cheaper way to reach more and more sleep patients, facilitating diagnostic approach and therapeutic follow-up.

The use of the internet and wearable technologies to facilitate diagnosis are under development and not ready for clinical application.

MAIN AREAS OF BASIC AND CLINICAL SLEEP RESEARCH

Portugal has several sleep researchers and some of them are organized in small groups. The research is mainly focused on clinical approach and treatment, especially in OSA, insomnia and chronobiology. Basic sleep research is scarce.

The main areas for continuing basic and clinical research should be as follows: improving classification and diagnosis of sleep disorders based on more epidemiological studies involving different countries; predicting disease and treatment prognosis by creating clinical algorithms; characterizing disease subtypes, phenotypes and endotypes, to construct a practical personalized medicine; improving sleep scoring *via* automation to reduce time-consuming exams; leveraging nightly PAP downloads for improved adherence support and intervention. Additionally, an important area to invest in is to reduce the gap between the number of people with sleep disorders and those appropriately treated.

In terms of research, the focus should be better understanding the basic functions of sleep, modulation of sleep as a clinical intervention for improving cognition, mood, and longevity, the role of artificial intelligence in Sleep Medicine and the role and regulation of telemedicine.

CHALLENGES AND FINAL CONSIDERATIONS

The challenges of Sleep Medicine for this century will be at clinical, educational and research levels.

At the clinical level, the most challenging is to diagnose and treat most patients with sleep disorders. For that accomplishment will be necessary certified and qualified sleep professionals working at certified and qualified sleep centers, without major limitations in human and physical resources. Also, it is necessary to develop cheaper and friendlier diagnostic tools with less timing consuming applications and reading. Also, it is urgent to bet on preventive sleep medicine, based on population education. The "voice" of sleep professionals should reach the governments to review some critical issues such as shift work, rest-protected time, school and work schedules, teleworking jobs, among others.

At the education level, it is important to bet on pre- and post-graduate in Sleep Medicine with UpToDate programs, more diversified and certified courses accessible for all health sleep professionals.

At the research level, the focus for this century should be on better understanding the basic mechanisms of sleep, the pathophysiological processes of sleep disorders, biomarkers of sleep and its disorders and respective application for diagnosis and treatment response and follow-up, personalized medicine with real clinical application.

Sleep science and sleep medicine should have no frontiers. A multi and an interdisciplinary approach are the necessary options for knowledge and practical evolution in the sleep field.

CONCLUSION

Although the current perspective of sleep medicine should be viewed as integrative within a broad field of action, an essential matrix should exist requiring infrastructures, human resources, education and qualification standards as well as health policies converging on preventive measures against common sleep disruptors often prevailing in modern societies.

By its history, geography, culture and socio-economic status within Europe and the standards comparable to the global developed countries, Portugal should manage in order to achieve major goals regarding the successful implementation of sleep medicine practice. This would involve major educational and strategic political interventions and would be required in the near future.

LIST OF ABBREVIATIONS

NHS   National Health Service

RHA   Regional Health Administrations

LHS   Local Health System

SMC   Sleep Medicine Center

PSG   polysomnography

MSLT Multiple Sleep Latency Test

CONSENT FOR PUBLICATION

Not applicable.

CONFLICT OF INTEREST

The authors declare no conflict of interest, financial or otherwise.

ACKNOWLEDGEMENT

Declared none.

REFERENCES

[1]   Kołodziejski M. Research for REGI Committee - Economic, social and territorial situation of Portugal. 2019.   Available   at: https://www.europarl.europa.eu/RegData/etudes/BRIE/2019/629190/IPOL_BRI(2019)629190_EN.pdf

[2]   Rodrigues LAC, Ed. Compreender os Recursos Humanos do Serviço Nacional de Saúde. Lisboa: Edições Colibri Publishing 2002.

[3]   2018.https://www.ine.pt/xurl/pub/277095050

[4]   Johns MW. A new method for measuring daytime sleepiness: the Epworth sleepiness scale. Sleep 1991; 14(6): 540-5.
        [http://dx.doi.org/10.1093/sleep/14.6.540] [PMID: 1798888]

[5]   MacLean AW, Fekken GC, Saskin P, Knowles JB. Psychometric evaluation of the Stanford Sleepiness Scale. J Sleep Res 1992; 1(1): 35-9.
        [http://dx.doi.org/10.1111/j.1365-2869.1992.tb00006.x] [PMID: 10607023]

[6]   Netzer NC, Stoohs RA, Netzer CM, Clark K, Strohl KP. Using the Berlin Questionnaire to identify patients at risk for the sleep apnea syndrome. Ann Intern Med 1999; 131(7): 485-91.
        [http://dx.doi.org/10.7326/0003-4819-131-7-199910050-00002] [PMID: 10507956]

[7]   Patel D, Tsang J, Saripella A, *et al.* Validation of the STOP questionnaire as a screening tool for OSA among different populations: a systematic review and meta-regression analysis. J Clin Sleep Med 2022; 18(5): 1441-53.
        [http://dx.doi.org/10.5664/jcsm.9820] [PMID: 34910625]

[8]   Bastien C, Vallières A, Morin CM. Validation of the Insomnia Severity Index as an outcome measure for insomnia research. Sleep Med 2001; 2(4): 297-307.
        [http://dx.doi.org/10.1016/S1389-9457(00)00065-4] [PMID: 11438246]

[9]   Yang M, Morin CM, Schaefer K, Wallenstein GV. Interpreting score differences in the Insomnia Severity Index: using health-related outcomes to define the minimally important difference. Curr Med Res Opin 2009; 25(10): 2487-94.
        [http://dx.doi.org/10.1185/03007990903167415] [PMID: 19689221]

[10]   Buysse DJ, Reynolds CF III, Monk TH, Berman SR, Kupfer DJ. The Pittsburgh sleep quality index: A new instrument for psychiatric practice and research. Psychiatry Res 1989; 28(2): 193-213.
        [http://dx.doi.org/10.1016/0165-1781(89)90047-4] [PMID: 2748771]

[11]   Horne JA, Ostberg O. A self-assessment questionnaire to determine morningness-eveningness in human circadian rhythms. Int J Chronobiol 1976; 4(2): 97-110.
        [PMID: 1027738]

[12]   Kohnen R, Allen RP, Benes H, *et al.* Assessment of restless legs syndrome—Methodological approaches for use in practice and clinical trials. Mov Disord 2007; 22(S18) (Suppl. 18): S485-94.
        [http://dx.doi.org/10.1002/mds.21588] [PMID: 17534967]

[13]   Walters AS, LeBrocq C, Dhar A, *et al.* Validation of the International Restless Legs Syndrome Study Group rating scale for restless legs syndrome. Sleep Med 2003; 4(2): 121-32.
        [http://dx.doi.org/10.1016/S1389-9457(02)00258-7] [PMID: 14592342]

[14]   Beck AT. WARD CH, MENDELSON M, MOCK J, ERBAUGH J. An inventory for measuring depression. Arch Gen Psychiatry 1961; 4(6): 561-71.
        [http://dx.doi.org/10.1001/archpsyc.1961.01710120031004]

[15]   Spitzer RL, Kroenke K, Williams JBW, Löwe B. A brief measure for assessing generalized anxiety

disorder: the GAD-7. Arch Intern Med 2006; 166(10): 1092-7.
[http://dx.doi.org/10.1001/archinte.166.10.1092] [PMID: 16717171]

[16]   Smith MT, McCrae CS, Cheung J, *et al.* Use of Actigraphy for the Evaluation of Sleep Disorders and Circadian Rhythm Sleep-Wake Disorders: An American Academy of Sleep Medicine Systematic Review, Meta-Analysis, and GRADE Assessment. J Clin Sleep Med 2018; 14(7): 1209-30.
[http://dx.doi.org/10.5664/jcsm.7228] [PMID: 29991438]

[17]   Krahn LE, Arand DL, Avidan AY, *et al.* Recommended protocols for the Multiple Sleep Latency Test and Maintenance of Wakefulness Test in adults: guidance from the American Academy of Sleep Medicine. J Clin Sleep Med 2021; 17(12): 2489-98.
[http://dx.doi.org/10.5664/jcsm.9620] [PMID: 34423768]

[18]   Kazemi R, Motamedzade M, Golmohammadi R, Mokarami H, Hemmatjo R, Heidarimoghadam R. Field Study of Effects of Night Shifts on Cognitive Performance, Salivary Melatonin, and Sleep. Saf Health Work 2018; 9(2): 203-9.
[http://dx.doi.org/10.1016/j.shaw.2017.07.007] [PMID: 29928535]

[19]   Mathis J, de Lacy S, Roth C, Hill EA. Measuring: Chapter B3: Monitoring sleep and wakefulness.Sleep Medicine Textbook. 2nd ed. European Sleep Research Society 2021; pp. 181-200.

[20]   Berry R, Quan S, Abreu A, *et al.* AASM Manual for the Scoring of Sleep and Associated Events Version 2.6. AASM 2020.

[21]   Bassetti C, McNicholas W, Paunio T, Peigneux P, Eds. Sleep Medicine Textbook. 2nd ed., European Sleep Research Society 2021.

CHAPTER 23

Sleep Medicine in Austria

Rainer Popovic[1,*], **Michael T. Saletu**[2] and **Reinhold Kerbl**[3]

[1] *Department of Internal Medicine, Franziskusspital, 1050 Wien, Austria*

[2] *Department of Sleep Medicine, State Hospital Graz II, Location South, 8036 Graz, Austria*

[3] *Department of Pediatrics and Adolescent Medicine, LKH Hochsteiermark, 8900 Leoben, Austria*

Abstract: Austria has had a long tradition of sleep and dream science since Sigmund Freund published his psychoanalytic theory of personality at the turn of the twentieth century. Sleep medicine today, however, is a multidisciplinary specialization and training in Austria lasts about 18 months. Exploring the impact of sleep on daily activity, Austrian scientists are especially interested in the role of sleep disorders as an independent risk factor for neurological, psychiatric, and vascular diseases and their therapeutic management.

When the Austrian Sleep Research Association (ASRA) was founded in 1991, CPAP therapy for sleep apnea had already celebrated its 10th birthday and had become a standard therapy covered by all public health insurance. Quite in contrast, in the field of insomnia, cognitive behavioral therapy for insomnia (CBT-I) has been established in international therapy guidelines, but for sleep-disturbed patients, affordable rapid access to this therapeutic option is still a challenge in our country.

Since 1998, the ASRA has been offering voluntary accreditation based on a quality check process to sleep centers. More recently, a sleep training plan was introduced to obtain a sleep physician diploma by the Austrian Medical Chamber.

Keywords: Board certification, Cognitive behavioral therapy (CBT-I), CPAP adherence, Home sleep apnea testing (HSAT), Insomnia, LORETA, Neuroimaging, Quality management, Memory consolidation, Narcolepsy, Parasomnia, Practice guidelines, Reimbursement, SIESTA project, Sleep apnea, Sleep center, Sleep coaching, Sleep specialist, Sleep staging, Telemedicine.

INTRODUCTION

Sleep Medicine is a heterogeneous area that plays a role in a number of clinical disciplines such as neurology, psychiatry, pulmonology, pediatrics, internal medicine, ENT, and psychology.

* **Corresponding author Rainer Popovic:** Department of Internal Medicine, Franziskusspital, Nikolsdorfer Gasse 32, 1050 Wien, Austria; E-mail: office@medis.at

Hrayr P. Attarian, Marie-Louise M. Coussa-Koniski & Alain Michel Sabri (Eds.)

Compared to Germany and other western European states, Austria is a small country, which counts approximately 9 million inhabitants and covers an area of about 84.000 square kilometers. The capital is Vienna with about 1.7 million inhabitants. Statistics show that about 14.4 percent of Austria's total population is between 0 and 14 years of age, and 19 percent are 65 years and older. Life expectancy at birth is roughly 82 years. In 2016, on average some 1.898 million people (~ 22.1% of the population) with foreign background were living in Austria. The gross domestic product (GDP) per capita is about 50 000 USD, constantly increasing.

CURRENT PRACTICE OF SLEEP MEDICINE

Patients face three main problems in sleep medicine. First, they don't know what is normal, and what can be done. Second, they get used to their problems and accept them by ignoring the symptoms, or regarding them as age-dependent. And finally, especially nonorganic insomnia needs to be treated individually by cognitive behavioral therapy. This is often a very time-consuming process, which is not adequately covered by insurance. Thus, patients often just receive symptomatic hypnotic drug therapy. However, GPs are not very well educated in sleep medicine. They generally do not attend sleep meetings, which are designed for specialists. The reason is not a lack of interest, but a lack of time, as their daily routine is very time-consuming, especially in rural areas. GPs usually prescribe medication for acute insomnia or continue prescribing drugs following a specialist's recommendations.

If serious problems persist, the patient will be assigned to a specialist. If the primary sleep complaint is insomnia, hypersomnia, or a sleep-related movement disorder, they will be referred to a psychiatrist or neurologist. The situation is quite different with sleep-related breathing disorders. In case of snoring or signs of sleep-disordered breathing, patients are mainly sent to a pulmonologist or an ENT specialist. If polysomnography (PSG) is necessary, the patient will be referred to a specialized sleep center. But there are long waiting lists for PSG. Although CPAP is an efficient therapy, some patients do not consider it an attractive option and require motivation/coaching to get used to it.

As most diagnostic and therapeutic procedures are covered by the public health insurance system, access to medical testing and treatment is no problem in Austria. The bottleneck, however, is to find the best specialist and to be patient if you are on a waiting list. It is obvious that specialists are concentrated in big cities and there is a lack of them in rural areas. And considering being a farmer who cannot leave his place when it is time to harvest or feed the cows, there are still limitations concerning access to health care and considerable differences between employees and self-employed or between people living in the country and the urban population.

Currently, we have around sixty sleep centers in Austria. They are usually run by a public hospital, and investigations are covered by public health insurance. Most of them focus mainly on the management of sleep-disordered breathing. About half of them have voluntarily undergone a quality check procedure and have been accredited by the ASRA. Direct referral by GPs is not intended, but possible. As waiting lists for a PSG are very long, the ASRA primarily recommends patients to see a specialist, who then decides if a PSG is necessary. If sleep apnea is suspected, a home sleep apnea testing (HSAT) is recommended, also to assess the urgency of treatment needed. Waiting time for a polysomnography (PSG) is 4-6 months or more.

Due to Covid 19 restrictions, all patients must be tested before admission to a hospital. The patient referred for PSG shows up in the afternoon and leaves the next morning. Results are then discussed with the patient later by phone, telemedicine, or in person if necessary. As many patients do not speak German quite well, the biggest problem is language barriers. Thus, it is much easier to explain the results and therapeutic options in person.

To become a sleep technician, you have to undergo specific training and acquire also technical knowledge at College for Biomedical Analytics, whereas nurses working in sleep centers do not have this special education and need to be trained onsite.

The cooperation with homecare providers (HCP) in Austria is quite good. Nevertheless, therapy options for sleep apnea like oral appliances or hypoglossal nerve stimulation are not covered on a regular base.

Home sleep apnea testing is provided by a number of specialists like pulmonologists, ENT or sleep medicine specialists and is thus more easily accessible compared to standard inpatient polysomnography. Sleep laboratories are usually centered in cities, whereas outpatient HSAT can be conducted almost anywhere. Actigraphy is available only in specialized sleep centers and is not covered by health insurance.

CPAP devices can only be prescribed by a sleep center and are covered by public health insurance. They can be bought or rented. However, for continued coverage, healthcare providers ask for compliance data. Compliance is usually very good once the patient has come to accept the device, and people feel better using the CPAP on a regular basis. In my office, the non-responder rate over time is less than 5%, and low responders are between 10% to 20%. The reasons for this good compliance are regular patient visits and cost coverage by health insurance. Moreover, it also has to do with the correct indication and clinical symptoms before starting therapy.

HEALTH CARE SYSTEM

Austria has a two-tier health care system in which virtually all individuals receive publicly funded care, but also have the option to purchase supplementary private health insurance. In the international ranking by the WHO in the mid-2000s, the Austrian healthcare system earned the 9th place. In 2015, the cost of health care was 11.2% of the GDP -the fifth highest in Europe. Still, one of the key weaknesses of the Austrian healthcare system is the prevention of illness.

The Austrian health care system provides universal coverage for a wide range of benefits and high-quality care. Free choice of providers and unrestricted access to all care levels (general practitioners, specialist physicians and hospitals) are characteristic features of the system. Hospitals and clinics can be either state-run or privately run. Care involving private insurance plans (sometimes referred to as "comfort class" care) can include more flexible visiting hours and private rooms and doctors. Some individuals choose to completely pay for their health care privately [1].

Enrollment in the public health care system is generally automatic and is linked to employment. However, insurance is also guaranteed to co-insured persons (i.e. spouses and dependents), pensioners, students, the disabled, and those receiving unemployment benefits. Enrollment is compulsory, and it is not possible to cross-shop the various social security institutions. Employers register their employees with the correct institution and deduct the health insurance fee from employees' salaries. Some people, such as the self-employed, are not automatically enrolled but are eligible to enroll in the public health insurance scheme. The cost of public insurance is based on income and is not related to individual medical history or risk factors.

Prescription medication is commonly available and, if indicated, paid for by health insurance. Quite in contrast to medication, cognitive behavioral therapy (CBT) as a therapeutic option for insomnia and/or comorbid psychiatric disorders is much less easily accessible. Health apps for CBT are becoming increasingly popular but are not covered by insurance.

AUSTRIAN SLEEP RESEARCH ASSOCIATION

The Austrian Sleep Research Association (ASRA, ÖGSM) is the only professional society in Austria aiding and offering education in the management of sleep disorders. Sleep medicine is not an established (sub)specialty by the Austrian Medical Chamber (AMC). Our association is therefore constituted as a nonprofit organization. The body is formed by an executive committee and a scientific board, where all disciplines are represented.

The ASRA was founded in October 1991, shortly after the first founding meeting of the World Federation of Sleep Research Societies in Cannes. The scientific goal was to explore sleep and its disturbances. The first scientific meeting dealt with the „Diagnosis and Treatment of Patients with Sleep Apnea-Syndrome". At this time, we were counting 20 members.

The following scientific meetings were held annually, with one exception: Our meeting in 2020 was cancelled due to the Corona SARS-CoV-2 pandemic. In 2021, we performed our first virtual annual meeting. Starting in 2018, our most ambitious aim was to modernize the structure of our society. First, we had to completely renew our internet presence, starting with member administration, then we increased the scientific and administrative content, and finally started offering e-learning. Shortly, accreditation terms for sleep labs will be adapted, and structured training for sleep medicine will be established.

Currently, we have about 120 members with growing numbers including physicians, psychologists, dentists, and sleep technicians. Membership costs are low (about 40 €/year), depending on the training status.

The first initiatives for a special "day of sleep" were observed in the German-speaking countries as early as in 1999. In Austria (as well as in Greece or China) it was celebrated on March 21 (keyword "spring fatigue"). In order to achieve a greater international impact, the internet platform "World Sleep Day" (http://Worldsleepday.org) was created. Since 2008, all national activities related to the "Day of Sleep" can be reported and presented there. Since 2011, the ASRA has been holding regular press conferences in Vienna on "World Sleep Day". The broad media coverage of these events proves again and again how great the public's interest in sleep-related topics is.

The regulation concerning driving licenses in Austria for persons with moderate or severe obstructive sleep apnea syndrome (OSAS) (apnea/hypopnea frequency >15/h associated with sleepiness) was changed and became effective on September 1, 2016, as fatal accidents due to fatigue or falling asleep at the wheel were associated with OSAS.

This had been preceded by a project of the European Sleep Research Society (ESRS) initiated at a meeting of the Assembly of National Sleep Societies (ANSS) in 2013. A "WAKE-UP BUS" was launched in Portugal on October 3,

2013, which drove through nine European countries, passed Vienna on October 11, 2013, and finally reached the European Parliament in Brussels on October 15, 2013. The aim was to inform about the dangers of sleepy driving [2].

Within the Austrian health care system, quality assessment has been introduced at various levels. After a training time of 6 years, every specialist must take an exam to get his license. To keep their license, physicians must participate in a continuous medical educational program monitored by the AMC. They are required to gather a total of 250 points over a time of five years by attending scientific meetings or medical courses, or by e-learning.

In Austria, the Medical Chamber is responsible for guidelines. However, sleep guidelines from other sleep societies (German, European and the AASM) are accepted as well.

Board certification for sleep medicine has not been introduced so far, although like in many other countries worldwide, sleep medicine represents an important field in medicine. In contrast to many other countries, however, in Austria sleep medicine had not even been accredited as a subspecialty by the AMC and the Ministry of Health until recent years. Starting in 2007, the ASRA tried to accommodate the different interests of all disciplines involved in sleep medicine, and to reach a consensus about a common curriculum. This goal could finally be achieved in 2017. Consequently, sleep medicine was approved as a subspecialty by both the AMC and the Ministry of Health in December 2018. The duration of training was defined as 18 months, a curriculum describes the knowledge, experience, and skills to be achieved during training. Furthermore, a board was created to check the application of candidates, both from individual persons and training centers. This approval process is currently being implemented. The subspecialty „sleep medicine" is open to the following disciplines: ENT, internal medicine, neurology, pediatrics and adolescent medicine, psychiatry, and psychotherapy, and pulmonology.

Since 1998, the ASRA has been offering a voluntary accreditation process to sleep medical facilities, performing polysomnography. Offering an out-patient clinic is obligatory, although performed with different ambitions. The evaluation process includes a site visit by three sleep specialists selected by our executive board. Achieving accreditation demonstrates a sleep medicine provider's commitment to high-quality standards.

CHALLENGES TO PRACTICE SLEEP MEDICINE

Adult people with sleep complaints usually consult their primary care physician (as a gatekeeper). Cultural differences or a migration background is generally not a great obstacle in the management of organic sleep disorders, except for the language barriers. Patients who speak neither German nor English (besides other languages), will not be able to explain their complaints. A good example is the ESS (Epworth Sleepiness Scale). If you do not understand the questions, you will not be able to answer them correctly. And to explore symptom-based diseases in sleep medicine, the patient needs to describe his or her problems adequately.

Pediatric sleep medicine in Austria evolved from a working group dealing with sudden infant death syndrome (SIDS) in the 1970ies. Around 1990, the first full pediatric sleep lab was established in Graz, followed by another institution in Vienna. Since then, several hospitals have established sleep labs for children, not all, however, are fully equipped for the whole panel of pediatric sleep disorders. At present, there are four pediatric sleep labs (Vienna, Leoben, Graz, Villach) that have been accredited by the ASRA. Investigations in pediatric sleep labs cover the age group from newborns (including premature babies) to adolescents (usually 18 years of age) and include diagnostic and therapeutic procedures for all sleep disorders occurring in this age group. Sleep staging is mostly done in accordance with AASM criteria. Multichannel EEG recording, sampling of common physiological variables and video recording are mandatory. Typical examples of investigations are those for CSA, OSA, hypoventilation syndromes, sleep-related seizures, narcolepsy, and others. In pediatric sleep medicine, parental counselling represents an important part of daily routine. Colleagues dealing with pediatric sleep medicine in Austria collaborate not only under the roof of the ASRA, but also with the Austrian Society of Pediatrics and Adolescent Medicine (ÖGKJ) and form their own working group in this society.

CLINICAL AND RESEARCH KNOWLEDGE

Although Austria is only a small country, it has many universities and is scientifically very active in many areas of sleep medicine. Epidemiological studies have been performed since 1994. Josef Zeitlhofer [3, 4] was a founding member of the ASRA. He has published numerous epidemiological papers on sleep disorders in Austria and was an important member of the SIESTA project focusing on the creation of an automatic sleep classification system and a normative database.

Bernd Saletu founded the first sleep laboratory at the General Hospital (AKH)/the Medical University of Vienna in 1975. Since his training at the University of Missouri, USA, his scientific interest has focused on biological psychiatry, neuropsychopharmacology and neurophysiology. For imaging the microstructure of sleep, he used EEG mapping and low-resolution brain electromagnetic tomography (LORETA) [5], thereby providing evidence for a key-lock principle in the diagnosis and therapy of sleep disorders. He passed the first international examination of the ESRS in Paris in 2012 and was conferred the title of "Somnologist/Expert in Sleep Medicine". The study group of Michael Saletu published studies on independent surrogate markers of cerebrovascular disease in obstructive sleep apnea [6] and showed recently that proactive telemedical monitoring of sleep apnea treatment improves CPAP adherence in people with sleep apnea [7].

At the Medical University of Vienna, Stefan Seidel and colleagues have focused on the treatment of RLS [8], parasomnias, narcolepsy, hypersomnia, and circadian arrhythmias and conducted clinical studies in hypersomnia, RLS and fatigue in neurological diseases [9], whereas Doris Moser, a clinical and health psychologist and psychotherapist (behavioral therapy) has concentrated on CBT-I, sleep and memory, and sleep disorders in neurological patients [10, 11].

Sleep, dreaming [12], lucid dreaming, nightmares, sleep-coaching [13] and recently the effects of COVID-19 on sleep and (lucid) dreams and nightmares have been among the interests of Brigitte Holzinger, who is also a founding member of the ASRA. Brigitte Holzinger and Gerhard Klösch developed and teach "Medical Sleep-Coaching". Gerhard Klösch, who was also very active in the SIESTA project [14] and investigated different kinds of sleeping arrangements (sleeping in pairs, sleeping with pets).Peter Anderer played a major role in the creation of an automatic sleep classification system [14 - 17] and a normative database, including polysomnographic (PSG) and psychometric measurements (European SIESTA project).

Rainer Popovic, currently president of the Austrian Sleep Research Association, explored the gender difference of upper airway dilator muscle activity [18, 19] preventing airway collapse during sleep. Guided by his mentor David White he won the first prize of the Young Investigator Award at the AASM Meeting in Boston 1993.

The Medical University of Innsbruck holds the largest academic interdisciplinary Sleep Center in Austria. The director of the Sleep Center is Birgit Högl [20], who is a full Professor of Neurology with a specific emphasis on Sleep Medicine and has contributed more than 300 MedlinePubMed publications and has a Hirsch Index of 59 in Web of Science. The scientific team of the Innsbruck Sleep Center consists of several internationally recognized sleep clinicians and researchers. Here, 3 team members shall be named, to represent the whole larger team of board -ertified sleep specialists and researchers: Ambra Stefani (RBD and neurodegeneration, RLS, secretary of the international RBD study group, secretary of the European RLS study group, member of the sleep-wake disorders scientific panel of the European Academy of Neurology) [21], Anna Heidbreder (hypersomnias, who is a board member of the German sleep society and in charge of the guideline committee of RLS for the German sleep society and the German Society for Neurology) [22], and the biomedical engineer Matteo Cesari (Artificial intelligence). Innsbruck team members have been awarded with multiple national and international recognitions and prizes. Birgit Högl has served as a president of the Austrian Sleep association from 2006-2010 and 2016-2018 currently past-president and is the current president of the World Sleep Society (Worldsleepsociety.org) (2019-2022).

The study group around Manuel Schabus and Kerstin Hödlmoser has focused on sleep spindles in connection with memory and intelligence [23, 24], also across age, and investigated the impact of using smartphones at night time before going to bed [25] as well as of blue light and sleep.

CONCLUSION

Although there is always space for improvement, sleep medicine is well-represented in Austria. Research is historically a big part of the growing knowledge about sleep and sleep disturbances. However, the interest of physicians in practicing sleep medicine is somewhat lacking activity as there are so many other fields to be covered. So, constant and ambitious input is necessary to get physicians interested in the field of clinical sleep medicine.

CONSENT FOR PUBLICATION

Not applicable.

CONFLICT OF INTEREST

The authors declare no conflict of interest, financial or otherwise.

ACKNOWLEDGEMENT

The authors would like to express their gratitude to the entire ASRA executive committee and scientific board at present or in the past (Peter Anderer, Anna Heidbreder, Kerstin Hödlmoser, Birgit Högl, Brigitte Holzinger, Gerhard Klösch, Wolfgang Mallin, Doris Moser, Bernd Saletu, Stefan Seidl, Ambra Stefani, Josef Zeitlhofer) for their precious assistance in this project, as well as to Elisabeth Grätzhofer for editorial assistance.

REFERENCES

[1]   Hofmarcher MM, Quentin W. Austria: health system review. Health Syst Transit 2013; 15(7): 1-292.
       [PMID: 24334772]

[2]   Bonsignore MR, Randerath W, Riha R, *et al.* New rules on driver licensing for patients with obstructive sleep apnoea: EU Directive 2014/85/EU. Eur Respir J 2016; 47(1): 39-41.
        [http://dx.doi.org/10.1183/13993003.01894-2015] [PMID: 26721963]

[3]   Zeitlhofer J, Rieder A, Kapfhammer G, *et al.* [Epidemiology of sleep disorders in Austria]. Wien Klin Wochenschr 1994; 106(3): 86-8.
        [PMID: 8053210]

[4]   Zeitlhofer J, Seidel S, Klösch G, *et al.* Sleep habits and sleep complaints in Austria: current self-reported data on sleep behaviour, sleep disturbances and their treatment. Acta Neurol Scand 2010; 122(6): 398-403.
        [http://dx.doi.org/10.1111/j.1600-0404.2010.01325.x] [PMID: 20298492]

[5]   Saletu B, Anderer P, Saletu-Zyhlarz GM, Pascual-Marqui RD. EEG topography and tomography in diagnosis and treatment of mental disorders: evidence for a key-lock principle Methods Find Exp Clin Pharmacol 2002; 24 Suppl D: 97-106

[6]   Saletu M, Nosiska D, Kapfhammer G, *et al.* Structural and serum surrogate markers of cerebrovascular disease in obstructive sleep apnea (OSA). J Neurol 2006; 253(6): 746-52.
        [http://dx.doi.org/10.1007/s00415-006-0110-6] [PMID: 16511651]

[7]   Kotzian ST, Saletu MT, Schwarzinger A, *et al.* Proactive telemedicine monitoring of sleep apnea treatment improves adherence in people with stroke– a randomized controlled trial (HOPES study). Sleep Med 2019; 64: 48-55.
        [http://dx.doi.org/10.1016/j.sleep.2019.06.004] [PMID: 31670004]

[8]   Seidel S, Garn H, Gall M, *et al.* Contactless detection of periodic leg movements during sleep: A 3D video pilot study. J Sleep Res 2020; 29(5): e12986.
        [http://dx.doi.org/10.1111/jsr.12986] [PMID: 32017288]

[9]   Seidel S, Dal-Bianco P, Pablik E, *et al.* Depressive Symptoms are the Main Predictor for Subjective Sleep Quality in Patients with Mild Cognitive Impairment—A Controlled Study. PLoS One 2015; 10(6): e0128139.
        [http://dx.doi.org/10.1371/journal.pone.0128139] [PMID: 26090659]

[10]   Moser D, Anderer P, Gruber G, *et al.* Sleep classification according to AASM and Rechtschaffen & Kales: effects on sleep scoring parameters. Sleep 2009; 32(2): 139-49.
        [http://dx.doi.org/10.1093/sleep/32.2.139] [PMID: 19238800]

[11]   Moser D, Kloesch G, Fischmeister FP, Bauer H, Zeitlhofer J. Cyclic alternating pattern and sleep quality in healthy subjects—Is there a first-night effect on different approaches of sleep quality? Biol Psychol 2010; 83(1): 20-6.
        [http://dx.doi.org/10.1016/j.biopsycho.2009.09.009] [PMID: 19786065]

[12]   Holzinger B, Saletu B, Klösch G. Cognitions in Sleep: Lucid Dreaming as an Intervention for Nightmares in Patients With Posttraumatic Stress Disorder. Front Psychol 2020; 11: 1826.
        [http://dx.doi.org/10.3389/fpsyg.2020.01826] [PMID: 32973600]

[13]   Holzinger B, Mayer L, Levec K, Munzinger MM, Klösch G. Sleep coaching: non-pharmacological treatment of non-restorative sleep in Austrian railway shift workers. Arh Hig Rada Toksikol 2019; 70(3): 186-93.
        [http://dx.doi.org/10.2478/aiht-2019-70-3244] [PMID: 32597126]

[14]   Klosh G, Kemp B, Penzel T, *et al.* The SIESTA project polygraphic and clinical database. IEEE Eng Med Biol Mag 2001; 20(3): 51-7.
        [http://dx.doi.org/10.1109/51.932725] [PMID: 11446210]

[15]   Anderer P, Klösch G, Gruber G, *et al.* Low-resolution brain electromagnetic tomography revealed simultaneously active frontal and parietal sleep spindle sources in the human cortex. Neuroscience 2001; 103(3): 581-92.
        [http://dx.doi.org/10.1016/S0306-4522(01)00028-8] [PMID: 11274780]

[16]	Anderer P, Moreau A, Woertz M, *et al.* Computer-assisted sleep classification according to the standard of the American Academy of Sleep Medicine: validation study of the AASM version of the Somnolyzer 24 × 7. Neuropsychobiology 2010; 62(4): 250-64.
[http://dx.doi.org/10.1159/000320864] [PMID: 20829636]

[17]	Danker-Hopfe H, Anderer P, Zeitlhofer J, *et al.* Interrater reliability for sleep scoring according to the Rechtschaffen & Kales and the new AASM standard. J Sleep Res 2009; 18(1): 74-84.
[http://dx.doi.org/10.1111/j.1365-2869.2008.00700.x] [PMID: 19250176]

[18]	Popovic RM, White DP. Influence of gender on waking genioglossal electromyogram and upper airway resistance. Am J Respir Crit Care Med 1995; 152(2): 725-31.
[http://dx.doi.org/10.1164/ajrccm.152.2.7633734] [PMID: 7633734]

[19]	Popovic RM, White DP. Upper airway muscle activity in normal women: influence of hormonal status. J Appl Physiol 1998; 84(3): 1055-62.
[http://dx.doi.org/10.1152/jappl.1998.84.3.1055] [PMID: 9480969]

[20]	Högl B, Stefani A, Videnovic A. Idiopathic REM sleep behaviour disorder and neurodegeneration — an update. Nat Rev Neurol 2018; 14(1): 40-55.
[http://dx.doi.org/10.1038/nrneurol.2017.157] [PMID: 29170501]

[21]	Stefani A, Iranzo A, Holzknecht E, *et al.* Alpha-synuclein seeds in olfactory mucosa of patients with isolated REM sleep behaviour disorder. Brain 2021; 144(4): 1118-26.
[http://dx.doi.org/10.1093/brain/awab005] [PMID: 33855335]

[22]	Gaig C, Compta Y, Heidbreder A, *et al.* Frequency and Characterization of Movement Disorders in Anti-IgLON5 Disease. Neurology 2021; 97(14): e1367-81.
[http://dx.doi.org/10.1212/WNL.0000000000012639] [PMID: 34380749]

[23]	Schabus M, Gruber G, Parapatics S, *et al.* Sleep spindles and their significance for declarative memory consolidation. Sleep 2004; 27(8): 1479-85.
[http://dx.doi.org/10.1093/sleep/27.7.1479] [PMID: 15683137]

[24]	van Schalkwijk FJ, Hauser T, Hoedlmoser K, *et al.* Procedural memory consolidation is associated with heart rate variability and sleep spindles. J Sleep Res 2020; 29(3): e12910.
[http://dx.doi.org/10.1111/jsr.12910] [PMID: 31454120]

[25]	Höhn C, Schmid SR, Plamberger CP, *et al.* Preliminary Results: The Impact of Smartphone Use and Short-Wavelength Light during the Evening on Circadian Rhythm, Sleep and Alertness. Clocks Sleep 2021; 3(1): 66-86.
[http://dx.doi.org/10.3390/clockssleep3010005] [PMID: 33499010]

CHAPTER 24

Practice of Sleep Medicine in the United Kingdom (UK)

Timothy G. Quinnell[1,*]

[1] *Royal Papworth Hospital NHS Foundation Trust, Cambridge, UK*

Abstract: The practice of sleep medicine in the UK has made considerable progress over the past 3 decades. This has been driven by the invention of CPAP and the development of OSA services, but other factors related to National Health Service innovations and healthcare professional developments have also been important. Key challenges remain in service provision, education and research, and in resolving regional equalities in access to care.

Keywords: Association for Respiratory Technology and Physiology, ARTP, BLF, British Thoracic Society, British Sleep Society, BSS, BTS, British Lung Foundation, Continuous positive airway pressure, CPAP, Getting It Right First Time, GIRFT, Marmot, National health service, NHS, Obstructive sleep apnoea, OSA, Regional Inequality, Sleep medicine.

INTRODUCTION

The healthcare services in the United Kingdom (UK) are provided by the National Health Service (NHS) and funded by the taxpayer. Only around 11% of the population have private health insurance [1]. Private policies often provide limited coverage and sleep medicine can be overlooked. Therefore this chapter will focus on sleep medicine provided by the NHS. The NHS was created in 1948 and brought together a heterogeneous collection of local and regional healthcare providers into one organisation. It has gone through a number of changes and restructuring since its inception. However, two of the NHS's founding principles have not changed: to make healthcare equally accessible to all and free at the point of care [2]. Each devolved nation (Wales, Scotland and Northern Ireland) has its own NHS (Health and Social Care for N. Ireland). Each has its own governance and varies slightly in its organisation and policies. Unfortunately, while there will be NHS data available for each nation, much of the available inf-

---
* **Corresponding author Timothy G. Quinnell:** Royal Papworth Hospital NHS Foundation Trust, Cambridge, UK; Tel: +44 1223 639718; E-mail: tim.quinnell@nhs.net

Hrayr P. Attarian, Marie-Louise M. Coussa-Koniski & Alain Michel Sabri (Eds.)

ormation regarding sleep medicine is limited to England. A detailed breakdown of the similarities and differences of each country's sleep medicine 'scene' is not possible. However, it will be made clear in this chapter where data and other information refer to England alone or to the UK. Even then there are significant gaps. In those cases the author has given his own impression formed through personal experience and professional networking.

CURRENT PRACTICE OF SLEEP MEDICINE IN THE UK

When it comes to considering the current state of sleep medicine obstructive sleep apnoea (OSA) is an obvious starting point. The prominence of OSA might overshadow other sleep disorders, but the development of highly effective treatment for this prevalent and impactful condition has undoubtedly fuelled the growth of sleep medicine. For the UK the publication of guidance by the National Institute for Health and Care Excellence (NICE) in 2008 [3] that recommended continuous positive airway pressure (CPAP) for moderate to severe OSA was probably a key driver for the development and expansion of sleep services.

Most OSA services in the UK are provided by respiratory departments within secondary and tertiary care hospitals. Lead clinicians usually work in partnership with respiratory physiology laboratories, although some units have evolved to operate separately. As in other countries, sleep services in the UK are not the exclusive preserve of respiratory physiology or its parent speciality. Many services have been founded by pioneering enthusiasts, sometimes from other clinical backgrounds, such as anaesthesia, neurology or otolaryngology. While some services are truly multidisciplinary, in other areas there are separate services operating for respiratory and non-respiratory sleep, although collaboration is common.

Much of the data regarding UK sleep services has been gathered from surveys conducted by various stakeholders. They give useful insights into UK sleep medicine at different timepoints but it is important to recognise their limitations. Any survey is only as good as the response rate and the representative accuracy of the population targeted. For example the Association for Respiratory Technology and Physiology (ARTP) is the national professional body for respiratory and sleep physiologists [4]. From time to time, it conducts surveys of its members. Registration with the ARTP is not mandated for sleep labs or individuals. When reporting their findings, the ARTP has recognised that they will have missed some services operating outside of respiratory physiology departments, particularly those concentrating on non-respiratory sleep.

The last two ARTP surveys relevant to this topic were published in 2012 [5] and 2018 [6]. Results from the 2012 ARTP survey indicate a significant amount of

OSA service provision being undertaken by clinical physiologists. The survey received responses from 156 of 251 respiratory function labs known to the ARTP. Most of these (143) were based in England and 109 reported undertaking sleep diagnostics, although this was limited to oximetry in just under a third of those labs.

In 79 labs, clinical physiologists were undertaking autonomous sleep diagnostics. Almost all autonomous practitioners were deemed 'regulated'. It is not clear from the 2012 report what that meant. However, the vast majority had postgraduate qualifications in healthcare science, albeit not in sleep medicine. Simple overnight oximetry was much more likely to be carried out by sub-degree level staff, presumably deferring interpretation to higher grades and medical colleagues. Slightly fewer labs (76) in the 2012 survey reported physiologists working as autonomous CPAP providers. However, most of these were 'regulated' and the large majority (74%) had postgraduate healthcare science qualifications. Much of the remaining activity from those labs reporting sleep activity was probably still undertaken by respiratory function lab staff at various grades, but presumably under medical oversight.

Those labs and sleep services not captured by ARTP surveys are likely to be run in a variety of ways. It is not unusual for CPAP to be provided by nurses or physiotherapists, probably influenced by local service set-up including non-invasive ventilation provision. The 2018 ARTP workforce report (survey undertaken in 2015-16) had a different focus and a much lower response rate (28%) than the 2012 survey. However, it gave anecdotal examples of units where various disciplines including nurses, physiotherapists and doctors delivered both diagnostic and therapeutic aspects of their sleep services [6].

Surveys carried out by other stakeholder organisations may have gained a fuller picture of UK sleep services. In 2012, the British Lung Foundation (BLF) explored the availability of sleep services. They worked with the ARTP but also the British Thoracic Society (BTS), which is the national professional society for respiratory medicine. They also linked with other relevant professional and charitable organisations and patient groups. They created a cross-country working group including all devolved states. The BLF survey identified 289 sleep units. Of these, 50 were reported to be undertaking polysomnography (PSG) [7].

More recently, the GIRFT (Getting it Right First Time) NHS England improvement program reported on respiratory medicine services [8]. GIRFT aims to improve the quality of care and deliver efficiencies by sharing the best practices and identifying variations between NHS services. The report includes respiratory sleep services within NHS England. GIRFT data sources were heterogeneous and broader than the ARTP reports. They sent questionnaires to NHS trusts and visited many of them. They accessed various other official data sources, covering hospital episodes, mortality, medicine use and diagnostic and therapeutic activity. By cross-referencing these sources, the GIRFT report aimed to build a picture of the extent and state of respiratory medicine services. A major finding, which was also a limiting factor in the analyses, was of significant discrepancies between the data sources. Questionnaire findings suggested there were 107 NHS trusts providing a diagnostic sleep service, whereas NHS England activity returns identified only 98 trusts performing over 50 limited sleep studies a year (including oximetry). Twenty-seven trusts were found to perform more than 50 PSGs a year, in contrast to only 4 being captured by an ARTP activity database.

Although medical specialists usually lead sleep services, there is no formal sleep medicine training programme in the UK. Training is sporadic and largely experiential, with limited mandated formal assessment. Some specialist training programmes require trainees to obtain an understanding of the basics but the curricula are limited. The shortcomings of medical sleep training will be discussed in more detail later. However, while formal training in the UK may be patchy and inadequate, high-quality hands-on training is available to interested trainees if they are fortunate enough to be in the right place or motivated enough to overcome obstacles in order to access it. Some pioneers were self-taught, with others perhaps spending time with existing services in the UK or abroad. New colleagues may be recruited from in-house trainees or those who have trained in other sleep services. Some will have undertaken extended bespoke clinical or research fellowships outside of their standard specialist training programme, where they will have acquired greater expertise in sleep medicine and perhaps completed a doctorate. Others will have moved to the UK having undertaken more structured sleep training overseas.

In contrast to sleep training for medical graduates, significant progress has been made in the training of respiratory and sleep physiologists and other healthcare scientists [9]. Graduate, postgraduate (*e.g.* MSc) and doctorate training programmes have been developed, with scopes that include and sometimes focus on sleep medicine. At the top end of the scale, there is now the Higher Specialist Scientist Training (HSST) programme which is a taught doctorate and leads to consultant clinical scientist roles. The programme is entirely bespoke to the individual healthcare scientist and their previous experiences. It is unlike other training programmes under the MSc umbrella in that it requires the trainee and their employer to develop an appropriate job plan against the demands of the specialism-specific curriculum. Therefore those scientists specialising in sleep medicine have the option for it to be a major focus. When originally devised those taking the HSST were supposed to be in leadership roles already and/or leading a department, or at least in a position where the leadership role would be available at the end of the programme. All of these training developments have been associated with an extension of the roles of clinical physiologists into therapeutics and increasing autonomy in service provision.

Although there is no formal UK based clinical sleep qualification for medical graduates, there is now a European 'somnologist' certification. This is run by the European Sleep Research Society (ESRS) and is not limited to doctors. It involves 3 levels of examinations, for medical graduates, psychologists and sleep scientists. In order to qualify to sit the exam applicants must provide evidence of having undertaken a certain amount of clinical sleep training [10]. Neither this nor any other sleep medicine certification obtained through course attendance is required to practice sleep medicine in the UK. However, it will help in a competitive job market.

While there is no formal UK sleep credentialing process, there are numerous training resources. These are provided by various organisations, which serve and reflect an active, if uncoordinated sleep medicine community.

The British Thoracic Society (BTS) is a registered charity and professional society for all who work in respiratory healthcare [11]. It runs 2 annual meetings, one focussed on training and the other on research and service provision. The BTS produces position statements and clinical guidelines. It has a strong sleep apnoea section that has its own Specialist Advisory Group (SAG). The SAG promotes and supports education and research in sleep apnoea and has a liaison role with other organisations including the government. It is a key stakeholder in relevant NICE publications including those relating to sleep medicine [3].

As already explained, sleep scientists with a respiratory physiology background are eligible to join the ARTP [4]. It develops and provides training programmes, sets standards and publishes clinical practice guidelines. It liaises with governmental healthcare bodies, other professional societies and charities. Sleep medicine has received increasing recognition within the ARTP. There is now a sleep section (ARTP-Sleep) which sleep physiologists without a respiratory background are also eligible to join. ARTP-Sleep works closely with the British Sleep Society (BSS).

The BSS was founded in 1989 and is the nation's largest charity for people working in sleep. The society recently published a 5-year strategic plan. Its vision statement is to 'be at the heart of a vibrant sleep health community in the UK'. Its renewed mission is to 'support excellence in multidisciplinary practice across the field of sleep science and medicine' [12]. The society holds a biennial scientific meeting and runs other educational events, including as a tripartite host for the annual International Sleep Medicine Course (focussed on the ESRS somnologist exam). The BSS might indeed be considered to be at the heart of respiratory and non-respiratory sleep, bringing together sleep professionals from all disciplines working in the UK and seeking to raise awareness of sleep and its disorders in the wider medical and lay community.

There are no regulatory bodies specific to sleep medicine for either services or individual practitioners. However medical graduates are registered with the General Medical Council (GMC) [13] and their postgraduate training is determined and overseen by Royal College Training Boards which link closely with the GMC. Aside from broad postgraduate examinations (*e.g.* membership of the Royal College of Physicians) many specialties these days have an exit exam. Once signed off as a fully-fledged specialist (consultant) this is added to the doctor's status on the GMC register. All fully trained doctors in the UK must undergo annual appraisal by a senior colleague trained in the process. Every 5 years, a doctor must undergo revalidation with the GMC, which mainly requires a complete appraisal portfolio and sign-off by the employing organisation. Sleep medicine is not a specialty recognised by the GMC, so doctors are registered under their mainstream specialty (*e.g.* respiratory medicine). The appraisal process sets professional development goals and documents their attainment, monitors probity and has pastoral care aspects. The process is general and broad rather than being a detailed review of an individual's expertise. Assessors work within the same healthcare organisation but usually in a different area. However, the requirements of appraisal include proof of continuing professional development (CPD) and maintenance of safe and current practices.

Other NHS healthcare workers must engage with similar appraisal processes. For example, nurses must do so in order to maintain their registration with the Nursing and Midwifery council and they too undergo periodic revalidation. In common with their medical colleagues there is nothing formal that is specific to sleep. However, the appraisal process requires evidence of CPD and maintenance of safe and current practices within whatever area the individual is working in.

There is no mandatory registration system for sleep services within the NHS. In 2008 the BSS developed a sleep centre accreditation process that was adapted from European guidelines [14]. However accreditation required the full range of respiratory and non-respiratory sleep services, including inpatient polysomnography, so the vast majority of UK sleep services were not eligible. There were no formal incentives for undertaking the accreditation process and there were no sanctions for not engaging. Two UK centres achieved accreditation. While the recognition and kudos which accreditation brought may have benefited those centres, nothing was lost by those who did not engage.

There is a broader service accreditation process that may ultimately become mandatory. The IQIPS (Improving Quality In Physiological Services) scheme is managed by the government-appointed UK Accreditation Service (UKAS) [15]. IQIPS is designed to ensure that patients receive high-quality care from competent staff in safe environments. Respiratory and Sleep Physiology is one of the 8 disciplines that IQIPS covers. The IQIPS Standard is intended to ensure that services are delivered accurately, safely and efficiently, and are accessible and sustainable. The standard aims to provide the correct infrastructure, culture and environment for high-quality service provision. The domains it covers are broad and generic (*e.g.* leadership and management). The standard does not provide detailed guidance on specific service provision (*e.g.* practice parameters for conducting a polysomnogram). However, it requires services to make sure they have policies in place that ensure adherence to relevant clinical guidelines. Therefore IQIPS accreditation may have merit for sleep services, provided specialty-specific detail is available from other sources. For sleep medicine, these sources are varied. There are some UK guidelines (*e.g.* NICE on CPAP) but there are huge gaps (*e.g.* clinical practice guidelines for disorders other than OSA, performing sleep diagnostics, *etc.*). However, where there are gaps there are often good alternatives (*e.g.* American and European) that could be adopted and adapted for the UK and NHS. It should be possible for the IQIPS assessors and professional stakeholders to take a view of these resources and develop pragmatic requirements for adherence by an NHS service. Although IQIPS is not yet mandatory, it is endorsed by the Care Quality Commission (CQC), which is the independent regulator of health and social care in England. The CQC regulates all hospitals and conducts mandatory inspections. A Respiratory and Sleep laboratory with IQIPs accreditation would be viewed favourably by the CQC. NHS England has also thrown its support behind the process as a means for local healthcare commissioners to select healthcare providers.

Treatment under the NHS is supposed to be free to all at the point of care. Patients do not have to pay to undergo sleep studies and CPAP therapy is free. The availability of diagnostic services has already been touched upon. Regional inequalities exist and will be discussed later. The 2008 NICE CPAP guidelines [3] obliged local NHS commissioners to fund CPAP services. The guidance recognised the associated need for OSA diagnostics but details were lacking. This is reflected in the variability of sleep diagnostics offered by individual services. In the UK, there has been a pragmatic minimum standard for confirming clinically suspected OSA and therefore eligibility for CPAP, through the use of overnight oximetry. While this makes access to diagnosis and treatment better than it might otherwise be, the limited availability of more complex sleep investigations has already been described. Respiratory polygraphy is increasingly available but far fewer centres have the expertise and facilities to provide a polysomnography

(PSG) service, or to manage the non-respiratory case-mix. The 2008 guidelines did not consider alternatives to CPAP such as oral appliances. Access to oral appliance therapy on the NHS is consequently poor and subject to local variation. New NICE guidance regarding sleep diagnostics and alternatives to CPAP therapy are currently being developed. Their recommendations are yet to be released and therefore impacts cannot be anticipated.

Sleep relevant medications, provided funding approval is forthcoming, are supposedly free although there are monthly prescription charges (currently £9.15 per item with exemptions for eligible groups). Prescribing medicines within the NHS is strictly managed. Drugs are licensed centrally for specific indications according to evidence based findings of clinical effectiveness and safety. For example, modafinil is licensed only for adults with narcolepsy. Its licensing used to be broader but was restricted by the Medicines and Healthcare products Regulatory Agency (MHRA) several years ago due to safety concerns initially recognised by the European Medicines Agency. Separately, NICE assesses and makes recommendations on whether treatments (pharmaceutical and other) should be funded by the NHS. Clinical and cost effectiveness are considered.

Payment systems within the NHS in England change fairly frequently. In 2012 the Health and Social Care Act introduced competitive tendering by service providers (*e.g.* hospitals) to NHS commissioners. Service providers were paid pro rata ('Payment by Results') according to a national tariff system. This has changed over subsequent years to block contracts with individual providers and has continued to be in flux as new, area-wide payment systems were due to be introduced. However everything may change again. A proposal for a new Health and Care Bill was released in February 2021. It proposes radical but controversial changes that are likely to be translated into law by a majority government. Details are yet to emerge. Broadly speaking it seems that central governmental control will be increased and NHS independence decreased. The competitive market will cease to exist with the stated aim being to improve integration of health and social care [16].

CHALLENGES TO PRACTICE OF SLEEP MEDICINE

Accessing sleep services first requires patients and their primary care team to be aware of sleep disorders. While there is always more to be done to increase public awareness of sleep disorders, sleep itself is increasingly popular as a media topic in the UK. Sleep and lifestyle articles, including the impact of smartphones and other IT, are fairly common. Now and again sleep disorders also have a platform in the lay media. The rising number of Apps that monitor sleep, whether standalone or as part of health and fitness monitoring with the use of wearables, should also be serving to increase public awareness in the UK and in many other countries. The quality and consistency of the advice or the science behind these unregulated resources is less certain.

Medical awareness of sleep disorders will vary according to discipline, interest and exposure. Despite curriculum limitations, those doctors specialising in respiratory, neurology and certain other disciplines should be aware of the common and relevant sleep disorders, even when they don't have the expertise or resources to deal with them. Awareness of OSA is now probably fairly good among primary care teams in the UK. However, this is a personal impression of the author based on his experience fielding primary care referrals in a region well served by an established sleep service. Awareness of sleep disorders probably varies according to area, influenced by local educational programmes and the extent of sleep service provision.

Primary care awareness of other sleep disorders is probably poorer and more variable. Sometimes doctors are educated by their patients, who recognise features of a condition (*e.g.* REM sleep behaviour disorder) in a media piece and seek a referral. Insomnia is likely to be the exception. Most people will have a reasonable idea what this is, often from personal experience. This is not the same as having expertise to manage it and it is probably true to say that availability of face to face cognitive behavioural therapy for insomnia (CBT-I) is very limited. However the NHS website has useful common medical conditions from A – Z where it describes key features of insomnia and treatments, including the role of self-help [17]. There are now also NHS approved online insomnia treatment programmes.

REGIONAL DIFFERENCES

In principle, there shouldn't be any differences in patients' access to sleep services within the NHS, but there do exist. These should be considered in the broader context of national health and social inequalities. Whenever healthcare services are more stretched, one might expect the gap between sleep medicine demand and supply to widen in association. Other social and health problems might be prioritised over sleep disorders although higher prevalence of shared risk factors will mean that OSA, for example, will be more common too.

In 2010, the independently commissioned Marmot report provided strong evidence of regional health inequalities in England and linked them with social determinants of health [18]. The report made recommendations to policymakers for redressing the balance. Unfortunately, the 2020 update found that things had deteriorated [19]. Health had improved in some areas, such as London and the Southeast of England, but worsened in others such as the North of England. Life expectancy, increasing in England since 1900, had stalled, and it had fallen in some of the most deprived areas in the Northeast of England. Although focussed on England, the report acknowledged similar problems in the devolved nations. The deterioration of the nation's health and the progression of inequality attributed to policy gaps and wealth differences. Funding cuts imposed in response to the global financial crash of 2008 were greatest outside London and the Southeast of England. The report made updated recommendations to the UK government on how to address these inequalities. Its publication could not foresee the socioeconomic and health impacts of COVID-19, and the departure of the UK from the European Union will have its own uncertain consequences.

Regional inequalities in access to sleep services are considered in England. In 2012, the British Lung Foundation explored differences between OSA service supply and demand [7]. By systematically surveying and analysing 5 factors associated with OSA (obesity, gender, age, diabetes and hypertension), they calculated relative predicted prevalence estimates of OSA according to NHS administrative area. The findings were mapped to sleep service distribution data which were described earlier. The survey gathered data for 239 NHS areas (mean population 261,604). There was significant regional variability in predicted OSA prevalence, with higher prevalence areas tending to be more rural (*e.g.* Wales and East Anglia). Large urban areas in Scotland and England, and areas around London, had the lowest prevalence. Diagnostic capabilities varied considerably. Fifty of 289 sleep services reported undertaking PSGs. This was calculated to be roughly equivalent to 1 PSG service per 1.25 million people, compared at that time with 2461 centres for 310 million people in the USA. For the remaining centres, standalone oximetry was not uncommon. Even more variable was the availability of sleep centres. Sixty six NHS areas had no sleep service while a single urban area had 9. The average was 1.2 per area. Populations most in need (*i.e.* those in more rural areas) were least well provided for.

These findings were consistent with formal NHS data. In 2011, the number of sleep studies carried out per head of population varied hugely across English Primary Care Trusts (healthcare areas), from 0.2 to 8.6 per 1000 population. This 57-fold variation, the highest of any respiratory service, was attributed to the lack of awareness among patients and clinicians and regional variability of service availability [20]. By 2016, the variability range had reduced to 3.6 studies per 1000 population but some areas still undertook no studies. In truth, the 5-year comparison was confounded by healthcare boundary changes. In 2013, the NHS in England was re-divided for funding purposes into Clinical Commissioning Groups (CCGs) [21]. Redefining healthcare areas may have altered statistics but probably would not have improved regional disparities. These groups are autonomous, clinically led bodies responsible for planning and commissioning health and community care for their local population. The populations covered (100,000 to over a million) are diverse with varying care needs and priorities. There are currently 135 CCGs. Each has its own budget and is independently accountable to the Secretary of State for Health and Social Care for how they use that budget to achieve the best outcomes for their population. Although there are some centrally commissioned services, CCGs are responsible for around 2/3 of the total NHS England budget, and practically all sleep services fall within their remit. Each CCG must decide what it can and should fund and commissions services from NHS providers within their area. This and demographic differences mean that geographical inequality is almost inevitable in a financially pressurized system.

The recent GIRFT report [8] identified ongoing regional and interservice variability in the nature and extent of sleep service provision. The number of sleep studies (all types) reported to be carried out annually by NHS trusts ranged from none by 20 trusts to between 2,000 and 10,000 per year for the top 15 performers. Access to CPAP therapy was similarly varied. Some clinical pathways continue to run along traditional lines, with clinical assessment being followed by sleep study and then leading to CPAP as appropriate. However, most services who responded to the survey now see patients after sleep studies. There are examples of other innovative practices which aim to deal with large workloads as efficiently as possible. The variety of clinical pathways is perhaps an example of necessity being the mother of invention. Whether these innovative practices always lead to better access to higher-quality care is unclear. However the wide range of waiting times for CPAP implementation described in the GIRFT report (1 to 36 weeks) indicates there is room for improvement. CPAP provision across the country might be improved if the most effective services were presented as models for others to learn from. Not all performance variation will be due to how services are run. Factors are likely to be multiple and varied. Some will be historical and influenced by local factors but broader geographical inequalities are also probably at play.

While there is more work to be done to improve and equalise access to sleep services, the national picture is far from discouraging. Data collected by NHS England suggest that there has been progress over the past 15 years. Referral to treatment is a governmental initiative that was launched in 2008 to reduce waiting times across the NHS. The NHS Constitution now gives patients the legal right to receive treatment within 18 weeks [22]. Within that, they should not have to wait more than 6 weeks to undergo diagnostic testing. NHS trusts must aim for over 92% of their patients to have their sleep study on time. The demand for sleep studies increased by 70% from 2006 to 2017 but so did activity [6]. Just prior to June 2006, 3900 sleep studies were being carried out in England every month [5].

By March 2012, around 8,500 studies were being undertaken a month and in August 2019, 10,370 studies were carried out. Despite this, the vast majority of patients were tested within 6 weeks. In August 2006 58.1% of patients were waiting over 6 weeks whereas in August 2019 this had dropped to 7.8% [23]. There are several possible reasons for the activity increase. Awareness of OSA probably has grown among the public and clinicians. The number of respiratory physicians has increased and so there may be more capacity to see patients. The introduction of RTT doubtless had an impact, causing trusts to undertake waiting list initiatives. Less positive is that increasing obesity may be another contributing factor [6].

Another area of inequality is access to medications for sleep disorders. If a treatment is recommended by NICE, then the local commissioners are obliged to support funding. However not all UK-licensed drugs receive NICE support. Each CCG is autonomous in having its own drug formulary. Their funding decisions are based largely on central licensing but they are not obliged to fund a medicine simply because it is licensed. This can lead to geographic inequalities, with access to sodium oxybate being a good example. Patients living in an area under one CCG may have relatively straightforward access to sodium oxybate provided its prescription is recommended and supervised by a sleep medicine specialist. The same doctor treating a patient from a neighbouring CCG may be required to apply for oxybate funding through a more complex route and still fail to secure funding approval. There are now Regional Medicines Optimisation Committees (RMOCs) that have the remit of trying to address national inequalities in medicines access [24]. The RMOCs can only publish recommendations and have no power to enforce them. Each medicine associated with unequal access must be considered individually and separately against each condition, so progress may be slow, but hopefully RMOCs will help even out access to key sleep medications over time.

CLINICAL AND RESEARCH KNOWLEDGE GAP

Within the UK, there are various data sources that help give a sense of the epidemiology of many of the mainstream medical disorders, including OSA. The sources do not necessarily provide direct incidence and prevalence data on OSA. However they allow extrapolations to be made from, for example, the number of sleep studies undertaken or the number of patients being commenced on CPAP. In 2012, the NHS North of England Specialised Commissioning Group concluded from the available evidence that 85% of people with OSA in the UK were undiagnosed [25]. In 2014, a health economics report commissioned by the British Lung Foundation (BLF) estimated the prevalence of OSA in the UK to be 1.5 million, with around 330,000 receiving treatment [25]. In 2019, investigators used a previously validated online system to survey a representative sample of

UK adults. They obtained estimated OSA prevalence of 8.7% and 5.6% for men and women, respectively. Comparison of these findings with published data from the 1990s suggested a highly significant increase in prevalence rates. The investigators reported an associated increase in obesity rates that was in keeping with data obtained by the NHS and Public Health England [26]. While the 2012 BLF study identified gross regional inequality in sleep service provision, the GIRFT and Marmot reports suggest little progress has been made in correcting this, and indeed gaps may have widened [7, 8, 19]. Although discouraging, the reports provide insights into the nature and scale of the problem, and a basis for making improvements. Some of these measures are specific to sleep medicine, while others are more general.

The 2020 Marmot report made a number of recommendations for addressing what it identified as the deteriorating health situation in the UK. The report outlined a 6-point action plan and placed the responsibility for implementing this policy firmly with the central government. The Marmot report did not deal specifically with sleep medicine. However, given the recognised association between OSA, in particular, and other lifestyle-impacted conditions, it seems reasonable to consider their findings and recommendations entirely relevant to it [19]. If the Marmot recommendations were to be successfully implemented and lead to the improvements predicted in the report then one might expect this to positively impact several risk factors for the development of OSA and some other common sleep disorders.

Whether improvements in healthcare provision in the UK would benefit sleep medicine in part depends on overcoming the existing obstacles specific to sleep medicine.

The limitations of medical sleep training in the UK have already been mentioned. There is no sleep curriculum, so trainees are limited to curricula from parent specialties. The curriculum of the main 'parent', respiratory medicine, is the remit and responsibility of the Joint Royal Colleges of Physicians Training Board. A new curriculum was created in 2010 and updated in 2014 [27]. The curriculum is extensive and robust but it explicitly covers the training requirements of a general respiratory physician. The curriculum does list 5 'special interest' areas. This falls short of subspecialty recognition but acknowledges the need for additional training of trainees hoping to focus on one of these areas. Unfortunately, sleep is not on the so-called 'credentialing' list. Instead in the sleep medicine section of the general curriculum, it states that trainees are expected to become 'competent to undertake specialist assessment and management of patients with sleep breathing disorders'. To achieve competency they 'must care for sufficient inpatients and outpatients with sleep breathing disorders during clinical placements', although 'sufficient' is not defined. In order to demonstrate competency in various areas (*e.g.* 'interpretation of sleep studies') the trainee must complete formalised clinical assessments. The assessment tools are generic and brief, so cannot truly assess specific competency. Respiratory medicine trainees must undertake 6 years of approved respiratory training and pass a Specialty Certificate Examination. The exam comprises 200 multiple choice questions, of which 5 cover sleep related breathing disorders and hypoventilation [28]. Ultimately whether a trainee is on track to achieve sufficient competency in respiratory medicine is decided at a penultimate interview. This is conducted by senior clinician-trainers, who may not have a sleep medicine background. Sometimes trainees are asked to strengthen their experience in a subspecialty by, for example, undertaking a limited attachment with a clinical service or attending a few clinics. The need for, nature and duration of this is a matter of judgement. It may be influenced by the supervisors' expertise and interests, local access to sleep training and the trainee's career focus.

Despite the plethora of non-respiratory sleep disorders, the neurology specialist training curriculum is even more limited when it comes to sleep medicine [29]. Like the respiratory curriculum, its requirements are open to interpretation.

While sleep training for healthcare scientists is probably ahead of medical training, there is more to be done. Attracting healthcare scientists to sleep medicine remains challenging. There are some excellent educational initiatives, but they don't lead to mandated sleep-specific qualifications. There is no degree-level qualification that focuses solely on sleep.

Despite the challenges there is increasing focus on improving the provision of sleep medicine in the UK, either directly through specific and wider health service changes, or through educational initiatives. What they achieve remains to be seen. Policymakers need to be persuaded of the importance of sleep medicine in the wider health service context. Stakeholders need to coordinate their efforts to develop a programme of education and service improvements that is scientifically rigorous yet pragmatic and flexible.

The UK is fortunate when it comes to clinical sleep research because it is often conducted in Westernised developed countries. A lot of the high-quality research is not only accessible through English language publications but is potentially translatable to NHS practice. Nonetheless, healthcare services and funding systems vary substantially between countries, so when it comes to convincing policymakers (*e.g.* NICE) of treatment effectiveness than UK derived data, particularly for health economics, is often required. The sleep community has a track record of conducting high-quality pragmatic clinical trials within the NHS, at least for OSA. Their results are tailor-made for translation into UK practice. Funding is always a challenge for researchers. However governmental and charitable research bodies have been supportive over the years, and hopefully this will continue. Commercial interests are fairly active in promoting their international research evidence and sponsoring UK-based studies for devices and pharmacotherapeutics, for OSA and other sleep disorders. This is naturally a controversial area and conflicts are to be navigated, but without their involvement progress would almost certainly be slower.

CONCLUSION

Sleep medicine in the UK faces challenges. Some of these are shared with the whole of health and social care provision, while others are specific to sleep medicine. However, there are many positives. Although it may have its problems and critics, the NHS provides an extensive, established infrastructure and ethos for engineering improvement. It is also an excellent laboratory for real-life clinical research. As in many other countries, sleep medicine has come a long way in the UK since the invention of CPAP. Despite the obstacles, the future depends on the growing body of enthusiastic professionals working in the field of sleep continuing to champion its cause in a coordinated, robust and pragmatic fashion. Hopefully, policymakers will play their role in making the right choices when it comes to healthcare in general and sleep medicine in particular.

CONSENT FOR PUBLICATION

Not applicable.

CONFLICT OF INTEREST

The authors declare no conflict of interest, financial or otherwise.

ACKNOWLEDGEMENT

Declared none.

REFERENCES

[1]   Commission on the Future of Health and Social Care in England: The UK private health market. King's Fund 2014. Available at:. https://www.kingsfund.org.uk/sites/default/files/media/commission-appendix-uk-private-health-market.pdf Accessed February 2021.

[2]   Rivett G. 1948-1957: Establishing the National Health Service. [Online book]. Available at:. https://www.nuffieldtrust.org.uk/health-and-social-care-explained/the-history-of-the-nhs/

[3]   National Institute for Health and Care Excellence. Continuous positive airway pressure for the treatment of obstructive sleep apnoea/hypopnoea syndrome. Lond. National Institute for Health and Care Excellence. TA139. Available at:. https://www.nice.org.uk/guidance/ta139

[4]   ARTP.org.uk [homepage on the Internet]. Available at:. https://www.artp.org.uk/ Accessed February 2021

[5]   Butterfield AK, Cooper BG, Bucknall M, Sylvester K. ARTP 2012 survey of respiratory and sleep services [online pdf]. January 2014. Available at 2014. https://www.artp.org.uk/reports Accessed February 2021

[6]   Bucknall M, Butterfield AK. ARTP workforce and workload survey [online pdf]. January 2018. Available at https://www.artp.org.uk/reports Accessed February 2021.

[7]   Steier J, Martin A, Harris J, Jarrold I, Pugh D, Williams A. Predicted relative prevalence estimates for obstructive sleep apnoea and the associated healthcare provision across the UK. Thorax 2014; 69(4): 390-2.
        [http://dx.doi.org/10.1136/thoraxjnl-2013-203887] [PMID: 24062427]

[8]   Allen M. Respiratory medicine; GIRFT national specialty report. First draft July 2020.

[9]   An Overview of Modernising Scientific Careers [Independent report (pdf) on Gov.uk website]. Available at https://www.gov.uk/government/publications/an-overview-of-modernising-scient-fic-careers Accessed February 2021.

[10]   European Sleep Research Society: Sleep research and sleep medicine in Europe. Available from:. https://www.esrs-examination.eu/ Accessed February 2021.

[11]   British Thoracic Society About Us' [homepage on BTS website]. Available at https://www.brit-thoracic.org.uk/about-us/ Accessed February 2021.

[12]   British Sleep Society Strategic Plan "Healthy Sleep for All" 2020-2025 [online pdf]. Available at:. https://www.sleepsociety.org.uk/bss-strategy/ Accessed February 2021

[13]   General Medical Council [homepage on website]. Available at: https://www.gmc-uk.org/ Accessed February 2021.

[14]   Pevernagie D. European guidelines for the accreditation of sleep medicine centres. J Sleep Res 2006; 15(2): 231-8.
        [http://dx.doi.org/10.1111/j.1365-2869.2006.00524.x] [PMID: 16704580]

[15]   https://www.ukas.com/accreditation/standards/iqips/

[16]   Godlee F. NHS reorganisation: We don't need a big bang. BMJ 2021; 372(464): n464. [online Article].
        [http://dx.doi.org/10.1136/bmj.n464]

[17]   https://www.nhs.uk/conditions/#I

[18]   Marmot M, Allen J, Boyce T, *et al.* Fair Society, healthy lives. The Marmot Report: Strategic review of health inequalities in England post-2010 [monograph (pdf) on the Internet]. Sponsored by The Institute of Health Equity. Available at: http://www.instituteofhealthequity.org/resources-reports/fair-society-healthy-lives-the-marmot-review/fair-society-healthy-lives-full-report-pdf.pdf Accessed February 2021.
        [http://dx.doi.org/10.1093/acprof:oso/9780199931392.003.0019]

[19]   Marmot M, Allen J, Boyce T, Goldblatt P, Morrison J. Health Equity in England: the Marmot review 10 years on [monograph (pdf) on the Internet]. Sponsored by The Institute of Health Equity. Available at: www.instituteofhealthequity.org/the-marmot-review-10-years-on

[20]   Right Care NHS. Map 16 from Atlas of Variation in Healthcare for People with Respiratory Disease 2012.http://www.rightcare.nhs.uk/index.php/atlas/respiratorydisease/

[21]   https://www.nhscc.org/ccgs/

[22]   https://www.gov.uk/government/publications/the-nhs-constitution-for-england

[23]   https://www.england.nhs.uk/statistics/statistical-work-areas/diagnostics-waiting-times-and-activity/

[24]　https://www.england.nhs.uk/medicines-2/regional-medicines-optimisation-committees/

[25]　Rejon-Parrilla JC, Garau M, Sussex J. Obstructive Sleep Apnoea Health Economics Report 2014.https://www.blf.org.uk/support-for-you/osa/health-care-professionals

[26]　Lechner M, Breeze CE, Ohayon MM, Kotecha B. Snoring and breathing pauses during sleep: interview survey of a United Kingdom population sample reveals a significant increase in the rates of sleep apnoea and obesity over the last 20 years - data from the UK sleep survey. Sleep Med 2019; 54: 250-6.
[http://dx.doi.org/10.1016/j.sleep.2018.08.029] [PMID: 30597439]

[27]　Specialty Training Curriculum for Respiratory Medicine. August 2010 (Amended May 2014). Joint Royal College of Physicians Training Board [Online pdf]. Available at:. https://www.jrcptb.org.uk/documents/2010-respiratory-medicine

[28]　SCE in Respiratory Medicine blueprint 2018 [Online pdf]. Available at:. https://www.jrcptb.org.uk Accessed March 2021.

[29]　Specialty Training Curriculum for Neurology. August 2010 (Amended August 2013). Joint Royal College of Physicians Training Board [Online pdf]. Available at:. https://www.jrcptb.org.uk/documents/2010-neurology-amendment-2013 Accessed March 2021.

CHAPTER 25

Sleep Medicine in Iceland – The Challenges of a Subarctic Small Nation

Erna Sif Arnardottir[1,2,*] and **Jordan Cunningham**[2]

[1] *Reykjavik University Sleep Institute, School of Technology, Reykjavik University, Reykjavik, Iceland*

[2] *Landspitali University Hospital, Reykjavik, Iceland*

Abstract: The practice of sleep medicine within Iceland has been shaped by its position as a sub-arctic Nordic nation with a small population and a strong tradition of sleep research.

The major facility providing clinical diagnostic and therapeutic sleep services is the Landspitali - The National University Hospital of Iceland. Sleep studies are mainly conducted as home sleep apnoea testing with video hook-up instructions and electronic questionnaires. In the context of the COVID-19 pandemic, the majority of positive airway pressure therapy initiation took place at the home of the patient with auto settings and remote follow-up.

Sleep medicine service challenges include inferior access for rural areas, funding limitations, the COVID-19 pandemic and low sleep education at a national level for both the general population and specifically healthcare staff.

The unique clinical and research knowledge gap of Iceland requires studies on the health effects of living at such a northern latitude. The high hypnotic and antidepressant use of Icelanders as well as the high prevalence of restless legs syndrome symptoms may be at least in part contributed by latitude. The 1-1.5 hour discrepancy between the solar clock and the local clock may also cause social jet lag in Icelanders but this needs to be studied further. Finally, social factors such as the high energy drink consumption of Icelandic teenagers and the high screen time made possible by the 99% internet penetration and a mobile connection percentage that exceeds the total population level may contribute to the short sleep length found in Icelandic teenagers.

Keywords: Auto--positive airway pressure (AutoPAP), COVID-19, Daylight savings time (DST), Delayed sleep time, Height, Home sleep apnea testing (HSAT), Iceland, Icelandic Sleep Research Society, Insomnia, Light exposure,

[*] **Corresponding author Erna Sif Arnardottir:** Reykjavik University Sleep Institute, School of Technology, Reykjavik University, Reykjavik, Iceland; Email: ernasifa@ru.is

Hrayr P. Attarian, Marie-Louise M. Coussa-Koniski & Alain Michel Sabri (Eds.)

Obstructive sleep apnea (OSA), National electronic health records, Remote short sleep, Restless legs syndrome (RLS), Rural, Seasonal affective disorder (SAD), Social jet lag, Subarctic, Telemedicine, Video instructions.

INTRODUCTION

The Icelandic environment to study sleep is unique in many aspects. This includes our sub-arctic latitude (64-66° North) with light exposure varying highly from ~4 hours in December to ~21 hours in June [1, 2]. The relatively isolated population of 370.000 inhabitants has a high willingness to participate in research and longitudinal follow-up, high educational status, and a very high level of digital knowledge [2, 3]. When coupled with the national electronic health records, this allows for state-of-the-art quality research studies on different topics related to sleep and health. *e.g.* a recent publication showing that obstructive sleep apnoea (OSA) is an independent risk factor for having a poor outcome due to COVID-19 after adjustment for age, gender and importantly, body mass index [4]. In this study, all adult community-dwelling Icelanders who had been diagnosed with COVID-19 were cross-referenced against OSA diagnosis from the centralized national registries and the original clinical sleep studies checked for accuracy.

The Icelandic Sleep Research Society was officially founded in 1991 [5]. The society is very active both within Iceland and within the Assembly of National Sleep Societies of Europe (ANSS) with ~100 members which is per capita the highest number of members among the Associated National Sleep Societies in Europe [6]. The members are a mixture of medical doctors of different specialties, psychologists, biologists, nurses, engineers, computer scientists, sports scientists, and others with a sleep focus in their work.

Icelandic sleep researchers have for many years participated in international research projects, including research supported by the National Institute of Health in the United States and the European Union, with an emphasis mostly on clinical sleep research as well as some basic sleep research [7]. The utilisation of clinical sleep services especially for OSA is high, with one study showing about 4% of Icelanders, 40 years and older on current treatment [8].

THE CURRENT PRACTICE OF SLEEP MEDICINE

The health system is primarily publicly funded, delivered between public hospitals and private clinical practices, with small co-contributions from individual patients. The majority of sleep studies are performed within the public system, although a substantial minority access sleep studies through either research institutions, or private medical clinics. Within the broader context of the 2019 Health Policy to 2030 (laying out a road map for all Icelandic health services), sleep medicine is undergoing a period of reorganisation to better unify services around the country, and to develop uniform quality standards for the Icelandic Health Insurance, the national insurance agency [9].

The major facility providing clinical diagnostic and therapeutic sleep services is at the Landspitali - The National University Hospital of Iceland [LSH], in the capital, Reykjavik [10]. The sleep unit falls under the broader Respiratory Medicine and Sleep Department, reflecting that from the early 1980s, respiratory physicians have taken the lead in sleep medicine within the unit. Iceland's small size requires most medical practitioners to undertake specialty training abroad, and medically the unit is currently headed by an Australian-trained sleep physician, and staffed by respiratory physicians and an ear-nose and throat [ENT] doctor, who variously undertook specialty training in the United States, the United Kingdom, Sweden, and Norway. LSH operates a three-bed lab for in-patient sleep studies including video polysomnography and multiple sleep latency tests [MSLT], as well as utilising home polysomnography and [much like our Nordic neighbours] heavily utilises home sleep apnoea testing [HSAT] [11]. LSH is also responsible for overseeing almost all positive airway pressure [PAP] therapy within Iceland, from continuous PAP through to home life support ventilators for ventilator-dependent patients. Finally, all sleep studies and treatment of children are performed at the Children's Hospital of LSH in collaboration with the sleep unit. A special service for children with behavioural and other sleep problems is available and very popular, especially with parents of children under the age of three.

HSAT is also available at numerous other sites throughout Iceland, whether through a direct partnership between LSH and local health stations, or overseen by regional hospitals. A number of studies are also performed in privately run centres, the majority of which are funded through the same public system as hospital studies. HSAT studies throughout Iceland are mainly performed with the use of video hook-up instructions, with an equally low failure rate and similar quality as the in-person instructions conducted previously [12]. This is an important step towards telemedicine-based way of diagnosing OSA, is less costly and time-demanding for sleep staff, and allowed these services to mostly continue despite the COVID-19 pandemic. Finally, all patients referred to the sleep unit, answer an extensive electronic questionnaire *via* the secure web application, REDCap [13], on their sleep and daytime functioning as well as risk factors, similar to the Sleep Apnea Genetics International Consortium [SAGIC] questionnaire described here [8].

PAP initiation and follow-up were done prior to 2019 mostly with one daytime visit to the hospital [either as an individual or group appointment – the latter having been both well accepted by patients, and effective in reducing waiting lists], typically with autoPAP pressure settings, followed by sleeping with the device at home for the first night and remote follow-up. Patients are followed up also with a minimum of one phone call after 2-3 months of treatment. This telemedicine development has been spurred further and for a broader spectrum of patients due to the COVID-19 pandemic, and now the majority of patients commence therapy at home [14]. The major health regulatory bodies within Iceland are the Directorate of Health [15], and the Icelandic Health Insurance. Assessment as to whether foreign basic and specialty medical qualifications meet Icelandic standards is performed by the Directorate of Health in partnership with the Faculty of Medicine at the University of Iceland [which oversees Iceland's only medical school] [16]. At present, no separate Icelandic qualification exists for sleep medicine. Medical specialties involved are sleep medicine, respiratory medicine, neurology, ENT, and to an increasing extent cardiology and dentistry as well as of course general practice.

The national insurer, however, holds responsibility for maintaining quality standards by controlling access to reimbursement for studies. Clinical guidelines for the diagnosis and treatment of sleep-related breathing disorders and other sleep disorders have been created by the LSH sleep unit, last updated in 2015 [17], although a replacement guideline influenced by the Swedish standards is in development.

The clinical management of sleep-related movement disorders, hypersomnia, and parasomnias is handled both at the LSH sleep unit and by a small number of private neurologists. The clinical management of insomnia and circadian rhythm disordersis done both at the LSH sleep unit and by a number of psychologists [largely working in the private sector]. Psychologists are the main providers of cognitive behavioural therapy for insomnia [CBT-I], both with individual and group therapy as well as by digital therapy in Icelandic [18]. Given current access issues around sleep psychological services, English language resources are utilised [*e.g.* CBT-I Coach from Stanford and the US Veterans Affairs, and metacognitive therapy [MCT] based resources from the Centre for Clinical Interventions in Western Australia] - the latter is in process of being adapted to Icelandic with kind permission. The main sleep surgeries currently performed are tonsillectomy and nasal passage surgeries for OSA. Uvulopalatopharyngoplasty and maxillary and mandibular advancement surgeries are infrequently performed.

CHALLENGES TO PRACTICE OF SLEEP MEDICINE

Access barriers in Iceland are numerous, despite the relative wealth of the country and the overall high educational status of the nation.

Sleep services are inferior for those living in rural areas compared to the capital region as the majority of service is performed in the capital and longer per capita waiting lists for rural areas. Bad weather in winter can also hinder travelling to the capital to obtain these services. These issues are being addressed in numerous ways to improve telemedicine pathways, such as for HSATs and PAP follow-up as described above as well as increased use of remote data collection at local healthcare facilities with central interpretation at the LSH sleep unit or by private expert sleep technologists.

Resource limitations are one of the major challenges as funding has not been able to grow as quickly as demand, one of a number of contributing factors to long waiting lists. Again, the use of technology and telemedicine pathways is being increasingly used to improve efficiency and this will be developed further in the coming years to reduce the needed healthcare staff hours per patient and still provide state-of-the-art services.

During the COVID-19 pandemic, despite the emphasis on remote sleep services, changes around infection control and closures of non-emergent activity during periods of crisis have led to increased wait list, particularly for inpatient studies, albeit not to the same extent as in many other sleep laboratories [19]. Home PSG studies and increased activity at peripheral centres [*e.g.* using secure video conferencing to oversee non-invasive ventilation initiations at other sites] will be developed further as a part of this vision.

Compared to PSG, HSAT will tend to underscore sleep disordered breathing, especially for a phenotype in patients with a low arousal threshold and therefore few oxygen desaturations, *e.g.* in women and the young [20]. A current clinical aim is to increase the utilisation of PSG for inconclusive HSAT studies of symptomatic patients [21] and to improve the clinical guidelines for when such a study is needed. The discrepancy between the apnoea-hypopnea index [AHI] as the major diagnostic index for OSA severity and the need for treatment has also been shown to be a limiting factor in Iceland as elsewhere [22], with little relationship between AHI and sleep-related symptoms in the Icelandic general population [8].

Another major challenge to improve sleep services in Iceland is the low sleep education at a national level, with little educational material available at any level from primary school to university. Even, medical students and students of health sciences receive only a few hours of sleep education during their education. Therefore, a major effort is needed to increase sleep awareness among different healthcare professionals and the general public of the many clinical faces of sleep disorders. These efforts have started with educational material being created for children and teenagers as well as more widespread efforts to educate the general public about sleep. These efforts are spearheaded by the Directorate of Health in collaboration with the major sleep experts of Iceland. At the university level, the Department of Sport Science at Reykjavik University has taken the largest step to include a sleep education for 2 ECTS units as a part of their core undergraduate program and extensive elective sleep courses are offered to students at Reykjavik University but needed at the other universities in Iceland. [23].

Major educational efforts are also needed among current healthcare staff to decrease the extensive use of hypnotics in Iceland [24, 25], which is twice as high as in other Nordic countries (Fig. **1**). A decrease in hypnotic use and increased referrals of patients to the recommended first-line treatment of cognitive behavioural therapy for insomnia [26] prior to prescribing hypnotics, is an ongoing effort by sleep specialists.

A

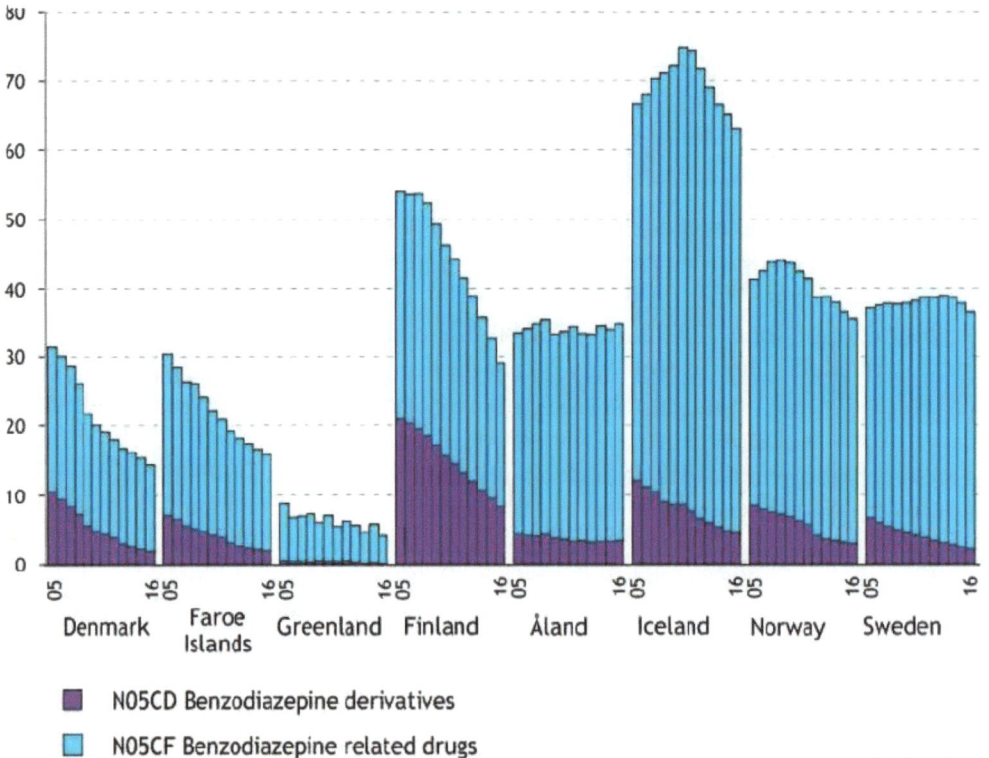

■ N05CD Benzodiazepine derivatives
☐ N05CF Benzodiazepine related drugs

(Fig. 1) contd.....

(B)

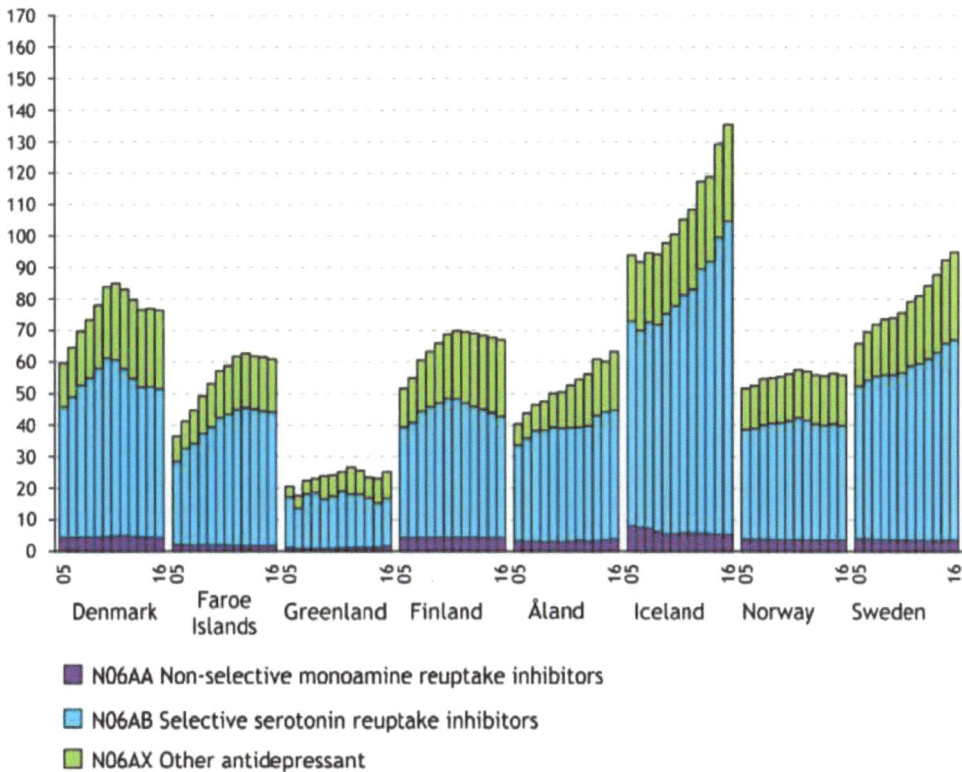

Fig. (1). Sales of (a) hypnotics and sedatives [Anatomical Therapeutic Chemical [ATC] groups N05CD and N05CF] and (b) antidepressants [ATC group N06A] in the Nordic Countries from 2005-2016 [25]. Defined daily dose [DDD]/1000 inhabitants/day.

CLINICAL AND RESEARCH KNOWLEDGE GAP

The unique needs of Iceland are numerous including the impact of the time zone which is not in synchrony with the sun time, potential high northern latitude impacts on circadian rhythm, sleep and mental health as well as behavioral components related to the high technology and caffeine use of Icelanders.

In 1968, the time zone of Iceland was fixed all year round at Greenwich Mean Time (GMT) +0 instead of only during daylight saving time (DST) in the summer [27]. This means that the sun is at its highest in the capital Reykjavik at approximately 13.30 and in the eastern part of Iceland at 13.00 instead of at 12.00 (Fig. 2). Parliament bills have been set forward four times since 2010 to move the delay clock time by one hour to GMT -1 to reflect more correctly the sun time [28]. However, after national-wide discussions and debates, in 2020, the prime minister of Iceland decided against a current change in clock time and stated that further research on the effects of such a clock change at Northern latitudes is needed. However, if the European Union dismisses daylight savings and moves to standard time all year round as recommended by sleep and circadian experts worldwide [29, 30], this would impact the time zone discussion in Iceland as well.

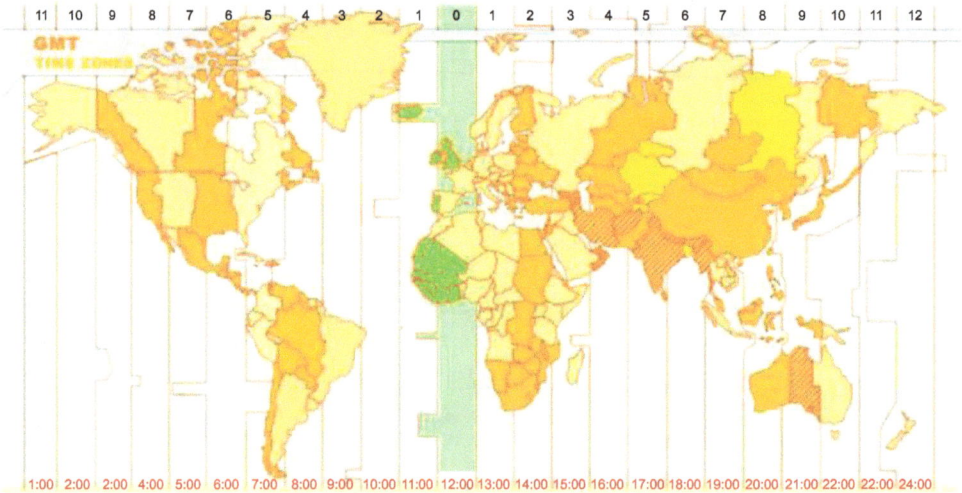

Fig. (2). Iceland is in the Greenwich Mean Time [GMT] +0 zone despite geographically being located in GMT-1 [28].

Current research strongly shows that a discrepancy between the solar clock and the local clock may cause social jet lag [31], a circadian mismatch leading to people having difficulties falling asleep and waking up at the necessary time for work and school. However, studies at Northern latitudes are indeed lacking. A Russian paper from longitudes 56-69° assessed the sleep times of 8000 individuals aged 10-24 years during nonDST, permanent DST and summer DST and found that during permanent DST, social jet lag was increased and an increase in winter seasonal affective disorder (SAD) symptoms was found as well [32].

Previous research on Icelanders indicates that they have a delayed circadian phase compared to other nations [33 - 35]. Studies have shown an average bedtime of elderly Icelanders close to midnight [36, 37] and that the majority of Icelandic teenagers have bedtimes after midnight, even on school days [38].

The high latitude of Iceland causes high variability in daylight hours by season, from about ~21 hours in June to ~4 hours in December (Fig. 3). This instability of light as a Zeitgeber for circadian rhythms and thereby sleep [39], may be one of the contributing factors to the high rates of antidepressants in Iceland compared to other Nordic countries (Fig. **1b**) [25], and hypnotics use as described above. Living at a northern latitude is a risk factor for seasonal affective disorder [SAD] [40, 41] and may be further affected by incorrect clock times as summarized above [32]. Interestingly, one Icelandic study on SAD levels from 1993 showed a similar level of SAD as on the East coast of the United States [42]. The hypothesis that this represents a population selection towards increased tolerance for winter darkness is supported by studies of people of Icelandic descent living in Canada showing lower levels of SAD than comparison groups [43, 44]. However, newer studies are needed to assess the current level of SAD and subsyndromal SAD levels in Iceland compared to other nations.

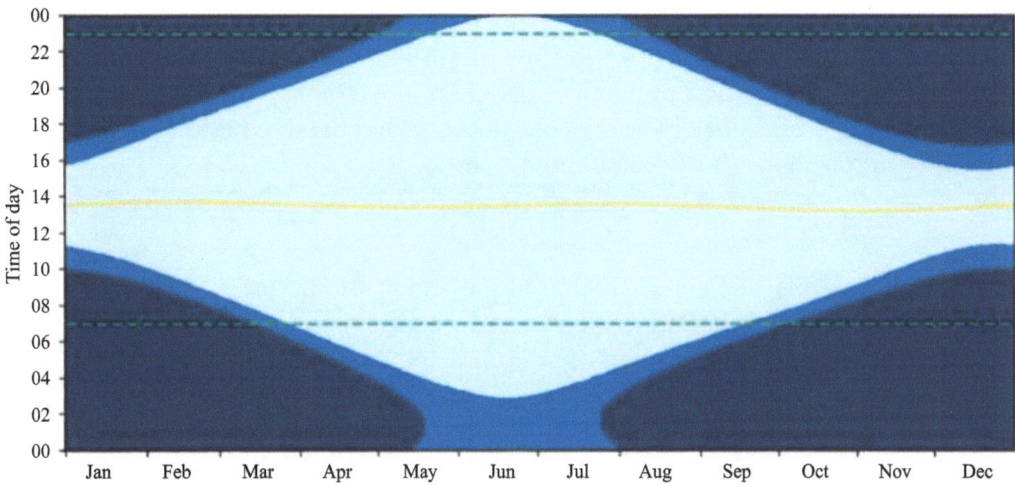

Fig. (3). The fluctuations in the number of daylight hours in Reykjavik, Iceland from January to December [1]. Daylight is shown in light blue, twilight hours in cobalt blue and darkness in dark blue. The yellow line shows when the sun is at the highest point. The green lines show the traditional wake times from 07-23.

A relationship between latitude and restless legs syndrome (RLS) prevalence has been reported with an increase in RLS symptoms the farther a country is from the equator [45]. The prevalence in Iceland as reported by a 2010 study is the highest in Europe, or 18.3% [45, 46]. Further studies are needed to determine the mediating factors for this relationship but may be related to ultraviolet radiation (impacting *e.g.* vitamin D) and ferritin levels [45].

A recent actigraphy study of 15-16 year old Icelanders showed an average ± standard deviation of 6.2 ± 0.7 hours on weekdays and 7.3 ± 1.1 hours on weekends [38], well below the recommended 8-10 hours' sleep time for this age group [47]. This short sleep length may be affected by the social jet lag and northern latitude as described above. Another major contributor is the high caffeine and energy drink consumption of Icelandic teenagers, as 30% of 13 year olds and 47% of 15 year olds consume energy drinks in a 2020 national wide survey of over 10,000 participants [48]. The same study showed a high correlation between high caffeine consumption and a report of both sleeping difficulties and short sleep times. The 99% internet penetration in Iceland and mobile connections equivalent to 145% of the total population [3] may also affect the sleep of Icelanders due to the negative associations found between screen time and sleep [49, 50].

Finally, Icelanders have specific PAP issues not encountered by many other nations. *e.g.* as one of the tallest countries on earth [51] even large full-face masks of leading brands are too small for a not-insignificant proportion of patients. Auto humidification also seems to be frequently uncomfortably warm and moist for Icelanders. Finally, the high proportion of sailors needs special consideration, with the unsuitability of humidification chambers for a North Atlantic swell. These clinical observations by one of the authors [JC] need to be followed up with clinical research studies to validate their claims.

CONCLUSION

The current position of sleep medicine in Iceland is strong, especially with regard to OSA and telemedicine approaches, but is challenged by resource limitations and relatively low sleep education of overall healthcare staff.

Icelanders face a unique set of challenges living at a very northern latitude with highly variable light exposure levels and an incorrect local clock time compared to sun time. A rich tradition of clinical sleep research and high levels of sleep medicine practises allow for a huge potential for future research studies on these topics, preferably using new tools of subjective and objective sleep measurements, including mobile applications and wearables for long-term data collection [52].

CONSENT FOR PUBLICATION

Not applicable.

CONFLICTS OF INTEREST

Dr. Arnardottir discloses lecture fees from Nox Medical, Philips and ResMed outside the scope of the work presented in the chapter.

Dr. Cunningham has no financial conflicts of interest to disclose.

ACKNOWLEDGEMENT

Declared none.

REFERENCES

[1]   Gauksson T. Ef við stillum klukkuna 2018.https://tandrigauksson.wordpress.com/2018/01/07/ef-vi--stillum-klukkuna/

[2]   Statistics Iceland [homepage on the Internet]. National Statistical Institute of Iceland; [Dec 9, 2021]. Available from:. https://www.statice.is/statistics/population/inhabitants/overview/

[3]   Kemp S. Kemp S. DataReportal 2020 [Dec 9, 2021]. Available from:. https://datareportal.com/reports/digital-2020-iceland

[4]   Rögnvaldsson KG, Eyþórsson ES, Emilsson Ö, Eysteinsdóttir B, Pálsson R, Gottfreðsson M, *et al.* Obstructive sleep apnea is an independent risk factor for severe COVID-19: a population-based study. Sleep (Basel) 2021.

[5]   The Icelandic Sleep Research Society [ISRS]. European Sleep Research Society [Dec 9, 2021]. Available from:. https://esrs.eu/iceland/

[6]   Affiliated National Sleep Societies: European Sleep Research Society; [Dec 9, 2021]. Available from: . https://esrs.eu/about/associate-national-sleep-societies/

[7]   PubMed search "[sleep] AND [Iceland[Affiliation]]" Bethesda, MD: National Library of Medicine; [Dec 9, 2021]. Available from:. https://pubmed.ncbi.nlm.nih.gov/?term=%28sleep%29+AND+%28Iceland%5BAffiliation%5D%29&sort=date

[8]   Arnardottir ES, Bjornsdottir E, Olafsdottir KA, Benediktsdottir B, Gislason T. Obstructive sleep apnoea in the general population: highly prevalent but minimal symptoms. Eur Respir J 2016; 47(1): 194-202.
[http://dx.doi.org/10.1183/13993003.01148-2015] [PMID: 26541533]

[9]   Icelandic Health Insurance https://www.sjukra.is/

[10] Landspitali- The National University Hospital of Iceland [Dec 9, 2021]. Available from:. https://www.landspitali.is/

[11] Arnardottir ES, Verbraecken J, Gonçalves M, *et al.* Variability in recording and scoring of respiratory events during sleep in Europe: a need for uniform standards. J Sleep Res 2016; 25(2): 144-57.
[http://dx.doi.org/10.1111/jsr.12353] [PMID: 26365742]

[12] Horne AF, Olafsdottir KA, Arnardottir ES. In-person vs. video hookup instructions: A comparison of home sleep apnea testingquality. [Submitted for publication];. 2021.

[13] REDCap consortium: Vanderbilt University; [Dec 9, 2021]. Available from: https://www.project-redcap.org/.. https://www.project-redcap.org/

[14] Schiza S, Simonds A, Randerath W, *et al.* Sleep laboratories reopening and COVID-19: a European perspective. Eur Respir J 2021; 57(3): 2002722.
[http://dx.doi.org/10.1183/13993003.02722-2020] [PMID: 33214202]

[15] The Directorate of Health [Dec 9, 2021]. Available from:. https://www.landlaeknir.is/

[16] Faculty of Medicine, School of Health Sciences, University of Iceland [Dec 9, 2021].. https://english.hi.is/school_of_health_sciences/faculty_of_medicine/front_page

[17] Gislason T, Arnardottir ES. Klínískar leiðbeiningar um greiningu og meðferð svefntengdra öndunartruflana/kæfisvefns [Icelandic: Clinical guidelines for the diagnosis and treatment of sleep related breathing disorders/obstructive sleep apnea]. 2nd edition ed. Landspitali - The National University Hospital of Iceland, Reykjavik, Iceland2015.

[18] Friðgeirsdóttir G, Jóhannsson G, Ellertsson S, Björnsdóttir E. Effectiveness of an online cognitive behavioral therapy for insomnia. Laeknabladid 2015; 101(4): 203-8.
[http://dx.doi.org/10.17992/lbl.2015.05.20] [PMID: 25894498]

[19] Grote L, McNicholas WT, Hedner J. collaborators E. Sleep apnoea management in Europe during the COVID-19 pandemic: data from the European Sleep Apnoea Database. Eur Respir J 2020. [ESADA].
[http://dx.doi.org/10.1183/13993003.01323-2020]

[20] Nerfeldt P, Aoki F, Friberg D. Polygraphy vs. polysomnography: missing osas in symptomatic snorers—a reminder for clinicians. Sleep Breath 2014; 18(2): 297-303.
[http://dx.doi.org/10.1007/s11325-013-0884-6] [PMID: 23942981]

[21] Kapur VK, Auckley DH, Chowdhuri S, *et al.* Clinical Practice Guideline for Diagnostic Testing for Adult Obstructive Sleep Apnea: An American Academy of Sleep Medicine Clinical Practice Guideline. J Clin Sleep Med 2017; 13(3): 479-504.
[http://dx.doi.org/10.5664/jcsm.6506] [PMID: 28162150]

[22] Pevernagie DA, Gnidovec-Strazisar B, Grote L, *et al.* On the rise and fall of the apnea–hypopnea index: A historical review and critical appraisal. J Sleep Res 2020; 29(4): e13066.
[http://dx.doi.org/10.1111/jsr.13066] [PMID: 32406974]

[23] Reykjavik University [Dec 9, 2021]. Available from:. https://www.ru.is/

[24] Linnet K, Sigurdsson JA, Tomasdottir MO, Sigurdsson EL, Gudmundsson LS. Association between prescription of hypnotics/anxiolytics and mortality in multimorbid and non-multimorbid patients: a longitudinal cohort study in primary care. BMJ Open 2019; 9(12): e033545.
[http://dx.doi.org/10.1136/bmjopen-2019-033545] [PMID: 31811011]

[25] MJ Health Statistics for the Nordic Countries 2017. Copenhagen: Nordic Medico-Statistical Committee 2017.

[26] Riemann D, Baglioni C, Bassetti C, *et al.* European guideline for the diagnosis and treatment of insomnia. J Sleep Res 2017; 26(6): 675-700.
[http://dx.doi.org/10.1111/jsr.12594] [PMID: 28875581]

[27] Iceland Go. Staðartími á Íslandi 2018.

[28] Server WT. https://www.worldtravelserver.com/travel/en/iceland/reykjavik/gmt_0.html

[29] [ESRS]. ESRS, [EBRS]. EBRS, [SRBR]. SfRoBR. Joint statement to the EU on DST.. 2019.

[30] Rishi MA, Ahmed O, Barrantes Perez JH, *et al.* Daylight saving time: an American Academy of Sleep Medicine position statement. J Clin Sleep Med 2020; 16(10): 1781-4.
[http://dx.doi.org/10.5664/jcsm.8780] [PMID: 32844740]

[31] Roenneberg T, Winnebeck EC, Klerman EB. Daylight Saving Time and Artificial Time Zones – A Battle Between Biological and Social Times. Front Physiol 2019; 10: 944.
[http://dx.doi.org/10.3389/fphys.2019.00944] [PMID: 31447685]

[32] Borisenkov MF, Tserne TA, Panev AS, *et al.* Seven-year survey of sleep timing in Russian children and adolescents: chronic 1-h forward transition of social clock is associated with increased social jetlag and winter pattern of mood seasonality. Biol Rhythm Res 2017; 48(1): 3-12.
[http://dx.doi.org/10.1080/09291016.2016.1223778]

[33] Thorleifsdottir B, Björnsson JK, Benediktsdottir B, Gislason T, Kristbjarnarson H. Sleep and sleep habits from childhood to young adulthood over a 10-year period. J Psychosom Res 2002; 53(1): 529-37.
[http://dx.doi.org/10.1016/S0022-3999(02)00444-0] [PMID: 12127168]

[34] Janson C, Gislason T, De Backer W, *et al.* Prevalence of sleep disturbances among young adults in three European countries. Sleep 1995; 18(7): 589-97.
[PMID: 8552930]

[35]   Gradisar M, Gardner G, Dohnt H. Recent worldwide sleep patterns and problems during adolescence: A review and meta-analysis of age, region, and sleep. Sleep Med 2011; 12(2): 110-8.
[http://dx.doi.org/10.1016/j.sleep.2010.11.008] [PMID: 21257344]

[36]   Brychta RJ, Arnardottir NY, Johannsson E, *et al.* Influence of Day Length and Physical Activity on Sleep Patterns in Older Icelandic Men and Women. J Clin Sleep Med 2016; 12(2): 203-13.
[http://dx.doi.org/10.5664/jcsm.5486] [PMID: 26414978]

[37]   Gíslason T, Reynisdóttir H, Kristbjarnarson H, Benediktsdóttir B. Sleep habits and sleep disturbances among the elderly-an epidemiological survey. J Intern Med 1993; 234(1): 31-9.
[http://dx.doi.org/10.1111/j.1365-2796.1993.tb00701.x] [PMID: 8326287]

[38]   Rognvaldsdottir V, Gudmundsdottir SL, Brychta RJ, *et al.* Sleep deficiency on school days in Icelandic youth, as assessed by wrist accelerometry. Sleep Med 2017; 33: 103-8.
[http://dx.doi.org/10.1016/j.sleep.2016.12.028] [PMID: 28449887]

[39]   Yamanaka Y. Basic concepts and unique features of human circadian rhythms: implications for human health. Nutr Rev 2020; 78(12) (Suppl. 3): 91-6.
[http://dx.doi.org/10.1093/nutrit/nuaa072] [PMID: 33259616]

[40]   Galima SV, Vogel SR, Kowalski AW. Seasonal Affective Disorder: Common Questions and Answers. Am Fam Physician 2020; 102(11): 668-72.
[PMID: 33252911]

[41]   Magnusson A, Partonen T. The diagnosis, symptomatology, and epidemiology of seasonal affective disorder. CNS Spectr 2005; 10(8): 625-34.
[http://dx.doi.org/10.1017/S1092852900019593] [PMID: 16041294]

[42]   Magnússon A, Stefánsson JG. Prevalence of seasonal affective disorder in Iceland. Arch Gen Psychiatry 1993; 50(12): 941-6.
[http://dx.doi.org/10.1001/archpsyc.1993.01820240025002] [PMID: 8250679]

[43]   Axelsson J, Stefánsson JG, Magnússon A, Sigvaldason H, Karlsson MM. Seasonal affective disorders: relevance of Icelandic and Icelandic-Canadian evidence to etiologic hypotheses. Can J Psychiatry 2002; 47(2): 153-8.
[http://dx.doi.org/10.1177/070674370204700205] [PMID: 11926077]

[44]   Magnússon A, Axelsson J. The prevalence of seasonal affective disorder is low among descendants of Icelandic emigrants in Canada. Arch Gen Psychiatry 1993; 50(12): 947-51.
[http://dx.doi.org/10.1001/archpsyc.1993.01820240031004] [PMID: 8250680]

[45]   Koo BB. Restless legs syndrome: relationship between prevalence and latitude. Sleep Breath 2012; 16(4): 1237-45.
[http://dx.doi.org/10.1007/s11325-011-0640-8] [PMID: 22210354]

[46]   Benediktsdottir B, Janson C, Lindberg E, *et al.* Prevalence of restless legs syndrome among adults in Iceland and Sweden: Lung function, comorbidity, ferritin, biomarkers and quality of life. Sleep Med 2010; 11(10): 1043-8.
[http://dx.doi.org/10.1016/j.sleep.2010.08.006] [PMID: 20961808]

[47]   Hirshkowitz M, Whiton K, Albert SM, *et al.* National Sleep Foundation's updated sleep duration recommendations: final report. Sleep Health 2015; 1(4): 233-43.
[http://dx.doi.org/10.1016/j.sleh.2015.10.004] [PMID: 29073398]

[48]   Halldorsson TI, Kristjansson AL, Thorisdottir I, *et al.* Caffeine exposure from beverages and its association with self-reported sleep duration and quality in a large sample of Icelandic adolescents. Food Chem Toxicol 2021; 157: 112549.
[http://dx.doi.org/10.1016/j.fct.2021.112549] [PMID: 34509583]

[49]   Wacks Y, Weinstein AM. Excessive Smartphone Use Is Associated With Health Problems in Adolescents and Young Adults. Front Psychiatry 2021; 12: 669042.
[http://dx.doi.org/10.3389/fpsyt.2021.669042] [PMID: 34140904]

[50]   Hrafnkelsdottir SM, Brychta RJ, Rognvaldsdottir V, *et al.* Less screen time and more physical activity is associated with more stable sleep patterns among Icelandic adolescents. Sleep Health 2020; 6(5): 609-17.
[http://dx.doi.org/10.1016/j.sleh.2020.02.005] [PMID: 32331863]

[51]   [NCD-RisC] NRFC. A century of trends in adult human height. Elife. 2016;5.
[PMID: 27458798]

[52]   Arnardottir ES, Islind AS, Óskarsdóttir M. The Future of Sleep Measurements. Sleep Med Clin 2021; 16(3): 447-64.
[http://dx.doi.org/10.1016/j.jsmc.2021.05.004] [PMID: 34325822]

CHAPTER 26

Practice of Sleep Medicine in Lithuania

Evelina   Pajėdienė[1,*],   Dalia   Matačiūnienė[2]   and   Eglė Sakalauskaitė-Juodeikienė[3]

[1] *Department of Neurology, Academy of Medicine, Lithuanian University of Health Sciences, Kaunas, Lithuania*

[2] *Kardiolita Hospital, Vilnius, Lithuania*

[3] *Department of Neurology and Neurosurgery, Institute of Clinical Medicine, Faculty of Medicine, Vilnius University, Vilnius, Lithuania*

Abstract: Lithuania is a small country with a relatively short (31 year) history of independence in the modern era. Complicated history and geopolitical situation determined gaps in many socioeconomic spheres compared to other western European countries 30 years ago. Nevertheless, the country's ambitious goals and direction towards democratic values resulted in high recent socioeconomic ratings and acknowledgment among other European Union, NATO and Organisation for Economic Co-operation and Development members. The chapter presents short Lithuania's geopolitical and healthcare system data, the current practice of sleep medicine, the practitioners involved, the availability of diagnostic tools and medications to treat common sleep disorders. It discusses challenges to the practice of sleep medicine: patient access to care, resource limitations and financial hardships, clinical and research knowledge gaps.

Keywords: Driving regulation, Insomnia, Lithuania, Research, Sleep apnea, Sleep disorders, Sleep medicine.

INTRODUCTION

Geopolitical Data

Lithuania, officially the Republic of Lithuania, is a small country (with area of 65.286 km^2) in the Baltic region of Europe. Situated on the eastern shore of the Baltic Sea, to the southeast of Sweden and Denmark, Lithuania is bordered by Latvia to the north, Belarus to the east and south, Poland to the south, and Kaliningrad to the southwest. The capital and largest city is Vilnius.

* **Corresponding author Evelina Pajėdienė:** Department of Neurology, Academy of Medicine, Lithuanian University of Health Sciences, Kaunas, Lithuania; Tel: +37065783809; E-mail: evelina.pajediene@lsmu.lt.

Hrayr P. Attarian, Marie-Louise M. Coussa-Koniski & Alain Michel Sabri (Eds.)

On 11 March 1990, a year before the formal dissolution of the Soviet Union, Lithuania became the first Baltic state to proclaim its independence, resulting in the restoration of the independent State of Lithuania. It is a republic based on parliamentary democracy. Lithuania joined the North Atlantic Treaty Organization (NATO) in 2004, European Union (EU) in 2004, Schengen in 2007 and Organization for Economic Co-operation and Development (OECD) in 2018. On 1 January 2015, the euro became the national currency [1].

Lithuania has an estimated population of 2.8 million people in 2020. One-third of the resident population lives in rural areas. Lithuanian life expectancy at birth was 76.4 (71.5 years for males and 81 for females) in 2019, the difference between rural and urban residents was not significant (74.8 and 77.3 respectively) [2].

Lithuania is a developed country with a high Human Development Index (HDI). A country scores a higher HDI when the lifespan is higher, the education level is higher, and the gross national income per capita is higher. The Human Development Report 2020 by the United Nations Development Program was released on 15 December 2020, and calculated HDI values based on data collected in 2019. Lithuania ranked in 34th place [3].

Lithuania provides free state-funded healthcare to all citizens and registered long-term residents. The Lithuanian health system is organized around a single insurance fund providing health coverage to nearly the entire population (98% in 2018) [4]. The Ministry of Health, which governs the National Health Insurance Fund (NHIF), formulates health policies and regulation and is responsible for licensing providers and health professionals, as well as for approving capital investment in healthcare facilities. Compulsory Health Insurance is obligatory for Lithuanian residents. Contributions for people who are economically active, are 9% of income. Emergency medical services are provided free of charge to all residents. Private healthcare is also available in the country. In 2003–2012, the network of hospitals was restructured, as part of wider healthcare service reforms. It started in 2003 with the expansion of ambulatory services and primary care. Decentralization of the healthcare system was achieved by segregating primary healthcare (family physicians), secondary healthcare (physicians-specialists), and tertiary healthcare levels (high specialization university clinics) [4].

Lithuania has a high number of doctors compared to the EU average (4.6 compared to 3.6 per 1000 population in 2017), of which slightly over one-fifth are general practitioners (GP). At the same time, the number of nurses is slightly lower than the EU average (7.7 *vs.* 8.5) [4].

Lithuania's spending on health care is among the lowest in the EU. In 2017, current health expenditure accounted for 6.5% of Gross Domestic Product (GDP), the fifth lowest in the EU and substantially lower than the EU average of 9.8%. In terms of spending per person, Lithuania spent 1605 Eur (adjusted for differences in purchasing power) in 2017 – slightly more than half the EU average of 2884 Eur per person. Furthermore, only about two-thirds (67%) of health expenditures are publicly funded, a significantly lower share than the EU average (79%). Out-of-pocket (OOP) payments cover the remaining third of healthcare spending [4].

The proportion of Lithuanians reporting unmet needs for medical examination and treatment is relatively small. Only 1.5% of the population reported barriers in access to care in 2017 due to waiting time, costs or distance to travel. In addition, the difference across income groups was relatively small [4]. In 2018, Lithuania ranked 28th in Europe in the Euro health consumer index (EHCI). EHCI is a comparison of European healthcare systems based on waiting times, results and generosity. The ranking included 37 countries measured by 48 indicators. It claims to measure the "consumer friendliness" of healthcare systems [5].

Nevertheless, some healthcare effectiveness measures are not satisfying in Lithuania. Lithuania has one of the highest mortality rates from preventable and treatable causes in the EU. Over 8500 deaths could have been avoided in Lithuania in 2016 through effective public health and prevention interventions, and a further 5000 through more effective and timely health care provision [4].

Lithuania's mortality rate by suicide in 2017 was still the highest reported in the EU. It remains an important cause of death, particularly among men. In recent years, the authorities have launched a number of suicide prevention campaigns that led to a 45% decrease in the number of deaths between 2000 and 2016.

In 2017, only 44% of the Lithuanian population reported perceiving themselves to be in good health – the lowest rate in the EU. As in other countries, people with higher incomes are more likely to report being in good health: two-thirds of those in the highest income quintile considered themselves to be in good health, compared with only one-quarter of those in the lowest quintile. This income gap in self-reported health is the second highest in the EU [4].

Historical Background

The origins of sleep medicine in Lithuania could be traced back to the early XIXth century [6]. It was the time when Lithuania was a part of the Russian empire, and Vilnius University (VU), founded in 1579, was the largest institution in the empire, based on student numbers and university departments. As czar Alexander I (1777–1825), a supporter of limited liberalism, wanted to transform Vilnius with its university into a gateway from the Russian Empire to an enlightened Europe, certain reforms were enacted. The number of departments at

VU was doubled and foreign professors were invited to lecture at the university. Prominent scholars and scientists from Austria, Germany, Italy, England, and France began to travel in increasing numbers to Vilnius. Joseph Frank (1771 – 1842) was one of them. A graduate of the University of Pavia, whose most famous teachers were Antonio Scarpa (1752 – 1832), Alessandro Volta (1745 – 1827), and his father Johann Peter Frank (1745 – 1821), J. Frank spent almost 20 years in Vilnius, being a Professor of Special Therapy and Clinical Medicine, an organiser, a reformer, a founder of clinics, institutes, and medical societies [7].

J. Frank wrote most of his *opus magnum*, a multivolume textbook titled *Praxeos medicae universae praecepta* ("Practical Textbook of General Medicine"), while living and working in Vilnius. In one of his volumes, devoted to nervous system diseases and published in 1818 in Leipzig, he also included chapters on sleep medicine [8]. Professor analyzed the phenomena and clinical cases of hypersomnia (*cataphora*), insomnia (*agrypnia*), snoring (*rhonchus*), restlessness with or without limb movements (*jactatio*), leg cramps, hot flushes (*ardor*), night terrors (*pavor in somno*), nightmares (*somnia terrifica*), breathlessness with feeling pressure on the chest (*incubus*), somnambulism, catalepsy and other sleep disorders. He analyzed the predisposing factors, causes and symptoms of the diseases, prognosis (for example, stated that snoring predisposes patients to apoplexy and headaches), and also discussed treatment options, mentioning the importance of antiphlogistic methods (bloodletting, leeches, cupping therapy, laxatives, diuretics), stimulating drugs (camphor, aether), opium, animal magnetism and sleep hygiene (recommended diet, safe environment, gymnastics, fast walks, to avoid long sitting and sleeping during daytime) [9].

The other scientific publication, devoted to sleep medicine in the XIXth-century Lithuania, was written by Joannes Adamus Schloezer and titled *Dissertatio inauguralis medico-practica de somnambulismo* ("Doctoral thesis on somnambulism", 1816). Somnambulism was perceived here as a sleep disorder, a disease of the brain, while this phenomenon for a long time was misunderstood as a weird, supernatural condition, "a miracle of nature", and "a labyrinth of the philosophers" [10]. Sleepwalking was stated to manifest during the night when an excited person woke up, stayed in the bed talking or walked around, performed simple or complex tasks, with eyes closed or opened, not responding to visual, auditory or tactile stimuli, avoiding obstacles, and finally returning to bed, knowing nothing of the episode. This sleep disorder was also treated using antiphlogistic methods, based on humoral theories that were still very popular at the time [11].

Patients with sleep disorders (some of them were admitted and treated in VU Therapy Clinic) were discussed by their physicians and university professors during Vilnius Medical Society (VMS) meetings. And when VU was closed by Russian imperial authorities in 1832 (following the suppression of a Polish and Lithuanian uprising), and Faculty of Medicine – a decade later, VMS remained the only scientific medical institution in the XIXth and beginning of the XXth centuries, still open for doctors, pharmacists, and veterinarians [12], and a place where complicated cases of patients with nervous system diseases and sleep disorders were discussed.

Training in Sleep Medicine: Physician and other Professionals

Higher education for biomedical sciences is mainly provided by two largest academic institutions – Vilnius University (VU) and Lithuanian University of Health Sciences (LUHS) in Lithuania.

Different faculties in VU receive approximately 20 000 students per year. Currently, the Faculty of Medicine is one of the largest and most significant faculties in Vilnius. Students of the Faculty of Medicine, residents and doctoral students also use different bases of VU, research institutes, and public and private healthcare institutions [13].

LUHS consists of two main academies: Medical Academy and Veterinary Academy. Students of medicine, odontology, and nursing gain their practical skills at the LUHS Hospital Kaunas Clinics, which is the largest medical institution in the Baltic States [14].

VU Faculty of Medicine and LUHS Medical Academy do not have any separate curriculum dedicated to sleep medicine, neither in master's, nor in residency programs. During medical studies, some theoretical and practical knowledge about sleep related breathing disorders is gained in pulmonology, otorhinolaryngology, and endocrinology cycles. Orthodontic and surgical treatment of bruxism and obstructive sleep apnea (OSA) is also briefly discussed during odontology and maxillofacial studies. Other sleep disorders, such as parasomnias (especially their differential aspects from epilepsy and REM sleep behavior disorder in neurodegenerative diseases), narcolepsy, restless legs syndrome, and periodic limb movement disorder are shortly discussed with medical students in neurology curriculum.

Regarding residency training, VU and LUHS physicians, specializing in sleep medicine, teach future child and adult neurologists about all main groups of sleep disorders, indications for further sleep diagnostics, interpretation of their results, and main treatment principles. Both adult and pediatric pulmonology residents rotating in sleep-lab mainly focus on sleep-related breathing disorders anamnesis, symptoms, diagnostics and treatment, while otorhinolaryngology residents can observe OSA-oriented diagnostic and surgical interventions.

Physicians and nurses who are specializing in sleep medicine are working in various public and private hospitals in Lithuania (cities of Vilnius, Kaunas, Klaipeda, and Palanga). These specialists have gained their knowledge *via* traineeships in sleep clinics abroad (Sweden, France, Denmark, Germany, *etc.*) and in Lithuania on the "peer-to-peer" learning basis. Till now there is one neurology physician that in 2016 became European Sleep Research Society Certified Expert Somnologist (E. Pajėdienė, MD).

The cognitive behavioral therapy for insomnia (CBT-I) course is integrated into the postgraduate studies of CBT, dedicated to medical professionals and psychologists, having a duration of 3-4 years and is organized by LUHS. The number of experienced CBT-I oriented psychotherapists is growing in recent years.

The main challenges regarding training in sleep medicine and possible solutions are as follows:

- Lack of sleep medicine-related training during master's studies; specified curriculum could be organized during neurology and pulmonology modules.

- Lack of sleep medicine-related training during residency programs for different specialties, starting from future family doctors, psychiatrists, various therapeutics and surgery specialists.

- Lack of training for nurses that could specialize in sleep lab as a sleep technologist, helping with sleep diagnostics and treatment.

- Need for defined agreements and requirements of sleep medicine training and practice in Lithuania, unified diagnostic and treatment guidelines for sleep disorders.

Type of Practitioners Involved in Sleep Medicine and Available Diagnostic Tools

General practitioners (GP) and mental health workers (in cases of insomnia) are the first line care providers to whom patients first address their sleep problems. In the Lithuanian healthcare system, primary care routinely acts as a first contact point for patients. Mental health practitioners are also accessible directly, without a referral. Primary care physicians play a gatekeeping function to more intensive levels of care. The average density of Lithuanian GPs per 100 000 population is 74, with the lower GP density in rural areas [2]. About 80% of patients find it easy to reach and gain access to GPs, while 10% of patients rate general practice care as not very or not at all affordable [15]. At the primary care level, services are delivered in 115 mental health care centers, which are sometimes co-located with primary care centers [4].

General practitioners recognize sleep problems, perform basic somatic screening and give sleep hygiene recommendations. They also prescribe initial treatment and refer to more specialized consultations and investigations if needed. The awareness about sleep problems among GPs is growing over the last few years, thanks to numerous conferences and seminars devoted to sleep problems.

Specialized sleep studies are performed in sleep centers. The first sleep laboratory in Lithuania was established in 1999 in LUHS Hospital Kaunas Clinics and was devoted to breathing disturbances during sleep [16]. Four years later, a semi-private neurologically oriented sleep center was opened in Vilnius and it covered diagnostics and treatment of the whole spectrum of sleep disorders. The network of sleep centers expanded in 2016, after the ratification of European Union directive 2014/85/EU on driver licensing in obstructive sleep apnea. At the beginning of 2021, there were five state-funded and three private sleep centers in Lithuania for adult patients and two sleep centers (in the biggest tertiary University hospitals) for children, together performing up to 1000 polysomnographies (PSG) per year. Five adult sleep centers are geographically distributed throughout Lithuania from the eastern to the western part of the country (Vilnius in the East, Kaunas-central region, and Klaipėda, Palanga in the West), and located in the public hospitals. The main two tertiary centers (in LUHS Hospital Kaunas Clinics and VU Hospital Santaros klinikos) have sleep beds both in pulmonology and neurology departments. A sleep center has from one to four PSG equipped beds. For the diagnosis of the most sleep disorders, PSG is the national standard. It is covered by the state health insurance as an in-patient investigation. Limited channel assessments are used by otorhinolaryngologists or pulmonologists only for screening purposes. Two neuro-oriented sleep centers (in tertiary University hospitals) perform multiple sleep latency tests (MSLT), and expanded electroencephalography channel PSG, if needed. Pulmonologists and neurologists are the main practitioners performing sleep studies in Lithuania, but there are also a few cardiologists involved. Specialized nurses (technicians) in sleep medicine centers are of great value and in high demand.

The main challenges regarding sleep diagnostics in Lithuania are as follows:

- Low GPs' awareness of sleep disorders and late referral to sleep centers (improving);

- Long waiting list for state funded PSG (up to 1.5 year, but with a tendency to decrease over the past 2 years);

- Laboratory weaknesses: no possibility to measure cerebrospinal fluid hypocretin, and to perform melatonin profile test.

There are no discrimination or difficulties in accessing care for patients on ethnic or gender basis in Lithuania.

Available Treatment Methods and Reimbursement

There are practically all up to date treatment possibilities for sleep disorders in Lithuania. But the greatest challenge is the reimbursement system.

Pulmonologists have more than 20 years of experience treating OSA with continuous positive airway pressure (CPAP) therapy. There are longtime working and reliable representatives of both Philips Respironics and ResMed companies in Lithuania. Unfortunately, CPAP treatment is not covered by state health insurance in typical OSA cases, and patients have to pay for CPAP devices and masks out of their pocket. Reimbursement is restricted only for central sleep apnea and cases where BiPAP or adaptive-servo ventilation is indicated.

As a member of the EU, Lithuania can use all drugs that are approved and registered by the European Medicines Agency (EMA) and are listed in the Register of Medicinal Products of the Republic of Lithuania or in the Community Register of Medicinal Products by the European Commission. For orphan drugs (as for narcolepsy), there were some supply and distribution difficulties for a small country with a small pharmaceutical market. Only in 2020, the first drug from the first line narcolepsy treatment recommendations (pitolisant) was approved and reimbursed for the treatment of narcolepsy. Sodium oxybate and modafinil are available, but not covered by health insurance, and methylphenidate is prescribed as an off-label drug, as narcolepsy was not included in nationally registered drug indications.

Treatment of insomnia for many years was drug-oriented as the availability and prices of hypnotics were unobstructed. Recent years show changes in this paradigm as psychotherapy evolves, cognitive behavioral therapy (CBT) is more and more available, and the network of CBT-I specialists increases. State health insurance covers 24 psychotherapy consultations per year in public mental health centers, but most psychotherapists work on a private basis. Mental health in Lithuania gained a lot of attention during the last 20 years, because of the leading position in the region by suicide rate. Despite constantly decreasing since its peak in 1995, the suicide rate in Lithuania remains among the highest in the EU and the

OECD. The suicide rate in 2018 was 24.4 suicides per 100,000. According to data, Lithuania has retained a high number of psychiatrists (225 per million inhabitants). Despite that fact, accessibility of services at mental health centers is uneven in Lithuania. Important efforts have been made in recent years to improve mental health services, which have contributed to initiate a reduction in the number of deaths by suicide. Many strategies have been developed not only to prevent suicide, but also to detect depression symptoms earlier and provide more appropriate treatment for other mental health diseases. Psychological help for those who are not willing or not able to seek out professional assistance of a psychologist or a psychotherapist due to financial restrictions is available through online or phone suicide prevention hotlines, there are nine phone numbers listed [17].

In summary, although few Lithuanians report unmet needs for medical care due to financial reasons (Table 1), reimbursement weaknesses and out of pocket payments are still the biggest challenge in ensuring optimal medical and CPAP treatment of sleep disorders. According to Lithuania Health Profile 2019, OOP represented almost one-third (32%) of health spending in Lithuania – more than twice the EU average. Most OOP spending (16.9%) is used to pay for pharmaceuticals. These high levels of OOP payments create financial hardship, especially in low-income households [4].

Table 1. Proportion of the population whose need for health care was not met because of their inability to pay for it (too expensive) [2].

Healthcare type	The proportion of the population whose need for health care was not met because of their inability to pay for it (%)	
-	2014	2019
Medical care (excluding dental care)	2.1	3.8
Dental care	5.3	15.5
Prescribed medicines	2.4	5.2
Mental health care	0.2	2.8

Scientific and Professional Societies

Sleep specialists come from different medical specialties, which have their own long-standing professional societies. In 2000, the Lithuanian Society of Sleep Medicine (LSSM) was founded by a professor Vanda Liesienė. The aim of the society was to support the development of sleep research and to facilitate the collaboration of different medical specialists in the diagnosis and treatment of sleep disorders. All members of the society are medical doctors, mostly pulmonologists and neurologists. LSSM is continuously growing, as new members from various fields of medicine, psychology and biosciences are joining the organization. LSSM is a member of The Assembly of National Sleep Societies (ANSS) which is a formal body of the European Sleep Research Society (ESRS) and represents the associate members from different European sleep societies [18].

Together with colleagues from other Baltic countries, LMMS in 2019 joined the initiative to launch regular Baltic Sleep meetings. The first Baltic Sleep meeting was hosted by Estonian colleagues and took place in Tallinn. The second Baltic Sleep Meeting is organized by LMMS in Kaunas in 2021.

There are no official patient-focused organizations or patient support groups for patients with sleep disorders in Lithuania.

Regulation of Driving Licenses and Practice Guidelines

The widespread recognition that obstructive sleep apnea represents an important risk factor for motor vehicle accidents has led to a revision of annex III of the European Union directive on driving licenses in 2014, which was implemented in Lithuania as an EU member state by the national law from December 31, 2015 [19]. The national regulation entirely met the EU directive text and stated that:

- Applicants or drivers in whom a moderate or severe obstructive sleep apnea syndrome is suspected, shall be referred for further authorized medical advice before a driving license is issued or renewed. They are advised not to drive until confirmation of the diagnosis;

- Driving licenses may be issued to applicants or drivers with moderate or severe obstructive sleep apnea syndrome, who show adequate control of their condition and compliance with appropriate treatment and improvement of sleepiness, if any, confirmed by authorized medical opinion.

Lithuania faced the same challenges as other EU countries with the practical application of the directive as it considerably increased the number of requests for specialist evaluation and lengthened waiting lists. An acceptable timeframe to obtain a new or renewed driving license becomes a challenge for OSA suspected patients and screening for OSA puts considerable strain on the healthcare system [20].

Even though there are no approved guidelines for narcolepsy management in Lithuania, sleep medicine specialists use international and especially European recommendations. Patients with narcolepsy, using medication(s) and achieving sufficient control of their symptoms (reduced both sleepiness and cataplexy episodes), confirmed by normal MSLT, can obtain or renew their driving license.

Lithuania follows international (especially European) practice guidelines for sleep disorders. Specialized national medical journals introduced and translated European guidelines for the diagnosis and treatment of insomnia [21, 22]. Up - to-date narcolepsy management recommendations are also discussed in the inner clinical diagnostic and treatment protocols and local professional press [23].

Official Lithuanian recommendations for diagnosis and management of OSA were produced and issued in 2018 by joint work of national societies of pulmonologists, allergists, otorhinolaryngologists and neurophysiologists [24]. It reflected international experience and competence and contributed to better implementation of driving license regulations.

Clinical and Fundamental Research

Sleep-related research is mainly done by specialists working in previously mentioned sleep labs of the two main medical universities – VU and LUHS.

One of the first articles published in sleep field by a Lithuanian author was "Effects of locus coeruleus lesions on heart rate during sleep in the cat" by the current professor Vanda Liesienė and her colleagues from the University Hospital Pitie Salpetriere in 1981 [25]. Professor has been leading many different doctoral works and international sleep research.

For many years, adult and children neurologists from VU Hospital Santaros klinikos have been performing research in sleep-related breathing disorders, sleep and circadian patterns among epilepsy patients [26 - 28]. Additionally, they have recently established collaborations with cardiology and nephrology specialists [29].

In 2014, pulmonologist Guoda Pilkauskaite (Vaitukaitiene) from LUHS Pulmonology Department defended her PhD thesis "Distinctive characteristics of metabolism and inflammation in men with obstructive sleep apnea", in which she had been investigating reactive oxygen species production in peripheral blood neutrophils and vascular adhesion molecules among OSA male patients [30, 31]. The department has few doctoral students who are continuing OSA-related research.

LUHS Behavioral Medicine Institute in Palanga has a strong group of neuroscience and sleep researchers focusing on behavioral, neuroendocrinological, metabolic patterns of sleep-related breathing disorders and insomnia among patients hospitalized for cardiovascular and stress rehabilitation [32 - 35]. The institute is collaborating with other European countries in the European Sleep Apnea Database (ESADA) and its research activities [36]. In 2018, psychologist and psychotherapist Alicja Juškienė, led by professor Giedrius Varoneckas, defended her PhD thesis about psychological and behavioral factors among OSA and ischemic heart disease patients [37].

LUHS Neurology Department has established a collaboration with Karolinska Institute (Stockholm, Sweden) and published a few articles about sleep patterns among chronic fatigue syndrome patients [38]. In 2018, neurologist and somnologist Evelina Pajėdienė started her PhD project "The patterns of sleep – wake rhythm disturbances and their metabolic and genetic markers among ischemic stroke patients and their impact on stroke outcome" [39]. Another neurologist from VU, Eglė Sakalauskaitė-Juodeikienė defended her PhD thesis "Nervous System Diseases in the First Half of the 19th Century in Vilnius" in 2019, also converting origins of sleep medicine in Lithuania [6].

The sleep research field in Lithuania is still very young and lacking continuous and longstanding translational experience. Additionally, there is a need for a bigger number of adapted and validated sleep-related questionnaires and scales that could be used both in scientific and clinical practice. International and local multidisciplinary collaboration, new funding opportunities and growing human resources could help to build scientifically strong sleep-oriented labs, working both on animal and human models, on molecular and clinical basis.

Use of Internet Technologies (Connected Objects)

Usage of internet technologies is rapidly growing in Lithuania, and the tendency is even more remarkable in the light of the COVID-19 pandemic. According to the Lithuanian Department of Statistics, in 2020 about 82% of Lithuanian households had internet access (mobile, wireless or connected) and 74% of 16-74 year-old inhabitants were using the internet every day for various purposes: learning, work, leisure, shopping, financial services, *etc* [2].

Tendency of health, physical activity and sleep-related mobile applications and wearable devices are also growing, especially among young and middle-aged Lithuanians. Specialists working with sleep medicine have noticed that patients are more commonly showing the reports from their smartphones or smartwatches about their sleep and sleep-wake rhythm. This additional information is not ignored, but still not replacing the "gold-standard" sleep diagnostics such as polysomnography, polygraphy and actigraphy.

The telemedicine situation in Lithuania is still slowly evolving because of indefinite legislation, reimbursement and organizational issues. For the past few years, teleconsultations were organized between healthcare professionals, *e.g.,* a radiologist and other physicians, or between an emergency medicine specialist and other physician. Remote patient consultations became more broadly available during the COVID-19 pandemic, when family doctors and specialists could consult patients *via* phone or internet-based call, and prescribe further diagnostic procedures and treatment. Hopefully, in the future, telemedicine services will be efficiently developing in the area of sleep medicine, as this field felt a remarkable lock-down during the pandemics, but could be flexibly adapted to teleconsultations, remote application and interpretation of sleep diagnostics, as well as treatment approaches.

CONCLUSION

Sleep medicine in Lithuania is evolving. In most regulatory matters Lithuania follows the EU guidelines, however, there is an independent Lithuanian Sleep Medicine society. Healthcare in general and sleep medicine in particular is embracing more and more telemedicine during the COVID-19 pandemic and hopefully beyond that as well.

CONSENT FOR PUBLICATION

Not applicable.

CONFLICT OF INTEREST

The authors declare no conflict of interest, financial or otherwise.

ACKNOWLEDGEMENT

Declared none.

REFERENCES

[1]   Bank of Lithuania website Available from https://www.lb.lt/en

[2]   The Lithuanian Department of Statistics website Available from: https://www.stat.gov.lt/en

[3]   The 2020 Human Development Report. Available from:. http://hdr.undp.org/sites/default/files/hdr2020.pdf

[4]   Country-Health-Profile-2019-Lithuania. Available from:. https://www.euro.who.int/__data/assets/pdf_file/0003/419466/Country-Health-Profile-2019-Lithuania. pdf

[5]   Health consumer powerhouse website Available from: https://healthpowerhouse.com/publications/

[6]   Sakalauskaitė-Juodeikienė E. Nervų ligos Vilniuje XIX-ojo amžiaus pirmoje pusėje. Daktaro disertacija [Nervous System Diseases in the First Half of the 19th Century in Vilnius. PhD

thesis].Vilnius: Vilniaus universiteto leidykla 2019.

[7]   Kondratas R. Joseph Frank (1771 – 1842) and the development of clinical medicine. A study of the transformation of medical thought and practice at the end of the 18th and the beginning of the 19th centuries. PhD thesis. Harvard University, Massachusetts; 1977.

[8]   Frank J. Praxeos medicae universae praecepta Partis secundae volumen primum, sectio prima, continens doctrinam de morbis systematis nervosi in genere et de iis cerebri in specie Lipsiae: sumptibus Bibliopolii Kuehniani; 1818.

[9]   Sakalauskaitė-Juodeikienė E, Jatužis D. Sleep disorders in *Praxeos medicae universae praecepta* by Joseph Frank (1771-1842). Journal of sleep research. Abstracts of the 24th Congress of the European Sleep Research Society. 25–28 September 2018; Basel, Switzerland. 2018.
[http://dx.doi.org/10.1111/jsr.12751]

[10]   Schloezer JA. Dissertatio inauguralis medico-practica de somnambulismo Vilnae: typis congregationis missionis; 1816.

[11]   Sakalauskaitė-Juodeikienė E, Jatužis D. The perception of somnambulism in the beginning of the nineteenth century in Vilnius. Sleep Med 2017; 40: e289.
[http://dx.doi.org/10.1016/j.sleep.2017.11.848]

[12]   Triponienė D. Prie Vilniaus medicinos draugijos versmės [At the Source of Vilnius Medical Society]. Vilnius: Vilniaus universiteto leidykla; 2012.

[13]   Lithuanian University of Health Sciences website Available from: https://lsmuni.lt/en/about-university/university-today/

[14]   Vilnius University website https://www.vu.lt/en/about-vu

[15]   Kasiulevicius V, Lember M. Lithuania. In: Kringos DS, Boerma WGW, Hutchinson A, et al, Eds. Building primary care in a changing Europe. Case studies. Copenhagen: European Observatory on Health Systems and Policies 2015; I.17.

[16]   Vaitukaitiene G. 20 years anniversary of Sleep laboratory of Pulmonology clinics. Pulmonologija ir alergologija 2018; 2(2): 88-9.

[17]   Liaugaudaite V, Zemaitiene N, Bunevicius A. Suicide and Depression: Epidemiology in Lithuania. Biological psychiatry and psychopharmacology 2020; 22: 3-10.

[18]   ESRS website Available from: https://esrs.eu/

[19]   European Union Commission Directive 2014/85/EU of 1 July 2014, amending Directive 2006/126/EC of the European Parliament and of the Council on driving licences OJ L 194, 272014, pp 10–13

[20]   Bonsignore MR, Randerath W, Riha R, *et al.* New rules on driver licensing for patients with obstructive sleep apnoea: EU Directive 2014/85/EU. Eur Respir J 2016; 47(1): 39-41.
[http://dx.doi.org/10.1183/13993003.01894-2015] [PMID: 26721963]

[21]   Riemann D, Baglioni C, Bassetti C, *et al.* European guideline for the diagnosis and treatment of insomnia. J Sleep Res 2017; 26(6): 675-700.
[http://dx.doi.org/10.1111/jsr.12594] [PMID: 28875581]

[22]   Sakalauskaitė-Juodeikienė E, Masaitienė R. Insomnia: definition, pathophysiological models, diagnosis, and treatment. Neurologijos seminarai 2018; 22(77): 164-173.

[23]   Sakalauskaitė-Juodeikienė E, Masaitienė R. Narcolepsy treatment: from exorcism and bloodletting to modern therapy with histamine receptor inverse agonists. Neurologijos seminarai 2020; 24(85): 189-201

[24]   Vaitukaitiene G, Miliauskas S, Danila E, *et al.* Lithuanian recommendations for diagnosis and management of obstructive sleep apnea. Pulmonologija ir alergologija 2018; 2(2): 92-108.

[25]   Liesiene V, Adrien J, Benoit O. Effects of locus coeruleus lesions on heart rate during sleep in the cat. Arch Ital Biol 1981; 119(2): 125-38.

[PMID: 7259394]

[26] Praninskiene R, Dumalakiene I, Mauricas M, *et al.* Circadian rhythm of melatonin secretion in children with epilepsy. Epilepsia 2005; 46(Suppl 6).

[27] Praninskienė R, Dumalakienė I, Kemežys R, Mauricas M, Jučaitė A. Diurnal melatonin patterns in children: ready to apply in clinical practice? Pediatr Neurol 2012; 46(2): 70-6.
[http://dx.doi.org/10.1016/j.pediatrneurol.2011.11.018] [PMID: 22264699]

[28] Praninskiene R, Dumalakiene I, Kemezys R, Mauricas M, Jucaite A. Melatonin secretion in children with epilepsy. Epilepsy Behav 2012; 25(3): 315-22.
[http://dx.doi.org/10.1016/j.yebeh.2012.08.012] [PMID: 23103303]

[29] Jakutis G, Juknevičius V, Barysienė J, *et al.* A rare case of REM sleep-related bradyarrhythmia syndrome with concomitant severe hypertension: a case report and a review of literature. Acta Med Litu 2018; 25(1): 1-6.
[http://dx.doi.org/10.6001/actamedica.v25i1.3697] [PMID: 29928151]

[30] Pilkauskaite G, Miliauskas S, Sakalauskas R. Reactive oxygen species production in peripheral blood neutrophils of obstructive sleep apnea patients. ScientificWorldJournal 2013; 2013: 1-6.
[http://dx.doi.org/10.1155/2013/421763] [PMID: 23766689]

[31] Pilkauskaite G, Miliauskas S, Vitkauskiene A, Sakalauskas R. Vascular adhesion molecules in men with obstructive sleep apnea: associations with obesity and metabolic syndrome. Sleep Breath 2014; 18(4): 869-74.
[http://dx.doi.org/10.1007/s11325-014-0958-0] [PMID: 24563330]

[32] Alonderis A, Varoneckas G, Raskauskiene N, Brozaitiene J. Prevalence and predictors of sleep apnea in patients with stable coronary artery disease: a cross-sectional study. Ther Clin Risk Manag 2017; 13: 1031-42.
[http://dx.doi.org/10.2147/TCRM.S136651] [PMID: 28860787]

[33] Lallukka T, Podlipskytė A, Sivertsen B, *et al.* Insomnia symptoms and mortality: a register-linked study among women and men from Finland, Norway and Lithuania. J Sleep Res 2016; 25(1): 96-103.
[http://dx.doi.org/10.1111/jsr.12343] [PMID: 26420582]

[34] Alonderis A, Raskauskiene N, Gelziniene V, Zaliunaite V, Brozaitiene J. Undiagnosed sleep apnoea in cardiac rehabilitation: Age-dependent effect on diastolic function in coronary artery disease patients with preserved ejection fraction. Eur J Cardiovasc Nurs 2020; 1474515120941373.
[http://dx.doi.org/10.1177/1474515120941373] [PMID: 33611367]

[35] Alonderis A, Raskauskiene N, Gelziniene V, Mickuviene N, Brozaitiene J. The association of sleep disordered breathing with left ventricular remodeling in CAD patients: a cross-sectional study. BMC Cardiovasc Disord 2017; 17(1): 250.
[http://dx.doi.org/10.1186/s12872-017-0684-1] [PMID: 28923022]

[36] Gunduz C, Basoglu OK, Kvamme JA, *et al.* Long-term positive airway pressure therapy is associated with reduced total cholesterol levels in patients with obstructive sleep apnea: data from the European Sleep Apnea Database (ESADA). Sleep Med 2020; 75: 201-9.
[http://dx.doi.org/10.1016/j.sleep.2020.02.023] [PMID: 32858361]

[37] Juskiene A, Podlipskyte A, Bunevicius A, Varoneckas G. Type d personality and sleep quality in coronary artery disease patients with and without obstructive sleep apnea: mediating effects of anxiety and depression. Int j behav med 2018; 25(2): 171-82.
[http://dx.doi.org/10.1007/s12529-017-9708-6] [PMID: 29327226]

[38] Pajediene E, Bileviciute-Ljungar I, Friberg D. Sleep patterns among patients with chronic fatigue: A polysomnography□based study. Clin Respir J 2018; 12(4): 1389-97.
[http://dx.doi.org/10.1111/crj.12667] [PMID: 28752613]

[39]   Pajediene E, Pajeda A, Urnieziute G, *et al.* Subjective and objective features of sleep disorders in patients with acute ischemic or haemorrhagic stroke: It is not only sleep apnoea which is important. Med Hypotheses 2020; 136: 109512.
[http://dx.doi.org/10.1016/j.mehy.2019.109512] [PMID: 31837521]

CHAPTER 27

Current Practice of Sleep Medicine in The Czech Republic

Sona Nevsimalova[1,*], **Ondrej Ludka**[2] and **Jana Vyskocilova**[3]

[1] *Department of Neurology and Clinical Sciences, 1st Faculty of Medicine, Charles University and General Teaching Hospital, Prague, Czech Republic*

[2] *Department of Internal Medicine – Cardioangiology, Faculty of Medicine, Masaryk University and Teaching Hospital St. Anna, Brno, Czech Republic*

[3] *EUC Clinic, Pilsen, Czech Republic*

Abstract: Prof. Bedrich Roth founded sleep medicine in our country 70 years ago. However, the inter- and multidisciplinary nature of sleep medicine developed several decades later, in the early 1990s, with the cooperation of pulmonologists, neurologists and psychiatrists. This led to the foundation of the Czech Sleep Research and Sleep Medicine Society (short title Czech Sleep Society) in 2001. At present, the Society includes 215 members and plays a leading role in the current practice of sleep medicine in the entire country. Activities include accreditation/certification procedures, educational programs, annual national meetings, the development of guidelines and recommendations for different sleep disorders, promoting research and many other endeavors. The society also collaborates with other medical societies in discussions with state health care authorities and health insurance companies. Health insurance companies cover sleep medicine care by means of a DRG system for hospitalizations, and a point system for outpatient care. The majority of sleep medicine care is centralized, and medications are largely covered (*e.g.* modafinil and natrium oxybate are available to patients free of charge). Positive airway pressure devices are lent to patients by health insurance companies if treatment criteria for sleep breathing disorders are met and compliance is fulfilled. The absence of acknowledged specialization or sub- specialization in sleep medicine by the Czech Ministry of Health is the main challenge to be overcome.

Keywords: Czech Sleep Society, accreditation process, education, certifications, guidelines, research, sleep medicine, health insurance.

---

* **Corresponding author Sona Nevsimalova:** Department of Neurology, Charles University, 1st Faculty of Medicine, Katerinska 30, 128 00 Prague 2, Czech Republic, Phone + 420-224965562, Mobile +420-607810139, Fax +420-224922678; E-mail: snevsi@lf1.cuni.cz

Hrayr P. Attarian, Marie-Louise M. Coussa-Koniski & Alain Michel Sabri (Eds.)
All rights reserved-© 2023 Bentham Science Publishers

INTRODUCTION AND HISTORY

Sleep medicine has a long history in our country [1 - 3]. The founder of this field was Prof. Bedrich Roth who started with clinical descriptions of narcolepsy and hypersomnia in the early 1950s and established the first polysomnographic lab in Central Europe in the early 1960s at the Department of Neurology in Prague. Prof. Roth collected the largest cohort of patients in the world suffering from excessive daytime sleepiness in the 1970s and 1980s. At the same time, Prof. Helena Illnerova from the Academy of Sciences became well-known for her experimental research in chronobiology and circadian rhythm, and Dr. Jaroslava Dittrichova from the Department for Mother and Child Care for clinical pediatric research. However, the evolution of true multidisciplinary sleep medicine began after falling of communism in the 1990s. Since 1991, Prague neurologists followed by other specialists including pulmonologists, ENT physicians and psychiatrists, have held annual meetings devoted to sleep disorders. The Czech Sleep Research and Sleep Medicine Society (short title Czech Sleep Society) was formed in 2001 [4]. In cooperation with the Slovak Sleep Society, the Society organizes annual Czech and Slovak Sleep Congresses and collaborates with other medical societies. In 2004, Prague hosted the 17th ESRS Congress with 1,300 delegates and in 2017, the World Sleep Congress was organized in Prague with 2,700 participants from 76 countries. The local convener of both events was Prof. Nevsimalova.

CURRENT PRACTICE OF SLEEP MEDICINE

The Czech Sleep Society plays a leading role in the current practice of sleep medicine in the Czech Republic. The society board has 7 members, and a further 3 members are elected as a Revision Commission. The online elections are repeated every 4 years. Dr. Vyskocilova has represented the Czech Sleep Society as a president for several voting periods, Prof. Nevsimalova is the Vice-President, and Prof. Ludka is the scientific secretary and a member of the Assembly of National Sleep Societies (ANSS) in ESRS.

The Czech Sleep Society presently has 215 members.

The accreditation process inspired by ESRS rules started in 2005 [5, 6]. The process is completely managed by the Society and the status of an accredited Sleep Center is recognized by health insurance companies but not by state authorities. The validity of accreditation is 5 years, and reaccreditation must be repeated every 5 years. According to ESRS recommendation, 3 main categories of Centers have been distinguished since 2019. Presently, 4 centers fulfill the highest requirements for Center type I, 13 workplaces fulfill requirements for Center type II, and 23 workplaces requirements for Center type III. ESRS recommendation was slightly modified for our practice (Fig. **1**). Referral centers for diagnosis and therapy of sleep disorder breathing with the highest specialization were ranged into Centers type II, while units of monitoring and therapy of sleep disorder breathing were ranged as sub-specialized Centers type III. A great majority of sub-specialized centers involve pulmonology or ENT units that are focused on sleep-breathing disorders. The density of Centers is not uniform; the highest network is located in the capital city – Prague.

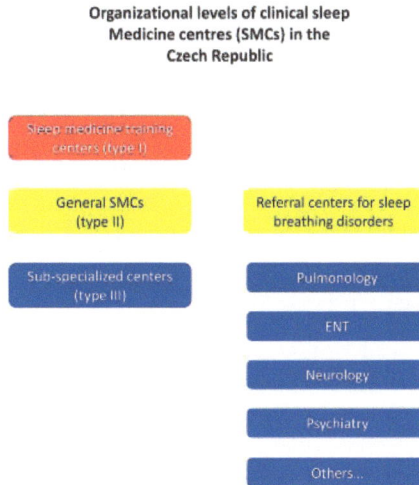

Organizational levels of clinical sleep Medicine centres (SMCs) in the Czech Republic

Sleep medicine training centers (type I)	
General SMCs (type II)	Referral centers for sleep breathing disorders
Sub-specialized centers (type III)	Pulmonology
	ENT
	Neurology
	Psychiatry
	Others...

Fig. (1). A modified scheme illustrating the organization levels of clinical sleep medicine centers in the Czech Republic.

Since 2006, the society has organized **_biennial theoretical courses_** in sleep medicine **_followed by theoretical and practical examinations_** [7, 8]. Successfully completing the examination is essential for attending accreditation. In the past 5 years, practical courses for technicians have begun to be organized as well, and there must be at least one certified technician at each accredited center who has completed this course and passed the exam.

The Sleep Society has submitted and published **_guidelines_** (or recommendations) for (1) issuing driving licenses to subjects with sleep apnea, (2) sleep breathing disorders in adults as well as in children (indication for CPAP, BiPAP, surgical options), (3) home non-invasive ventilation, and (4) clinical standards for the diagnosis and therapy of narcolepsy. ESRS and AASM standards were taken into consideration as a model when our guidelines were developed.

Several **_branches_** participate in the progress of our Sleep Society. The most effective is the surgical section that joined forces with ETN sleep specialists in the Czech Society of otolaryngology, head and neck surgery and assured a common diagnostic and therapeutic procedure for obstructive apnea in both societies. The branch for acute and home non-invasive ventilation supports not only patients with progressive lung diseases, but with neuromuscular diseases that include a wide spectrum of motor unit diseases from childhood to adulthood. Non-invasive care of ventilation improved very much their quality of life in recent years.

The society tries to **promote research** by awarding the best publication of the year [9] (with a separate award for young researchers), and by supporting presenters at ESRS, WSS or APSS meetings. More than 200 delegates participate in annual Czech and Slovak Sleep Congresses every year, internationally well-known speakers are invited, and awards for the best publications are presented. Several members of the Sleep Society are active beyond publication activities as reviewers of renowned sleep journals and assistant editors. The 3rd edition of the Czech monograph on the Disorders of Sleep and Vigilance (edited by S. Nevsimalova and K. Sonka) was published in 2020 [10]. The book may be used as a manual for examinations, and as a practical guide for the diagnosis and management of sleep disorders for sleep researchers, interested practitioners and physicians of allied medical fields.

Health insurance takes a leading role in the financial reimbursement of *sleep medicine health care*. They cover health care during hospitalizations by means of a DRG system and ambulatory care by point system according to different codes. The majority of sleep medicine care is centralized, and medication and/or equipment for breathing support are largely covered. Some prescriptions, - *e.g.* modafinil and natrium oxybate are available to patients free of charge. Positive pressure airway devices are lent to patients by health insurance agencies if the criteria for treatment of sleep breathing disorders are met and compliance is fulfilled. Patients pay only 10% for equipment accessory exchange every year. The situation is different in some psychological methods, – *e-g.* cognitive behavior therapy (CBT) is covered by the patient.

CHALLENGES TO THE PRACTICE OF SLEEP MEDICINE

Sleep medicine is a part of educational programs at the pre- and postgraduate level in several medical faculties in the Czech Republic, and the Society collaborates with other societies for scientific meetings, workshops and keynote lectures. However, the absence of acknowledged specialization or sub-specialization in sleep medicine by the Czech Ministry of Health is the main challenge to be overcome. Our application is still waiting for the ministry's approval.

Although the network of different centers appears to be relatively dense, there are regions in which centers are lacking. Despite the fact that the majority of type II and III Centers care (according to our modification) for patients with sleep breathing disorders, there are long waiting lists of patients who have to wait up to 6-9 months for examinations and therapeutic outcomes. Home-none-invasive ventilation needs also better financial evaluation from health companies. There is also a lack of centers caring for children. Only 5 Centers (type I-III) in the Czech Republic include care of infants, toddlers or young children, and only one is targeted exclusively at the pediatric population.

Another challenge to be overcome is related to telemedicine. Health companies will discharge these codes only from the next year (2022).

As regards the patients´ organizations, we surely need active patient-focused membership organization supporting services and advocacy for patients with all sleep disorders. Presently the only our patients´ organization is focused on narcolepsy, however, their activities should be greatly improved.

CLINICAL AND RESEARCH KNOWLEDGE GASP

Some clinical challenges have been described above. The main challenge with respect to research is the absence of almost any basic research. These scientists constitute less than 1% of our Sleep Society members.

CONCLUSION

Sleep medicine has a strong inter- and multidisciplinary character in the Czech Republic. The activity of our society is directed mainly to improve the quality of our work through the accreditation process, by organizing annual Czech and Slovak Sleep Medicine Congresses and biennial theoretical courses followed by theoretical and practical examinations. The society promotes research by awarding the best publication every year, and by supporting presenters at international meetings. Sleep medicine is a part of educational programs at the pre- and postgraduate level and tries to be an independent medical subspeciality acknowledged by the Czech Ministry of Health.

CONSENT FOR PUBLICATION

Not applicable.

CONFLICT OF INTEREST

The authors declare no conflict of interest, financial or otherwise.

ACKNOWLEDGEMENT

Declared none.

REFERENCES

[1]   Nevšímalová S. History of sleep study.Disorders of sleep and vigilance. Prague: Galen 2020; pp. 17-20. (in Czech)

[2]   Šonka K, Nevšímalová S. 60 years of sleep medicine at the Department of Neurology, First Faculty of Medicine, Charles University in Prague and General University Hospital in Prague. Prague Med Rep 2011; 112(3): 236-43.
        [PMID: 21978784]

[3]   European Sleep Research Society 1972-2012. 40th Anniversary of the ESRS. Bassetti CL. (ed.). Wecom Gesellschaft für Kommunikation mbH & Co. KG, Hildesheim/ Germany 2012 2012.

[4]   http://www.sleep-society.cz

[5]   Fischer J, Dogas Z, Bassetti CL, *et al.* Standard procedures for adults in accredited sleep medicine centres in Europe. J Sleep Res 2012; 21(4): 357-68.
        [http://dx.doi.org/10.1111/j.1365-2869.2011.00987.x] [PMID: 22133127]

[6]   Pevernagie D, Fischer J, Bassetti C. Organization of Sleep Medicine Centers. 2014.

[7]   International classification of sleep disorders. 3rd ed., Darien, IL: American Academy of Sleep Medicine 2014.

[8]   Berry RB, Brook R, Gamaldo CE, *et al.* The AASM scoring manual for the scoring of sleep and associated events: rules, terminology and technical specification Version 24 Darien, Il: American Academy of Sleep Medicine. 2017.

[9]   Nevsimalova s, Bruni O. (Eds.). Sleep disorders in children. Basel: Springer 2017.

[10]   Nevšímalová S, Šonka K, Eds. Disorders of sleep and vigilance (in Czech) Galen, Prague. 2020.

CHAPTER 28

Practice of Sleep Medicine in Russia

Mikhail Bochkarev[1,*], Lyudmila Korostovtseva[1], Mikhail Agaltsov[2], Natalya Leonenko[3], Valeria Amelina[1,3], Anatoly Alekhin[3] and Yurii Sviryaev[1]

[1] *Almazov National Medical Research Centre, St Petersburg, Russia*

[2] *National Medicine Therapy and Preventive Centre, Moscow, Russia*

[3] *Herzen State Pedagogical University of Russia, St Petersburg, Russia*

Abstract: Somnology in Russia is a competency area for medical doctors from different disciplines. Most of them are cardiologists involved in private clinics located in the central and western parts of the country in the major cities. Some factors limit the development of somnology: differences between the regions, absence of legislative and regulatory absence of documents, lack of sleep-related services in the medical standards of health care, no insurance reimbursement, undergraduate sleep-related programs, and high cost of diagnostic and treatment equipment. Several professional societies focus on the development of different fields - clinical, fundamental, pediatric somnology, chronobiology and dream research. The postgraduate activities for medical doctors include different lectures online, web-based interactive educational modules on sleep disorders within the continuing medical education system, regular seminars in the major medical centers; certified (within other medical specialties) short training courses on sleep-disordered breathing and non-invasive ventilation and longer 36-72 hours courses in sleep medicine. The members of sleep-related societies perform various public activities all year round and in relation to the World Sleep Day. Diagnostic features of sleep practice include the unique use of rheopneumogram in Holter monitoring for very rough screening of apneas during sleep. Initiation of non-invasive ventilation therapy is more often started at home with the use of auto-CPAP machines. Various instrumental methods developed in Russia for insomnia treatment lack strong evidence. Support of the governmental institutions would help to solve present issues with regulatory standards in education and treatment in sleep medicine.

Keywords: Sleep, Sleep Medicine, Sleep Disorders, Russia.

---

* **Corresponding author Mikhail Bochkarev:** Almazov National Medical Research Centre, St Petersburg, Russia; Email: bochkarev_mv@almazovcentre.ru

Hrayr P. Attarian, Marie-Louise M. Coussa-Koniski & Alain Michel Sabri (Eds.)

SLEEP MEDICINE IN THE RUSSIAN FEDERATION: STATE OF THE ART

Currently, somnology in Russia is recognized as a competency area (and not as a separate specialty or a subspecialty), and medical doctors specialized in different disciplines can provide medical care in the field of sleep medicine after additional training in the field (see *Education in somnology in the Russian Federation)*. The variety of different medical specialties involved in sleep medicine healthcare and services reflect the multidisciplinary nature of somnology. These specialties include internal diseases, neurology, psychiatry, cardiology, pulmonology; otolaryngology (ENT), endocrinology, psychology and others. Based on the variety of clinical specialties presented among the members of the sleep-related societies, the most common specialists involved in sleep-related health care are neurologists, cardiologists, general physicians, pulmonologists, ENT specialists, and endocrinologists. The characteristic feature of sleep medicine in Russia is a rather high number of cardiologists involved in sleep-related healthcare compared to other countries.

The development of sleep medicine in Russia is limited by a number of factors:

− No recognition of somnology as a separate specialty or subspecialty;

− The absence of legislative and regulatory documents;

− The inconsistencies in the current legislative documents;

− The lack of sleep-related services in the medical standards of health care;

− No insurance reimbursement;

− Low awareness of medical doctors and patients (the situation has been changing in the last decade);

− High cost of diagnostic and treatment equipment;

− Low interest of hospital administration and local authorities;

− Great differences between the regions.

Despite the absence of official recognition, sleep labs (the majority are medical offices of respiratory care providing continuous positive airway pressure (CPAP) therapy to sleep apnea patients) are widely spread throughout Russia mostly located in the central and western part of the country in the big cities and lacking in the small ones. Sleep-related health care is provided in more than 100 sleep labs located in more than 50 cities of the Russian Federation (Fig. **1**). In big cities, including Moscow, St, Petersburg, Novosibirsk, Rostov-on-Don, Yekaterinburg, Irkutsk and others, there are larger specialized, multidisciplinary clinical and research sleep centers and laboratories, while in the smaller cities and towns, sleep-related health care is usually provided in non-specialized clinics.

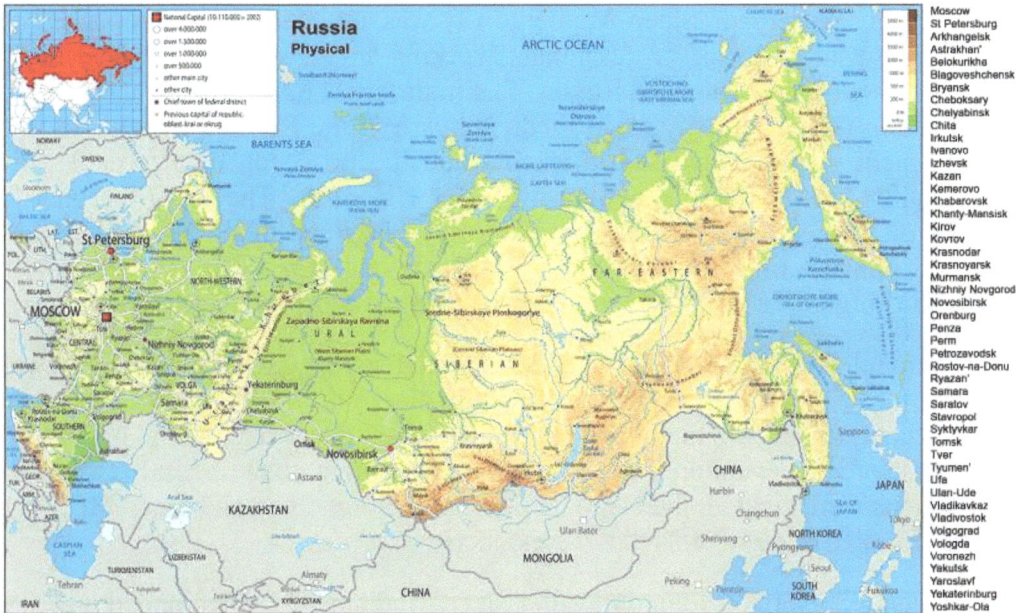

Fig. (1). The distribution of centers/clinics which provide sleep-related services in Russia.

PROFESSIONAL SLEEP-RELATED ASSOCIATIONS IN RUSSIA

There are several professional societies in the sleep field in the Russian Federation. Clinical sleep medicine in Russia has been developing since the 1980s (the biggest impact made by the Academician A.G. Chuchalin and Professor Alexander Vein and their medical schools), and the first somnological society was organized by Professor A. Vein in the late 1990s [1]. After his decease, the society disintegrated into several associations. The Russian Society of Somnologists [2] was reorganized from the Somnology Section of the Pavlov Physiology Society of the Russian Academy of Sciences. Currently, the RSS is the official member of the Assembly of National Sleep Societies (ANSS) which is affiliated with the European Sleep Research Society (ESRS) (since 2012). The main purposes of RSS include the consolidation of specialists in different fields and building a real bridge between fundamental and clinical science by promoting research on sleep and related areas, by improving professional education and health care for patients with sleep problems, by constant scientific exchange and spreading knowledge on sleep and sleep medicine among general population and implementation of novel technologies and achievements regarding sleep and related areas. The RSS combines both fundamental researchers and clinicians in the field of somnology and covers both clinical and scientific aspects of sleep medicine. The RSS holds an annual "Sleep Forum" which usually takes place in the middle of March, close to the vernal equinox date.

The Russian Society of Sleep Medicine [3] was founded in 2012 in order to represent the interests of professionals working in the field of clinical sleep medicine in various regions of Russia. The main goals of the RSSM include the organization of high-quality sleep medicine care in the Russian Federation, the advancement of domestic sleep medicine and the provision of affordable and high-quality healthcare for people with sleep disorders. The RSSM primarily focuses on clinical rather than scientific issues of sleep medicine. The RSSM currently consists of 45 regional units in the regions of the Russian Federation. The RSSM organizes an annual conference "Clinical Sleep Medicine".

The National Society of Pediatric Sleep Specialists on Children Sleep [4] was founded in 2007 with the main goal to study sleep in different periods of child development, to develop methods for pediatric sleep improvement and promotion of sleep disorder prevention in children. In partnership with the NSPSS, two other associations were created: the National Society of Somnology and Sleep Medicine and the Russian Society of Dream Researchers.

The National Society of Somnology and Sleep Medicine [5] was founded in 2008, and its main activity is the organization of professional meetings and conferences.

The Russian Society of Researchers of Dreams (RSRD) [6] was founded in 2014 and deals with the investigation of dreams. RSRD supports studies of psychic activity in sleep, development and implementation of innovative research projects in the field of the studies of dreams, promotion of professional development and training of specialists in researching psychic activity in sleep and dream work.

The Committee on Chronobiology and Chronomedicine (CCC) of the Russian Academy of Sciences, firstly, founded in 1981, aimed at the development of multidisciplinary and international collaboration in the field of biological rhythms, chronobiology and chronomedicine, coordination of chronobiology research in Russia, as well as the organization of professional conferences and meetings [7]. Since 2010, the CCC has organized regular educational courses on chronobiology and chronomedicine. Currently, the CCC coordinates the development of such subdisciplines as chronotherapy, chronoprevention, chronorehabilitation and others.

EDUCATION IN SOMNOLOGY IN THE RUSSIAN FEDERATION

Education in somnology differs from other medical training because it requires multidisciplinary knowledge (internal diseases, cardiology, pulmonology, otorhinolaryngology, neurology, psychiatry), as well as specialized training in novel diagnostics (polysomnography, polygraphy, actigraphy, tests for assessment of sleepiness and wakefulness *etc.*) and treatment of sleep disorders (including cognitive-behavioral therapy and pharmacotherapy of insomnia, noninvasive ventilation, chronobiological approaches for circadian disorders, *etc.*).

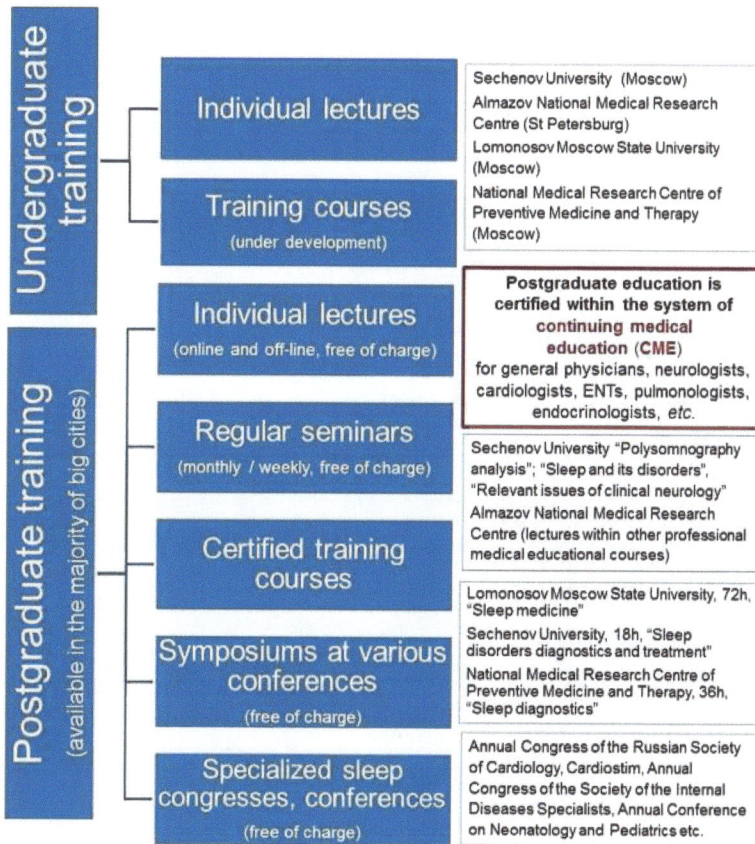

Fig. (2). Education in sleep field in Russia.

In the Russian Federation, education in the somnology field is multilevel (Fig. **2**) which is due to the existing barriers. The undergraduate sleep-related programs are under development and are planned to be implied into the regular education in the big medical universities (in Moscow and St Petersburg), currently, individual lectures or series of lectures are available within other courses.

The postgraduate activities for medical professionals (Fig. **3**) include individual lectures which are held almost throughout the country, regular seminars held in the big medical centers; certified (within other medical specialties) training courses. The professionals can choose between longer general courses on sleep disorders, and more specialized courses on sleep-disordered breathing, cognitive-behavioral therapy of insomnia (CBT-I), diagnostics of sleep disorders and others. They are provided by the largest research centers and the biggest universities. Usually, the duration of one course is 1-2 weeks. Medical professionals of different specialties may attend the courses. In the state educational and research centers/universities, the attendees get a state certificate (within another medical specialty) and credits within the system of continuous medical education (CME). The price varies from 50 to 150 euros per course. The fees can be covered either by the clinic referring the specialist for training or by the attendee him/herself.

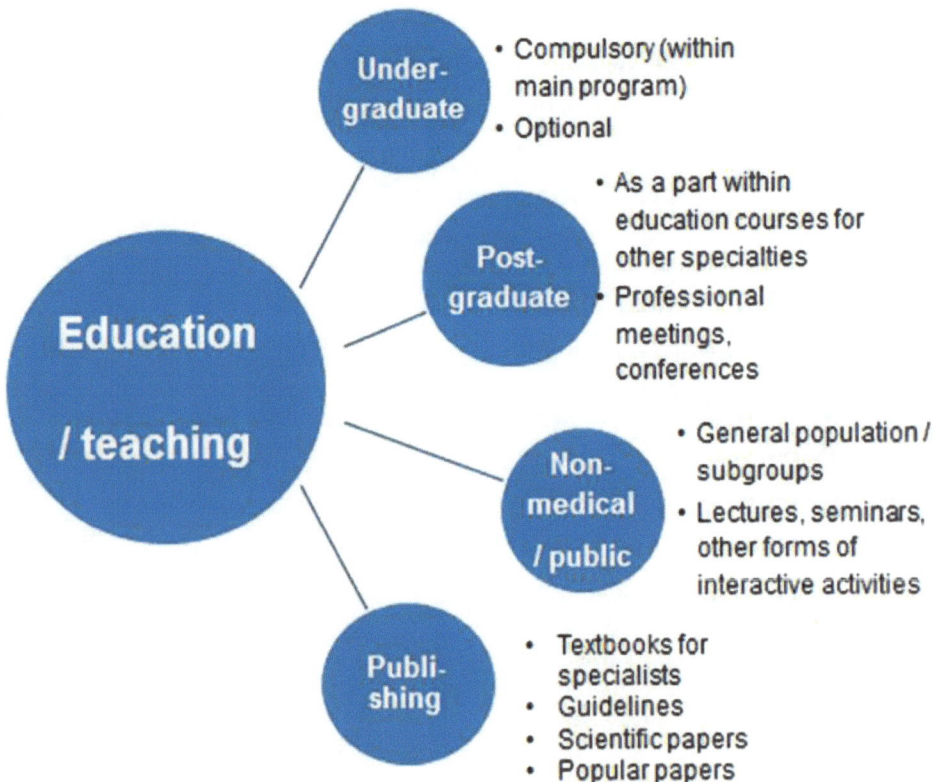

Fig. (3). Postgraduate education in sleep field in Russia.

For instance, National Research Medical Center on Therapy and Preventive Medicine offers a training course (since 2017) on diagnostics of sleep-disordered breathing including polysomnography, ambulatory (cardiorespiratory) sleep monitoring, and assessment of daytime sleepiness. During this course, the attendees take part in sleep studies and acquire practical skills including conducting the studies and composing the clinical report. Sechenov University and Moscow State University also provide training courses in sleep medicine. The Russian Society of Sleep Medicine organized different kinds of education opportunities: 9-hour training for new competencies in the diagnosis and treatment of sleep-disordered breathing, 72-hour online course on diagnostics and treatment of sleep disorders, internship in theory and practice of polysomnography.

Some big universities (Sechenov University, Moscow) and research clinical centers (Almazov National Medical Research Centre, National Research Medical Center on Therapy and Preventive Medicine) provide series of lectures and seminars on diagnosis and treatment of sleep-related disorders for residents and postgraduate students specialized in different specialties (mainly, neurology, cardiology, internal medicine *etc.*).

Some private education courses are provided, including courses from private psychology centers for CBT-I, and CBT for other sleep disorders.

In 2001, a highly successful initiative of the biennial International Youth Workshops "Sleep: a window to the world of wakefulness" was started. The main goal of the Workshops is the education of young specialists and reinforcement of their professional skills in the sleep field, as well as the integration of young specialists in a professional society, and the promotion of collaborative research and clinical projects. The main audience of the Workshops includes students, young researchers and clinicians. The 2-3-day agenda provides various sessions, i.e. lectures, interactive seminars, round tables, "brainstorming" sessions, presentation of own data by the participants, *etc.*

Since 2015, several web-based interactive educational modules on sleep disorders (mainly sleep-disordered breathing) have been developed and are available within the continuing medical education (CME) system (1-2 CME credits per 2-hour module) free of charge for medical professionals. During the COVID-19 pandemic, a few commercial online courses on general issues of sleep disorders have been developed.

Annually symposiums at the meetings of other medical associations are organized (*e.g.* Russian Society of Cardiologists, Society of the Specialists in Internal Diseases, Association of Pediatricians in Russia, Russian Respiratory Society, *etc.*). As currently we mainly conceive somnology as a competency area, it is important that all these educational training programs and meetings are certified within CME for various specialties. It should be noted, that although not officially recognized, the European certification in somnology remains important at an individual level.

Textbooks are an essential part of education in both undergraduate and postgraduate training. Currently, there are several official Russian textbooks registered for medical professionals in the sleep field which is important considering the rather low availability of professional literature for Russian speakers. In addition, several Russian medical journals regularly publish papers on sleep-related topics (Table **1**).

Table 1. Russian medical journals regularly publishing sleep-related materials.

Journal	Information (editor, ISSN, web-site, citation indices)	Regularity
Journal of Neurology and Psychiatry n.a. S.S. Korsakov [Zhurnal nevrologii i psikhiatrii imeni S.S. Korsakova]	Editor-in-Chief – E.I. Gusev (Moscow) ISSN 1997-7298 (Print), ISSN 2309-4729 (Online) Website: https://www.mediasphera.ru/issues/anesteziologiya--reanimatologiya/2019/6/1020175632019061005 Citation Indices: Scopus, Web of Science, eLibrary	Monthly (12 issues per year) Special regular Issue "Sleep disorders" is published once per year (responsible Editor: Dr. M. Poluektov)
Journal "Effective Pharmacotherapy"	Editor-in-Chief (Moscow) ISSN 2307-3586 (Print) Website: https://umedp.ru/magazines/ Citation Indices: eLibrary	36 issues per year Special regular Issue "Sleep disorders" is published once per year (responsible Editor: Dr. M. Poluektov)
Journal "Arterial Hypertension" [Arterial'naya Gipertenziya]	Editor-in-Chief – A. O. Konradi (St Petersburg) ISSN 1607-419X (Print), ISSN 2411-8524 (Online) Website: http://htn.almazovcentre.ru Citation Indices: Scopus, eLibrary	6 issues per year A special heading "The Somnologist's Page" is published regularly (at least 3 times per year)

(Table 1) cont.....

Journal	Information (editor, ISSN, web-site, citation indices)	Regularity
Journal of Chronomedicine	Editor-in-Chief – D.G.Gubin (Tyumen) ISSN 2712-7494 (Print), Website: https://jchrono.tyumsmu.ru/ Citation Indices: eLibrary	2 issues per year

The current professional education in the field of somnology has certain limitations, such as the lack of standard, uniform plan of education, centralized education system (lack of available training in small towns), low capacity due to irregular schedule of the courses and lack of teaching staff, and lack of training programs for sleep technicians/medical assistants. At the same time, there are various ongoing activities that offer some educational opportunities to those who are interested in.

Another side of education is the *public promotion* of healthy sleep and knowledge about sleep disorders among the general population (Fig. **4**). The members of the sleep-related societies perform various activities all year round and in relation to the World Sleep Day, including public consultations, popular and professional lectures, interactive seminars for the school and high-school students, and other actions such as postcard sending, interviews on social media, *etc.* In March 2020, an exhibition "About Sleep" was held together with the team of the Museum of Health in St Petersburg. The exhibition included several parts: 1) the lullaby-related part, where the visitors could listen to the lullabies from different regions of Russia, to know more about the traditions of lullabies and other sleep-related rituals; 2) the medical part where the visitors could get some medical information presented in a popular manner about sleep, sleep stages, *etc.*, as well as several interactive tests (reaction rate, myths about sleep *etc.*); 3) sleep-related technology part, where the visitors could see and try different devices and tools which are used to improve sleep quality and sleep-wakefulness cycle and to treat some sleep disorders (lamps, robots, pillows, CPAP-machines, oral appliances, light therapy glasses).

The activities aimed at popularization of sleep medicine and promotion of healthy sleep help to attract attention to this field and to increase the recognition of sleep medicine.

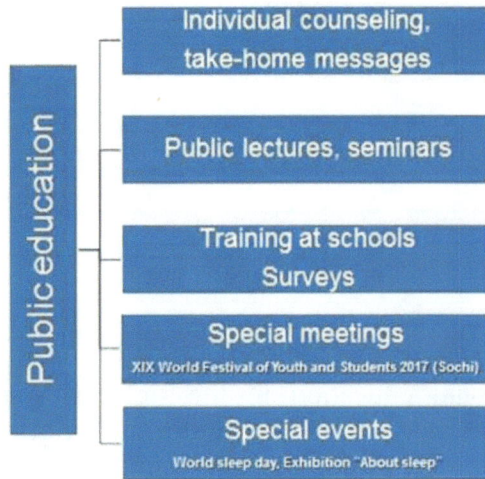

Fig. (4). Public promotion of sleep-related knowledge in Russia.

There is a lack of sleep-related competencies in the professional standards regulating the knowledge and skills of medical specialists. The diagnostics and treatment of a number of sleep disorders (insomnia, hypersomnia, parasomnias and others) fall within the competencies of psychiatrists and neurologists, however, the knowledge of specialized diagnostics (including polysomnography and other tests) is not included in the list of their competences. Pulmonologists must be able to assess sleep-disordered breathing in patients with bronchopulmonary pathology and to set the NIV-therapy and O_2-therapy. Specialists in functional diagnostics must be able to perform cardiorespiratory monitoring (polygraphy study) and to know the principles and opportunities of polysomnography. However, none of the existing professional standards regulates the performance of polysomnography, actigraphy or other sleep tests.

LEGISLATION IN THE FIELD OF SLEEP MEDICINE

Although generally Russian somnology is characterized by the absence of legislative and regulatory documents, there are several documents that regulate use and application of some of the sleep-related diagnostic and treatment procedures. Thus, a few orders and laws consider the application of sleep studies in certain pathologies, including bronchopulmonary and endocrinology diseases (Table **2**). When indicated, ambulatory devices for noninvasive ventilation are provided to patients with neurodegenerative diseases, and oxygen-therapy is provided to patients with bronchopulmonary disease and pulmonary hypertension. Other orders mainly consider the equipment of acute care units and in-patient clinics.

Table 2. Official documents regulating sleep-related services.

Sleep-related Procedure	Target population / Pathology	Order / Law	Statement
Diagnostics: pulse oximetry, sleep studies	Alcohol and tobacco users (healthy lifestyle promotion)	The Order of the Ministry of Health on the organization of "the Health Center for promotion of the Healthy Lifestyle among the Russian population, including the decrease of alcohol consumption and tobacco use" #597 19.08.2009	A Health Center must be equipped by a nocturnal pulse oximeter.
	Patients with endocrinology diseases	The Order of the Ministry of Health on the Health Care in patients with the Endocrinology Pathology #899н 12.11.2012	The Endocrinology Medical Center must be equipped by a polysomnography device (at least one device).
	Patients with bronchopulmonary Pathology	The Order of the Ministry of Health on the Health Care in patients with the Bronchopulmonary Pathology #222н 07.04.2010	The Pulmonology department must be equipped by a nocturnal pulse oximeter (at least two devices) and a device for sleep apnea screening (at least one device).
	Patients with hypertension	The order dated by 24.01.2003	Polysomnography is mentioned as a screening tool to rule out sleep apnea in suspected secondary hypertension.
		The order #708н dated by 09.11.2012	Only nocturnal pulse oximetry is mentioned.
	Patients with acute stroke	The Order of the Ministry of Health Care on "the Health Care in Patients with Acute Stroke" #389н 06.07.2009	Intensive care unit must be equipped by a portable nocturnal pulse oximeter (at least 3 devices). Early rehabilitation unit must be equipped by portable nocturnal pulse oximeter (at least one device per 12 beds).
	Special groups: Hoffmann's muscular atrophy	-	The patients must be provided by a nocturnal pulse oximetry, cardiorespiratory monitoring.* *in federal institutions, in case of the official counseling by a geneticist of a federal institution

(Table 2) cont.....

Sleep-related Procedure	Target population / Pathology	Order / Law	Statement
Treatment: Non-invasive ventilation (NIV) and O2-therapy	Patients requiring rehabilitation	The Order of the Ministry of Health Nº949 25.11.2016 on the Supply of the Special groups of patients by the rehabilitation devices	-
	Patients requiring palliative care (advanced respiratory diseases)	The Order of the Ministry of Health Nº345/372н 31.05.2019 on the Palliative care	NIV and oxygen (O2) therapy are included in palliative care for patients with respiratory diseases (respiratory failure 3 degree, required NIV/O2-therapy due to respiratory failure). The order regulates the organization, structure and equipment of respiratory centers.
	Patients with lateral amyotrophic sclerosis	The Order of the Administration of St Petersburg: (regional order has been put into force only in St Petersburg, since 2018)	The provision of patients with lateral amyotrophic sclerosis by NIV-devices
	Patients with acute stroke	The Order of the Ministry of Health Care on "the Health Care in Patients with Acute Stroke" #389н 06.07.2009	Intensive care unit must be equipped by a NIV device (at least 1 device per 3 beds)
	Patients with cardiovascular pathology	The Order of the Ministry of Health Care on "the Health Care in Patients with Cardiovascular Pathology" #599н 19.08.2009	Intensive care unit must be equipped by a NIV device (at least 1 device per 6 beds)
		The Order of the Ministry of Health Care on "the Health Care in Patients with Cardiovascular Pathology" #222н 07.04.2010	Intensive care unit must be equipped by a NIV device (at least 1 device per 10 beds)
	Patients with pulmonary hypertension	The Order of the Ministry of Health Care dated by 24.12.2012 #1446н "About the standard of primary medical care in pulmonary arterial hypertension"	When indicated, O2-therapy should be provided to the patients with pulmonary hypertension.

Driving licensing in Russia is regulated by several orders:

– The Order of the Ministry of Health 15.06.2015 Nº344н "On the obligatory medical assessment of the drivers",

– The Decree of the Government of the Russian Federation 29.12.2014 Nº1604 "On the list of medical contraindications, indications and limitations for driving",

– The Order of the Ministry of Health 12.04.2011 Nº302н on the preliminary and occasional medical examinations.

However, none of these documents provide a single word about diagnostics and/or treatment of sleep apnea, sleepiness / hypersomnolence, or any other sleep disorder.

Practice Guidelines for Somnology and Sleep Disorders in the Clinical Guidelines of Other Professional Societies

Specialized documents considering sleep disorders developed by the Russian experts include the following guidelines:

– Recommendations on diagnostics and treatment of chronic insomnia (Russian Somnology Society) [8].

– Recommendations on diagnostics and treatment of obstructive sleep apnea in adults (Russian Somnology Society) [9].

– National clinical guideline "Diagnosis and management of patients with resistant hypertension and obstructive sleep apnea" (Russian Scientific Medical Society of Physicians) [10].

However, it should be noted that these documents lack information on the peculiarities of diagnostics and treatment of sleep-related disorders in Russia and do not consider the existing barriers and limitations.

A number of current clinical guidelines focusing on various pathologies of internal medicine include recommendations on related sleep disorders. These include two documents published by the Ministry of Health of the Russian Federation and other guidelines:

– Bradyarrhythmias and heart conduction disorders. (Clinical guidelines of the Ministry of Health of Russian Federation) [11].

– Arterial hypertension in adults. (Clinical guidelines of the Ministry of Health of Russian Federation) [12].

– Guidelines on the diagnostics, treatment and prevention of obesity and associated diseases. (Russian Society of Cardiologists) [13].

– Clinical recommendations on conducting electrophysiological studies, catheter ablation and implantable antiarrhythmic devices. (All-Russian scientific society of specialists in clinical electrophysiology, arrhythmology and cardiac pacing) [14].

– Clinical guidelines on the management of patients with ischemic stroke and transient ischemic attacks (National Stroke Association) [15].

– Guidelines for Heart failure: chronic and acute decompensated (Russian Scientific Medical Society of Internal Medicine) [16].

– National clinical guidelines on the treatment of morbid obesity in adults. 3rd ed [17].

– Cardiovascular Prevention (Russian Society of Cardiology) [18].

DIAGNOSTICS AND TREATMENT OF SLEEP DISORDERS IN PRACTICE

Healthcare in Russia is free for citizens and covered by the Obligatory Medical Insurance. Private Health Insurance is an alternative option and gives access to medicine in private clinics and to a number of services which are not covered by the Obligatory Medical Insurance. However, neither of these options covers the majority of sleep-related diagnostics and treatment procedures.

As somnology is not recognized as a medical (sub)specialty, there is a lack of somnologists in state-budget clinics. Therefore, patients with sleep complaints usually refer to physician/general practitioners at the outpatient department. The latter can refer the patient to another specialist including neurologist/pulmonologist/cardiologist, *etc.* Many patients with snoring often refer directly to ENT doctors, and depending on the availability of ENT-surgery facilities quite often they can get surgery without preceding sleep diagnostics.

Diagnostic and Treatment Procedures of Sleep Apnea

In the last decades, the use of rheopneumogram during Holter monitoring has been implemented widely into clinical practice in Russia, which allows for a very rough screening of sleep apnea in cardiovascular patients who undergo a routine electrocardiography (ECG) monitoring based on the evaluation of thorax movements (sensitivity for obstructive sleep apnea detection 0,91 and specificity 0,85) [19]. Another widely available option is cardiorespiratory monitoring which includes 2 extra sensors – nasal cannulas and pulse oximeter, so together with the rheopneumogram it can be considered as a class IV device (based on AASM classification). It was validated against polysomnography showing rather good validity for sleep apnea detection [19]. Non-contact monitoring is being developed by Russian technologists [20], but it is mainly used in research and is not currently available on market (see also *Challenges in clinical somnology in Russia*).

The initiation of NIV therapy is more often started at home with the use of auto-CPAP machines. Few clinics offer in-lab titration procedures under online polysomnography monitoring. Currently, only foreign devices are available in Russia, which are not covered by the insurances, so patients have to purchase machines themselves at distributor sites or *via* online services. A few charity organizations provide CPAP-machines to those in need in several regions in Russia (see also *Challenges in clinical somnology in Russia*). However, few start-ups have emerged recently for the development of national CPAP-devices. Commonly, the latest versions of the devices and masks are becoming available later in Russia due to the complicated and long process of registration and licensing.

Oral appliances treatment of sleep apnea and snoring is limited due to the very few dentists/orthodontists familiar with specialized custom-made oral appliances for sleep problems. However, some simple, self-adjusted oral devices are available at the pharmacy and online shops.

Diagnostic and Treatment Procedures of Circadian Disorders, Insomnia and other Sleep Disorders

The diagnostics of circadian rhythm disorders, hypersomnolence disturbances is limited by the lack of specialists familiar with these pathologies as well as by the absence of diagnostic tools, *e.g.* DLMO assessment (which is available only within research but not in routine laboratories). Light therapy devices are available at shops for bedroom accessories and medical equipment providers. Drugs for the treatment of hypersomnia and narcolepsy (*e.g.* modafinil and armodafinil) are not available in Russia and are prohibited as they are listed as narcotic drugs and psychotropic substances.

In case of insomnia, most patients are referred to a neurologist or psychiatrist. Sedatives and hypnotics are widely used and prescribed in Russia. Many patients consider the treatment of insomnia only in terms of taking sleeping pills and are not ready for psychotherapy. The off-label use of drugs is common among some cohorts for insomnia treatment (*e.g.* elderly people). Some recent drugs for insomnia treatment like orexin inhibitors and melatonin receptor agonists are not approved in Russia yet (see also *Challenges in clinical somnology in Russia*).

On the other hand, various methods which lack strong evidence are common in the Russian Federation. As an example, brain music therapy was developed by the leading Russian sleep researcher Yakov Levin in the 1990s [21]. It is based on the transformation of electroencephalography (EEG) into music using a special algorithm. Small comparative studies showed sleep improvement after 2-week brain music therapy in more than 80% of the insomniac patients. Another method is electrosleep therapy which is based on the electric stimulation of the brain by low frequency (1-150 Hz) pulsed current, low power (up to 10 mA) and voltage up to 80 V. It has been used since late 1940s with the short-term effect in insomnia [22].

The psychological approaches and psychotherapy for insomnia treatment have been spreading in the recent decade.

Psychological Approaches to Treatment of Sleep Disorders in Russia

Among the nonpharmacological methods of treating insomnia, CBT-I, methods of self-regulation, psychoanalytic and existential-humanistic approaches, and method of clinical hypnosis are used in Russia. CBT is currently considered as the first-line treatment for insomnia, regardless of its form and clinical manifestations. It includes recommendations on sleep hygiene, stimulus control therapy, techniques targeting intrusive/ catastrophic thoughts and negative sleep beliefs.

The biofeedback method has been implemented into somnology practice in Russia. It allows patients to master and later independently use skills for controlling physiological processes. Since patients with insomnia tend to show sympathetic hyperarousal, diaphragmatic breathing and muscle relaxation techniques help to activate the parasympathetic system, reduce tension and facilitate the initiation and maintenance of sleep. In addition, self-regulation training with EEG, temperature, and skin-galvanic response sensors are also used. In addition to the skill of regulating functional state itself, the person receives positive reinforcement, which gradually increases his or her self-confidence and competence in coping with stress.

Depending on the approaches used by a specialist, it is possible to combine them in a comprehensive program of sleep disorders treatment, aimed at working both with symptoms of sleep disorders and with the personality, in particular, at developing his/her adaptive capabilities and resilience resources. According to the modern model of sleep reactivity, the risk of insomnia is increased by a high pre-morbid sleep reactivity to stress. In this context, the above mentioned programs may also have preventive and psychoeducational value for people predisposed to sleep disorders under stress.

The idea of regulated activity based on feedback in the psychological dimension is consonant with the understanding of the existential worldview of a psychologically mature individual who perceives reality as a total uncertainty into which certainty can be introduced only by him-/herself with the support of feedback [23].

The ideas in the field of psychology emerged in 20-21 centuries have been fully adopted and further developed in Russia, including psychology of uncertainty (Kahneman, I.M. Feigenberg, *etc.*), psychology of social instability (G.V. Soldatova), personology of maladaptive behavior (A.V. Petrovskii), psychology of self-organization of psychological systems (V.E. Klochko), psychology of complexity (A.N. Poddyakov) and others [24], theoretical construct of "hardiness". The latter was defined by Salvatore Maddi as a systemic ability of a personality to mature and complex forms of psychological and psychophysical self-regulation, allowing to overcome difficulties while maintaining internal balance, somatic health and successful activity [25, 26]. The ideas of developing hardiness skills (relaxation and emotional self-regulation skills; cognitive coping strategies; communication skills; healthy nutrition skills; physical exercise to maintain fitness and performance) and coping at all possible levels (somatic, psychological, social, existential) have been accepted by the Russian professional psychology society, including the field of sleep disorders.

The existential context of hardiness also determines the approach to its development. Conventionally we can distinguish two forms of approach to develop hardiness - individual (psychoeducation) and organized (group training). In the course of this psychological work, a participant is supposed to become the subject of his/her own development, strengthen inner resources, and have a responsible attitude to oneself including self-care, self-discipline, and self-determination. The value of developing hardiness within the scope of insomnia psychotherapy is determined by its systemic nature, the ability to maintain mental, somatic and psychological health in situations of stress. In the conditions of total uncertainty and lack of external reference points, hardiness as an internal point of support in coping with the challenges of complexity, represents reasonable means of preserving the well-being of the individual at all levels of functioning.

CHALLENGES IN CLINICAL SOMNOLOGY IN RUSSIA

Geographical and Epidemiological Challenges

Russia is the largest country in the world and stretches over a vast area of Europe and Northern Asia. The large extent of the Russian territory, heterogeneous distribution of the population and multi-ethnicity are significant barriers for medical healthcare organization. As a result, sleep medicine specialists are lacking in many regions [27]. Territory constitutionally consists of 85 federal subjects with significant differences in the size of the population. As example, the largest federal subject the Republic of Sakha (Yakutia) has population less than 1 billion people and a territory size similar to India or Argentina. Russia is a home to over 193 ethnic groups. Approximately 2 million people live in the Arctic covering 18% of territory. Russia includes 11 time-zones ranging from UTC+02:00 to UTC+12:00. After a period of debates, daylight saving time was canceled in Russia in 2014, although in some regions, issues of misalignment between astronomic time and artificial time zones remain unsolved.

Few epidemiological studies included the assessment of sleep and sleep disorders in Russia mainly by questionnaires. The earliest one was the "MONICA-psychosocial" study started in 1994 and included 2400 people 25-64 years old living in Novosibirsk and used Jenkins Sleep Scale. Results showed 48% prevalence of sleep disorders in males [28] and 65.3% in females [29]. The authors did not use the questions separately to assess the frequency and prevalence of insomnia symptoms. The prevalence of sleep disorders in citizens of Chuvash Republic was evaluated in 2011 in 1508 citizens 17-94 years old by interview. Mean sleep duration was 7.4 hours, prevalence of morning and evening chronotypes was 35.8% and 25.9%, respectively, frequent sleep disturbances were found in 20%, night awakenings in 62.7%, and long sleep latency in 48.4% [30]. By NoSAS scale, 13.7% respondents (21.4% males and 6.9% females) showed probable obstructive sleep apnea [31].

The ESSE-RF study addresses the epidemiology of cardiovascular risk factors and major cardiovascular diseases in Russian Federation (urban and rural population) and included 13 regions with a total of more than 22000 participants 25-64 years old during 2012-2014 years. Sleep module included questions about average sleep duration, complaints of snoring and sleep apnea, frequency of difficulties in sleep initiation, maintenance, sleepiness and sleep drugs. Studies showed that 58% of respondents had snoring and 7% had sleep apnea complaints [32], 18% had frequent sleep initiation difficulties, 13% had frequent sleep maintenance difficulties, and 6% had high daily sleepiness [33]. The prospective branch of the ESSE-RF study is ongoing in some cities. Epidemiology studies of sleep disorders conducted in Russia include only certain regions and only questionnaires without polysomnography or instrumental evaluation of sleep-disordered breathing. Unfortunately, possible regional and ethnic differences in the prevalence and susceptibility to sleep disorders have not been properly addressed yet. No annual sleep polls have been implemented till now.

Availability of Sleep-related Healthcare Services

In general, primary counseling for sleep-related problems (when suspected or identified by the general physician or any other relevant specialist) and primary screening diagnostics (screening questionnaires, ambulatory cardiorespiratory monitoring) can be provided within the system of obligatory medical insurance available for every single resident of the Russian Federation according to the Federal Law #323-F3 dated by 21.11.2011 (ed. 22.12.2020) "About health protection of the citizens of the Russian Federation".

Furthermore, the diagnostics of sleep disorders (both by polysomnography and polygraphy), as well as the treatment approaches (noninvasive ventilation for sleep apnea, CBT-insomnia and others) are approved for use in the Russian Federation and can be applied when necessary. These approaches should and can be performed by MDs of any specialty who have undergone additional training. Over 300 MDs are currently involved in the sleep field.

At the same time, one of the biggest limitations of sleep-related healthcare services in Russia is the centralization of an organization. The specialized, complex diagnostics and multidisciplinary treatment are mainly available in big cities in the Western and North-Western (European) regions of the Russian Federation while poorer access to the facilities is observed in the Eastern regions. Telemedicine services are being developed and spreading throughout Russia, however, there are some obstacles in the broader implementation of remote monitoring of NIV-adherence due to the strict regulations of personal data protection.

Small settlements often lack multidisciplinary medical centers. At its best, only a medical station with a general physician or only a medical assistant is available. In the latter cases, sleep disorders are unlikely to be diagnosed on the spot, but the patients can be referred to the medical center in the bigger town or in the referral regional center. The unequal distribution of sleep-related facilities leads to the underdiagnosis of sleep disorders in smaller cities and settlements.

Moreover, in big cities, multidisciplinary sleep centers are concentrated on large-scale medical research and educational centers or in the private clinics. Therefore, the availability of specialized diagnostic procedures (*e.g.* (video) polysomnography, multiple sleep latency test, maintenance of wakefulness test and others) and complex treatment is limited.

Other limitations include the lack of healthcare standards regarding sleep-related services, the lack of reimbursement of sleep diagnostics and treatment (including NIV, CBT insomnia which are not included in the obligatory health insurance), the lack of certain medications which are not registered in Russia (*e.g.* modern treatments for hypersomnia and narcolepsy are not available in the Russian Federation).

Patients with certain pathologies can obtain reimbursement of specialized sleep-related diagnostics and treatment procedures (*e.g.* NIV). These mainly include patients with disabilities requiring palliative care.

In the last decade, several charity organizations supply some categories of patients with the devices for ambulatory non-invasive ventilation or partially cover the expenses:

− The foundation "The Life Line" (together with the Ministry of Health it started a pilot program "NIV at home": in 2017 and 2018, 37 and 57 children were supplied with the NIV devices, respectively)

− The foundation "The memory of generations" (supports war veterans)

− The foundation "Medical brotherhood" (supports medical staff)

− The foundation "Actor" (supports theater employees)

− Others: Pravmir, Vera, AiF "Kind Heart" (provide support in some regions of Russia, and some additional criteria can be applied, *e.g.* age category)

In addition, patients with severe disabilities and indications for ambulatory NIV and/or O2-therapy can get governmental support within the program of individual rehabilitation, however, the procedure is rather complicated and time-consuming, and few patients fulfill the eligibility criteria.

Patient Organizations in the Russian Federation

Most patient organizations in the Russian Federation deal with oncological, neuromuscular, rare genetic diseases, and organ transplantation. However, there is no patient organization related to sleep disorders. The only patient organization which is somehow related to sleep disorders is the Association of Russian Families of Central Congenital Hypoventilation Syndrome (CCHS) which was founded in 2016 [34]. The main goal of this organization is providing information about CCHS and support to families with children with CCHS to improve early diagnosis and treatment. According to the data of this Association, 21 children are currently diagnosed with CCHS in Russia. The members (children's parents) of the Association take an active part in the promotion of knowledge about CCHS, in the organization of medical meetings, and in schools for parents. With the support of Almazov National Medical Research Center (Dr. N. Petrova, Head of the Research Laboratory of Neonatal Pathology) and several charity organizations, the association helps children with CCHS to obtain the required diagnostics, counseling (including the consultations of specialists from abroad), and treatment (NIV, phrenic nerve stimulation). In the last couple of years, the distributors of NIV-devices in Russia (Unimedica, official distributor of Resmed; Philips Respironics) have been developing web-portals where patients with sleep apnea and other sleep disorders can find relevant information and get information support regarding their disease.

Cultural and Psychological Barriers

According to the Russian folklore stories, the epical heroes (brave and strong men) always snored, which might have affected the perception and attitude to snoring in the general population which used to be recognized as a symbol of robust health. In recent decades, this situation has been changing slowly, also due to the promotion of healthy sleep and information about sleep disorders at population levels.

Generally, Russian citizens (and patients with sleep disorders) are reluctant to seek help from psychiatrists and psychologists, which limits the initial examination of patients with insomnia, hypersomnia, and other sleep disorders. Based on the survey conducted in 2009, over two-thirds of Volgograd citizens do not understand what psychotherapy is and whether there are any differences between a psychiatrist and a psychotherapist. Although the situation is changing for the better, the barriers still remain, and a distrustful and cautious attitude toward psychiatry and psychiatrists in Russian society is described [35].

Some authors suggest that the Russian culture is a Dionysian one according to Benedict's classification which should be considered when a psychotherapeutic approach is chosen [36].

Lack of Clinical and Scientific Knowledge

The use of different diagnostic and treatment methods which do not have strong validation is another barrier in Russia which can be also attributed to psychological and cultural aspects. Thus, the use of rheopneumography method during Holter monitoring became popular for sleep apnea detection, and many medical doctors rely on this method for sleep apnea diagnosis without further verification, although rheopneumography does not fulfill criteria for standard assessment according to the guidelines [9].

Non-proven methods to treat insomnia are also popular among the Russian population. Many patients, although reluctant to refer to psychologists and psychiatrists, would be highly compliant to various non-evidenced approaches (commonly available in private clinics). These include Xenon gas, electrosleep therapy, brain music therapy, *etc.* (see *Diagnostics and treatment of sleep disorders in practice*).

EDUCATION IN SLEEP MEDICINE: CHALLENGES AND WAYS OUT OF PROBLEMS

The education system in the Russian Federation lacks a structured program of undergraduate and postgraduate training for both medical doctors and medical assistants/technologists in the field of sleep medicine. Medical staff currently involved in sleep-related services have obtained knowledge and skills either at short-term training courses, or abroad, or on-site. In many cases, this training is not licensed, there is no final certification exam, or the certificate (foreign) is not valid in Russia. These factors impede the development of standard approaches, healthcare and sleep centers. The existing sleep labs experience staff shortages and difficulties with collaboration between the centers.

Moreover, there is no conception of a specialist who performs polysomnography and other specialized sleep diagnostics. None of the existing professional standards regulates this field. There is no term for such a specialty/profession. Therefore, a number of issues remain unsolved: who should perform these procedures (medical doctors, nurses, trained technologists)? Are they authorized for analyzing the data? Are they authorized for making and signing medical reports? Are they qualified for prescribing sleep-related treatment, *etc.*?

Another issue considers diagnostic equipment and treatment devices. The diagnostic tools applied in Russia are not defined in the official regulatory documents. Accordingly, no indications/contraindications are officially listed. Therefore, they are used depending on their availability [37]. Practical guidelines of medical associations could be an alternative regulatory document, however, they are lacking in the sleep field. These are basic, primary limitations in clinical sleep medicine in the Russian Federation. Other issues include lack of systematic literature, lack of teaching staff and the place of medical specialists who underwent training (is it a separate (sub)specialty, or a competency within the main medical specialty, in the latter case the subspecialty sleep-related competencies should be listed).

The following goals are the primary ones to be addressed in order to develop a systematic education in the field of somnology:

1. The development of regulatory statements/standards for medical doctors and medical assistants specialized in sleep medicine (or within other specialties);

2. The development of an examination system for medical specialists in the field of sleep medicine - medical doctors, nurses, and technologists (which considers the primary professional education and availability of diagnostic and treatment tools in the Russian Federation);

3. The development of undergraduate (medical doctors and nurses) education courses on basic knowledge of sleep and sleep disorders (high-school medical training).

4. The development of regulatory statements/standards on specialized sleep-related diagnostic equipment and procedures.

These goals can be achieved only with the support of governmental institutions (Ministry of Health and Ministry of Education).

CONCLUSION

Somnology in Russia faces many challenges: lack of recognition of somnology as a separate specialty, lack of doctors' training in medical institutes, doctors' low awareness of modern approaches in somnology, and lack of standards of medical care in somnology. The developed technologies of sleep disorder screening and insomnia treatment are used only locally. At the same time, physicians from different specialties work closely together to treat sleep disorders in Russia, sleep laboratories for screening sleep breathing disorders and selecting noninvasive ventilation are widespread in major cities. There are unique technologies for detecting apnea during sleep, psychologists are involved in cognitive behavioral therapy, and treatment standards for some diseases include international approaches in treating sleep-disordered breathing.

LIST OF ABBREVIATIONS

ANSS	Assembly of National Sleep Societies
CBT	cognitive behavioral therapy
CCC	Committee on Chronobiology and Chronomedicine
CCHS	Central Congenital Hypoventilation Syndrome
CME	continuous medical education
COVID-19	coronavirus disease 2019
CPAP	continuous positive airway pressure
EEG	electroencephalography

ENT	ear nose and throat
ECG	electrocardiography
ESRS	European Sleep Research Society
MDs	medical doctors
NIV	Non-invasive ventilation
O2	oxygen therapy
RSS	Russian Society of Somnologists
RSSM	Russian Society of Sleep Medicine
NSPSS	National Society of Pediatric Sleep Specialists on Children Sleep
NSSSM	National Society of Somnology and Sleep Medicine
RSRD	Russian Society of Researchers of Dreams

FUNDING

This work is supported by the Ministry of Science and Higher Education of the Russian Federation (Agreement No. 075-15-2022-301).

CONSENT FOR PUBLICATION

Not applicable.

CONFLICT OF INTEREST

The authors declare no conflict of interest, financial or otherwise.

ACKNOWLEDGEMENT

Declared none.

REFERENCES

[1]   Romanov AI, Belov AM, Kallistov DY, Romanova EA, Butkov N, Rafaelson M, Eds. Organization of a sleep center. Moscow: Management, Budget, Methodology 1997.

[2]   sleep.ru [homepage on the Internet]. The Russian Society of Somnologists.

[3]   rossleep.ru [homepage on the Internet]. The Russian Society of Sleep Medicine.

[4]   pedsleep.ru [homepage on the Internet]. The National Society of Pediatric Sleep Specialists on Children Sleep.

[5]   Sleep Medicine [homepage on the Internet]. The National Society of Somnology and Sleep Medicine [cited: 31 December 2020], Available from: http://medsna.ru/natsionalnoe-obshhestvo-po-somnologii/

[6]   The Russian Society of Researchers of Dreams [homepage on the Internet]. The Russian Society of Researchers of Dreams (page in English) [cited 31 December 2020], Available from: http://rsdr.ru/glavnaya/2-uncategorised/26-russian-society-of-dream-researchers-rsdr.html

[7]   chronobiology.ru [homepage on the Internet]. The Committee on Chronobiology and Chronomedicine of Russian Academy of Sciences.

[8]   Poluektov MG, Buzunov RV, Averbukh VM, *et al.* Project of clinical recommendations on diagnosis and treatment of chronic insomnia in adults. Consilium Medicum. Neurol Rheumatol 2016; 2 (Suppl.): 41-51.

[9]   Buzunov RV, Palman AD, Melnikov AY, *et al.* Diagnosis and treatment of obstructive sleep apnea syndrome in adults. Recommendations of the Russian Society of Somnologists. Effective Pharmacotherapy 2018; 35: 34-45.

[10]   Malyavin AG, Babak SL, Adasheva TV, Gorbunova MV, Martynov AI. Diagnosis and management of patients with resistant arterial hypertension and obstructive sleep apnea (Clinical guidelines). Therapy 2018; 1: 4-42.

[11]   Bradyarrhythmias and conduction disorders. Clinical guidelines of the Ministry of Health of Russian Federation 2020, viewed 31 December 2020.https://scardio.ru/content/Guidelines/2020/Clinic_rekom_Bradiaritmiya.pdf

[12]   Kobalava ZD, Konradi AO, Nedogoda SV, *et al.* Arterial hypertension in adults. Clinical guidelines 2020. Russian Journal of Cardiology 2020; 25(3): 3786.
        [http://dx.doi.org/10.15829/1560-4071-2020-3-3786]

[13]   Diagnosis, treatment and prevention of obesity and associated diseases. Saint Petersburg: National Clinical Guidelines 2017.

[14]   Clinical recommendations on conducting electrophysiological studies, catheter ablation and implantable antiarrhythmic devices. All-Russian scientific society of specialists in clinical electrophysiology, arrhythmology and cardiac pacing 2017, viewed 31 December 2020.https://vnoa.ru/upload/Recomendation_2017_30_10_2017_HR.pdf

[15]   Alferova BV, Belkin AA, Voznyuk IA, *et al.* Clinical guidelines on the management of patients with ischemic stroke and transient ischemic attacks. 2017.

[16]   Mareev VY, Fomin IV, Ageev FT, *et al.* OSSN-RCO-RNMOT clinical guidelines. Heart failure: chronic and acute decompensation. Diagnosis, prevention, and treatment. Cardiol 2018; 58(6S): 8-158.

[17]   Dodos II, Melnichenko GA, Shestakova MV, *et al.* Morbid obesity treatment in adults. Obes Metab 2018; 15(1): 53-70.

[18]   Boytsov SA, Pogosova NV, Bubnova MG, *et al.* Cardiovascular prevention. Russian national recommendations. Russ J Cardiol 2018; 6: 7-122.

[19]   Tikhonenko VM, Aparina IV. Possibilities of Holter monitoring in assessing the relationship between cardiac rhythm disturbances and cardiac conduction with apnea episodes. J Arrhythm 2009; 55: 49-55.

[20]   Anishchenko LN, Bugaev AS, Ivashov SI, *et al.* Determination of the sleep structure *via* radar monitoring of respiratory movements and motor activity. J Commun Technol Electron 2017; 62(8): 886-93.
        [http://dx.doi.org/10.1134/S1064226917080022]

[21]   Levin YI. "Brain music" in the treatment of patients with insomnia. Neurosci Behav Physiol 1998; 28(3): 330-5.
        [http://dx.doi.org/10.1007/BF02462965] [PMID: 9682240]

[22]   Feighner JP, Brown SL, Olivier JE. Electrosleep therapy. A controlled double blind study. J Nerv Ment Dis 1973; 157(2): 121-8.
        [http://dx.doi.org/10.1097/00005053-197308000-00004] [PMID: 4724809]

[23]   Leontiev DA, Osin EN, Lukovitskaya EG. Diagnostics of tolerance to uncertainty. Moscow: Smysl 2016.

[24]   Asmolov AG. Psychology of contemporary age: challenges of uncertainty, complexity and diversity.

Psychol Res 2015; 8(40): 1.

[25]   Leontiev DA, Rasskazova EI. Hardiness test. Moscow: Smysl 2006.

[26]   Maddi SR. Hardiness: An operacionalisation of existential courage. J Humanist Psychol 2004; 44(3): 279-98.
[http://dx.doi.org/10.1177/0022167804266101]

[27]   Catalog of sleep centers https://rossleep.ru/katalog-akkreditovannyih-tsentrov-2/

[28]   Gafarov VV, Panov DO, Gromova EA, Gagulin IV, Gafarova AV. Sleep disorders and the risk of arterial hypertension and stroke in open female population 25-64 year old in Russia/Siberia (Population study — WHO program "MONICA-psychosocial"). Cardiovasc Ther Prev (Fidenza) 2017; 16(5): 86-90.
[http://dx.doi.org/10.15829/1728-8800-2017-5-86-90]

[29]   Gafarov VV, Voevoda M, Gromova EA, *et al.* WHO program «MONICA-psychosocial»: insomnia and biological markers in the male population aged 25-64 years. Bekhterev Rev Psychiatry Med Psychol 2016; (1): 66-70.

[30]   Golenkov AV, Poluektov MG. Prevalence of sleep disorders among residents of Chuvashia (data from a complete questionnaire survey). Korsakov J Neurol Psychiatry 2011; 111(6): 64-7.
[PMID: 21905337]

[31]   Golenkov AV, Kurakina NG, Vecherkina MI, Naumova TV, Filonenko AV. Risk factors for obstructive sleep apnea syndrome in sociodemographic population groups in Chuvashia 2020.

[32]   Bochkarev MV, Korostovtseva LS, Filchenko IA, *et al.* Complaints on sleep breathing disorder and cardiovascular risk factors in Russian regions: Data from ESSE-RF study. Russian Journal of Cardiology 2018; 6(6): 152-8.
[http://dx.doi.org/10.15829/1560-4071-2018-6-152-158]

[33]   Bochkarev MV, Korostovtseva LS, Filchenko IA, *et al.* Socio-demographic aspects of insomnia in the Russian population according to the ESSE-RF study 2018.

[34]   cchs.ru [homepage on the Internet] Association of Russian Families of Central Congenital Hypoventilation Syndrome.

[35]   Gorbunov AA, Delaryu VV. Attitude towards psychotherapy in the Russian society (based on the results of a survey of primary health care professionals and the population) Medical Psychology in Russia: electronic   scientific   journal   2009;   1,   Available   from: http://medpsy.ru/mprj/archiv_global/2009-1-1/nomer/nomer03.php

[36]   Agarkov VA, Bronfman SA, Bozhko SA, Sherina TF, Gurtovenko IY. 2014. http://www.medtsu.tula.ru/VNMT/Bulletin/E2014-1/4993.pdf

[37]   Agaltsov MV. Polysomnography or cardiorespiratory monitoring: what is the best method to diagnose sleep-disordered breathing? "Arterial'naya Gipertenziya" ("Arterial Hypertension") 2019; 25(6): 604-12.

SUBJECT INDEX

www.ingramcontent.com/pod-product-compliance
Lightning Source LLC
Chambersburg PA
CBHW050758220326
41598CB00006B/54